AAHIVM
AMERICAN ACADEMY OF HIV MEDICINE

THE HIV MEDICINE SELF-DIRECTED STUDY GUIDE

2005

Overview of HIV Infection

Approach to the Patient With HIV

Clinical Manifestations of HIV Infection and Associated Conditions

Principles of Antiretroviral Therapy

A Continuing Education offering jointly sponsored by:
Medical Education Collaborative, Inc. and
The American Academy of HIV Medicine

Release date: July 1, 2005
Expiration date: June 30, 2006

This CME activity was planned and produced in accordance with the ACCME Essential Areas and Policies.

IMPORTANT NOTICE
AAHIVM STUDY GUIDE USE AND DISCLAIMER STATEMENT

The American Academy of HIV Medicine, Inc. (AAHIVM) has developed this Study Guide as part of its deep commitment to provide the latest, most comprehensive information available concerning HIV/AIDS-related health care. As part of this commitment, AAHIVM has made reasonable effort to ensure the accuracy and completeness of the information and materials contained herein.

However, please be aware that the materials contained herein may discuss therapies, protocols and/or therapeutic products that have not been approved by the U.S. Food and Drug Administration or other government agencies. A qualified health care professional should be consulted before using any therapeutic product or therapy discussed. Prescribers should carefully review all relevant materials concerning a medication, including all package insert information, before prescribing any medication.

AAHIVM disclaims any liability to any party for the accuracy and completeness of the information and material contained herein, or for any damages arising out of the use or nonuse of any of this material and information. Readers should directly consult all guidelines and textbooks cited herein, and should verify all information and data before treating patients or using the therapies or products identified in this publication.

Published by AAHIVM
Printed in the Unites States of America

For ordering or permission to reprint, please contact: AAHIVM – Self-Directed HIV Medicine Education Program; 1705 DeSales Street NW, 7th Floor, Washington, DC 20036; Phone: (202) 659-0699 or toll-free at (866) 241-9601; Fax: (202) 659-0976; E-mail: info@aahivm.org; www.aahivm.org

ISBN: 0-9726758-4-1
ISSN: 1543-5954

Suggested Citation: AAHIVM. [objective title.] HIV Medicine Self-Directed Study Guide – 2005 Update. Washington, DC: The American Academy of HIV Medicine; 2005[:inclusive pages].

For information about Study Guide updates, please go to http://www.aahivm.org

TABLE OF CONTENTS

CONTINUING EDUCATION ACCREDITATION

The 2005 Update to the *HIV Medicine Self-Directed Study Guide* is designed for use by physicians, physician assistants, nurse practitioners, registered nurses and pharmacists specializing in care for patients with HIV/AIDS throughout the United States.

CONTINUING EDUCATION CREDIT APPLICATION INSTRUCTIONS

1. Keep a record of the time required to complete each section.
2. Review the post-test at the end of this volume.
3. Complete application, activity evaluation, and post-test online at the AAHIVM Website at http://www.aahivm.org (click on "Study Guide") before the activity expiration date (June 30, 2006). You must score at least 70% to pass the post-test.

Computer System Requirements

Your web browser must support the following technologies:

- Cookies are enabled
- Support JavaScript
- Allow Popup Windows

You must be using the latest version of any of the following web browsers:

- Mozilla Firefox
- Internet Explorer
- Opera
- Safari

(Links are provided for free browser program upgrades if needed.)

Note: There is an application fee of $50 per submission. Certificates will be mailed by Medical Education Collaborative within 6 weeks of receiving your payment with successfully completed application, evaluation and post-test.

For questions regarding the accreditation of this program, please contact Medical Education Collaborative at (303) 420-3252.

ACCME

This activity has been planned and implemented in accordance with the Essential Areas and Policies of the Accreditation Council for Continuing Medical Education (ACCME) through the joint sponsorship of Medical Education Collaborative, Inc. (MEC) and the American Academy of HIV Medicine (AAHIVM). MEC is accredited by the ACCME to provide continuing medical education for physicians. MEC designates this educational activity for a maximum of 17.25 category 1 credits towards the AMA Physician's Recognition Award. Each physician should claim only those credit hours that he/she actually spent in the activity.

AANP

This program has been approved for 20.7 contact hours of continuing education by the American Academy of Nurse Practitioners (AANP). Program ID 0504191.

ANCC

This program qualifies for 20.7 contact hours. This activity is cosponsored with Medical Education Collaborative, Inc. (MEC) and the American Academy of HIV Medicine (AAHIVM). MEC is accredited as a provider of continuing nursing education by the American Nurses Credentialing Center's (ANCC) Commission on Accreditation. Provider approved by the California Board of Registered Nursing, Provider Number CEP 12990, for 20.7 contact hours.

ACPE

17.25 contact hours (1.725 CEUs) of credit for pharmacists. Approval of this course for pharmacists is under a cosponsorship agreement between Medical Education Collaborative, Inc. (MEC) and the American Academy of HIV Medicine (AAHIVM). MEC is approved by the American Council on Pharmaceutical Education (ACPE) as a provider of continuing pharmaceutical education. ACPE# 815-999-05-041-H01. The program is designed for all pharmacists.

CONTRIBUTORS

Special note:

AAHIVM also thanks all of the contributors to the HIV Medicine Self-Directed Study Guide: 2003 Edition and 2004 Update, as their work provided the basis for the 2005 Update.

PROGRAM CHAIR

Charles F. Farthing, MD, AAHIVS
Chief of Medicine
AIDS Healthcare Foundation

CO-CHIEF EDITORS

Ian Frank, MD
Director,
Antiretroviral Clinical Research
Director, Clinical Core
Penn Center for AIDS Research
Associate Professor of Medicine
University of Pennsylvania

Paul E. Sax, MD
Clinical Director
Division of Infectious Diseases
and HIV Program
Brigham and Women's Hospital
Associate Professor of Medicine
Harvard Medical School

AUTHORS

Stephen L. Becker, MD, AAHIVS
Associate Clinical Professor of Medicine
UCSF School of Medicine

Brian A. Boyle, MD, JD
Associate Professor, Division of
International Medicine and
Infectious Diseases
Weill Medical College of Cornell
University

Robert Catalla, MD, AAHIVS
Medical Director
AIDS Healthcare Foundation
Riverside Healthcare Center
Clinical Instructor
Mayo Clinic Jacksonville

Roberto B. Corales, DO
Medical Director
AIDS Community Health Center -
Rochester, New York

Gary M. Cox, MD
Associate Professor of Medicine
Duke University Medical Center

Eric S. Daar, MD, AAHIVS
Chief, Division of HIV Medicine
Harbor-UCLA Medical Center
Professor of Medicine
David Geffen School of Medicine at the
University of California Los Angeles

Joel E. Gallant, MD, MPH, AAHIVS
Associate Professor of Medicine
and Epidemiology
Associate Director,
Johns Hopkins AIDS Service
Division of Infectious Diseases
Johns Hopkins University School
of Medicine

Charles B. Hicks, MD
Associate Professor of Medicine
Division of Infectious Diseases
Duke University Medical Center

Homayoun Khanlou, MD, AAHIVS
Associate Director of Medicine
Regional Medical Director
AIDS Healthcare Foundation

Andrew Luber, PharmD
Consultant,
Division of Infectious Diseases
University of Pennsylvania

Kalvin Yu, MD
Co-Director
HIV/Hepatitis C Clinic
AIDS Healthcare Foundation

PEER REVIEWERS

Bisher Akil, MD
John A. Bartlett, MD
Diane E. Bennett, MD, MPH
Stuart M. Berman, MD, ScM
Bernard Branson, MD
Raphael Campo, MD
Calvin J. Cohen, MD
Kenneth L. Dominguez, MD, MPH
Charles F. Farthing, MD, AAHIVS
Ian Frank, MD
Wolfgang Hladik, MD, MSc
Richard K. Hsu, MD
Mark H. Katz, MD, AAHIVS
Andrew Luber, PharmD
Steve McDougal, MD
Robert Munk, PhD
Fred Poordad, MD
Raul A. Romaguera, DMD, MPH
Paul E. Sax, MD
Pablo Tebas, MD
Stefan Wiktor MD, MPH
Kim Workowski, MD
Benjamin Young, MD, PhD
Andrew Zolopa, MD

AAHIVM REVIEWERS

Rori B. Ferensic
Howard A. Grossman, MD, AAHIVS

PROJECT LEADER

Melanie Moore, MA

MANAGING EDITORS

David Gilden
John Hawes

MEDICAL WRITERS

Tracey Fine, MS, ELS
Alan Gambrell, MPA
David Gilden
John Hawes
Sean Hosein
Kristen J. Kresge, MA
Alyce Kuklinski, MSN, RN, NP
Lark Lands, MS
Priscilla Scherer, RN

TECHNICAL EDITORS

Alyce Kuklinski, MSN, RN, NP
Terri O'Quin
Laurie B. Rosenblum, MPH
Jill Shuman, MS, ELS

COPY AND PROOF EDITORS

Susanna Leuci
Cathy Neel Mills

GRAPHIC ARTIST

Roger Gragg

FACULTY DISCLOSURES

It is the policy of Medial Education Collaborative, Inc. (MEC) to ensure balance, independence, objectivity and scientific rigor in all of its educational activities. In accordance with the Essential Areas and Policies of the Accreditation Council for Continuing Medical Education (ACCME), faculty have been asked to disclose any affiliation or financial interest that may affect the content of their presentation, as well as any discussion that deals with investigational or off-label use of pharmaceutical or medical equipment products. Disclosures do not suggest bias but provide participants with information relevant to evaluating presentations.

The Authors, Program Chair, Co-Chief Editors, and Managing Editors for this program have disclosed the following information.

Stephen L. Becker, MD, AAHIVS
Financial interests: Abbott (research grant); Boehringer Ingelheim (research grant); Bristol-Myers Squibb (research grant); GlaxoSmithKline (research grant); Roche (research grant). No plans to discuss investigational or off-label uses of products.

Brian A. Boyle, MD, JD
Financial interests: Abbott (consulting agreement); Gilead (consulting agreement); GlaxoSmithKline (consulting agreement); Vertex (consulting agreement). No plans to discuss investigational or off-label uses of products.

Robert Catalla, MD, AAHIVS
Financial interests: Abbott (consulting agreement); Boehringer Ingelheim (consulting agreement); Bristol-Myers Squibb (consulting agreement); Gilead (consulting agreement); GlaxoSmithKline (consulting agreement); Merck (consulting agreement); Pfizer (consulting agreement); Roche (consulting agreement). No plans to discuss investigational or off-label uses of products.

Roberto B. Corales, DO
Financial interests: Boehringer Ingelheim (consulting agreement); Bristol-Myers Squibb (consulting agreement); Gilead (consulting agreement); GlaxoSmithKline (consulting agreement); Merck (consulting agreement); Pfizer (consulting agreement); Roche (consulting agreement).
No plans to discuss investigational or off-label uses of products.

Gary M. Cox, MD
No financial interests. Plans to discuss investigational use of tipranavir, and other agents in Phase I-III clinical trials.

Eric S. Daar, MD, AAHIVS
Financial interests: Abbott (clinical grant, consulting agreement); Boehringer Ingelheim (consulting agreement); Bristol-Myers Squibb (consulting agreement); Gilead (consulting agreement); GlaxoSmithKline (consulting agreement); Merck (clinical grant); Ortho Biotech (consulting agreement); Pfizer (consulting agreement); Roche (clinical grant); Serono (clinical grant, consulting agreement); Virologic (clinical grant, consulting agreement). No plans to discuss investigational or off-label uses of products.

Charles F. Farthing, MD, AAHIVS
Financial interests: Abbott (clinical grant, consulting agreement); Boehringer Ingelheim (clinical grant, consulting agreement); Bristol-Myers Squibb (clinical grant, consulting agreement); Gilead (clinical grant, consulting agreement); Roche (clinical grant). Plans for discussion to include investigational or off-label uses of multiple antiretroviral agents.

Ian Frank, MD
Financial interests: Abbott (consulting agreement and other financial interest); Boehringer Ingelheim (clinical grant); Bristol-Myers Squibb (clinical grant, consulting agreement, and other financial interest); GlaxoSmithKline (consulting agreement, and other financial interest); Roche (other financial interest); Tibotec (clinical grant); Virologic (other financial interest). Plans for discussion to include investigational or off-label uses of multiple antiretroviral agents.

Joel E. Gallant, MD, MPH, AAHIVS
Financial interests: Abbott (consulting agreement, honoraria); Boehringer Ingelheim (clinical grant); Bristol-Myers Squibb (clinical grant, consulting agreement); Gilead (clinical grant, consulting agreement, honoraria); GlaxoSmithKline (clinical grant, consulting agreement, honoraria); Roche (clinical grant, honoraria); Vertex (consulting agreement); Tanox (clinical grant, consulting agreement); Tibotec-Virco (clinical grant); Virologic (consulting agreement). No plans to discuss investigational or off-label uses of products.

David Gilden
No financial interests. Plans for content to include investigational or off-label uses of multiple antiretroviral agents.

John Hawes
Financial interests: Amgen (financial interest/stock ownership); Pfizer (consulting agreement). Plans for content to include investigational or off-label uses of multiple antiretroviral agents.

Charles B. Hicks, MD
Financial interests: Abbott (clinical grant, consulting agreement); Boehringer Ingelheim (clinical grant, consulting agreement); Bristol-Myers Squibb (clinical grant, consulting agreement); Gilead (clinical grant); GlaxoSmithKline (clinical grant); Merck (clinical grant); Virologic (clinical grant, consulting agreement). Plans to discuss investigational or off-label uses of products.

Homayoun Khanlou, MD, AAHIVS
No financial interests or plans to discuss investigational or off-label uses of products.

Andrew Luber, PharmD
Financial interests: Abbott (clinical grant, consulting agreement); Boehringer Ingelheim (clinical grant, consulting agreement); Gilead (clinical grant); GlaxoSmithKline (clinical grant, consulting agreement); Roche (clinical grant, consulting agreement); Vertex (agreement). Plans for discussion to include investigational or off-label uses of several antiretroviral agents, including tipranavir.

Paul E. Sax, MD
Financial interests: Abbott (consulting agreement); Bristol-Myers Squibb (consulting agreement); Gilead (consulting agreement); GlaxoSmithKline (clinical grant, consulting agreement); Merck (consulting agreement); Pfizer (clinical grant). Plans for discussion to include investigational or off-label uses of multiple antiretroviral agents.

Kalvin Yu, MD
No financial interests or plans to discuss investigational or off-label uses of products.

ABOUT THE AAHIVM

The American Academy of HIV Medicine (AAHIVM) is an independent organization of AAHIVM HIV Specialists™ (AAHIVS) and others dedicated to advancing excellence in HIV/AIDS care. Through advocacy and education, AAHIVM is committed to supporting health care providers in HIV medicine and to ensuring better care for those living with AIDS and HIV disease.

To promote best practices in the field of HIV medicine, AAHIVM offers a number of resources to its members, their patients, community organizations and government and policy makers. These programs, services and activities, many of which are listed below, have helped establish AAHIVM as an authority in HIV health care education and public policy as well as provide recognition of HIV specialists.

The AAHIVM Self-Directed HIV Medicine Education Program

AAHIVM established the Self-Directed HIV Medicine Education Program as a part of its commitment to frontline HIV health care providers to address these very issues. This program, which includes the Core Curriculum, the *HIV Medicine Self-Directed Study Guide,* and the "HIV Update - An Overview of the Recent Learning Objectives of the AAHIVM Core Curriculum" workshop program, establishes a standard in health care education and training that can improve the quality of life for HIV/AIDS patients, improve outcomes and contribute to a more coordinated approach to HIV care. Private practices, medical groups, specialty organizations and other institutions can use these tools to help their members keep up with recent changes in HIV knowledge.

Credentialing

AAHIVM gives HIV health care providers an opportunity to be nationally recognized as an AAHIVM HIV Specialist™ (AAHIVS). AAHIVM began its credentialing process in December 2001 using its definition of an HIV specialist. Since then, more than 2000 providers have obtained the AAHIVS designation, establishing AAHIVM's credentialing program as a proven and credible process.

AAHIVM's credentialing process is independent of membership and is provided as a free service to both members and nonmembers alike. Credentialing requirements must be met every 2 years to ensure that applicants maintain up-to-date knowledge in HIV medicine.

Public Policy

As a voice at national and state levels, the Academy advocates for the best interests of HIV patients and frontline HIV medical care providers. As part of its commitment to excellence in HIV/AIDS care, the Academy interacts with government agencies, AIDS service organizations and others in efforts to help shape legislation. Through public policy initiatives, the Academy is working to serve patient needs in an era of increased complacency around HIV issues and to bring together historical and present-day perspectives of thousands of HIV primary care providers to advocate for policies that represent their unique point of view.

Contact Us

For more information about AAHIVM, please visit our Website at www.aahivm.org or call us toll-free at 866-241-9601.

OVERVIEW OF HIV INFECTION

This section covers the most recent information developments in the epidemiology, transmission and detection of HIV.

Upon completion of this section, clinicians should be able to describe recent demographic trends in HIV disease; identify the various clades of HIV-1 and discuss the clinically relevant points that derive from that knowledge; describe factors predictive of HIV disease progression; describe accumulating evidence of superinfection; discuss the many diagnostic tests now available; and describe antibody and viral load test sensitivities to HIV variants.

At-a-glance

What's New – Overview

The HIV epidemic continues to expand, with the steepest increases in Eastern Europe and Asia and an increasing incidence among MSM here. Young African American men are at particular risk. The introduction of rapid HIV assays opens new avenues for testing and counseling, as has testing for acute infection through the use of RNA testing on pooled blood samples. Once infected, interpersonal variations in such host factors as CCR5 structure and density influence the course of disease.

Contents

(RLO-1)

I.1. U.S. EPIDEMIOLOGY

LEARNING OBJECTIVE: Describe current demographic trends in HIV disease in the United States, especially regarding gender, sexuality, race/ethnicity, age, injection-drug use, socioeconomic status, emerging subtypes and transmission of resistant virus.

According to the CDC, which reports annually on the prevalence and incidence of HIV and AIDS in the United States and its territories, there were an estimated 929,985 cumulative AIDS cases in 2003, of which an estimated 524,060 (56%) died through the end of that year (CDC 2004). CDC cautions that although the completeness of reporting of AIDS and HIV cases is estimated to be more than 85%, HIV surveillance may not reflect the true incidence of HIV infection because not all HIV-infected persons have been tested. Also, those who test positive through anonymous HIV testing and home testing kits are not automatically recorded in public health surveillance programs. Thus, the CDC estimates that there are currently 850,000 to 950,000 cases of HIV infection and AIDS in the United States, with one-fourth unaware that they are infected (Fleming et al. 2002). Each year, 40,000 new HIV infections occur in the United States

Since the beginning of the epidemic, certain ethnic and other minority groups have comprised a disproportionate number of HIV/AIDS cases in the United States, when measured against their representation in the overall population. This trend continues among persons currently living with AIDS (AIDS prevalence). As of December 2003, African Americans and Hispanics comprised 40% and 19% of persons living with AIDS, but comprise only 12% and 13% of the U.S. population. Whites accounted for 41% of the total number of persons living with AIDS in the United States (CDC 2004). In the 29 states with HIV reporting during 1999-2002, African Americans had an HIV prevalence rate of 75.6 per 100,000 in 2002, nearly 10 times the rate for whites and 2.5 times the rate for Hispanics (Hall et al. 2004). A New York City study including over 70,000 HIV-infected persons found the highest prevalence of HIV/AIDS among African American men ages 40 to 54 years (Wiewel et al. 2004).

Racial and ethnic minorities are overrepresented among all HIV risk groups. Among adult and adolescent men living with AIDS, 47% are men who have sex with men (MSM), 19% are injection-drug users (IDU) and 7% are MSM who use injection drugs (CDC 2004). Minority males represent a disproportionately high number of MSM cases compared with the number of minority males in the general population (CDC 2001). The New York City Department of Health calculated that in 2001, the HIV prevalence among sexually active MSM was 10.2%. It was 18.0% among African American MSM, 10.3% among white MSM and 7.9% among Hispanic MSM (Manning et al. 2004).

Among U.S. adult and adolescent women, who represent 18% of persons living with AIDS in the United States, 55% reported heterosexual sex as their primary risk for infection and 41% reported IDU (CDC 2004). Minority women comprise more than three-fourths of U.S. AIDS cases in women, with African American women representing well over half of these (CDC 2004). One factor driving the HIV infection rate in women appears to be transmission

What's New

Sexually active young men continue to be at high risk for HIV infection, particularly African Americans and men of mixed race. Bisexual young men appear to be a transmission bridge to the heterosexual population. An increase in HIV incidence among MSM appears to be occurring together with an increase in high-risk behavior and a rise in sexually transmitted diseases.

Key Points

- HIV/AIDS cases are greatest among certain at-risk populations, including men who have sex with men (MSM) and injection-drug users.
- HIV/AIDS cases are disproportionately high among racial/ethnic minority populations.
- A significant proportion of HIV-infected individuals in the United States is unaware of their infection. Another segment of the infected population is aware of their diagnosis but has not received medical care.
- Trends suggest a resurgence in cases among MSM, occurring with reports of increased high-risk sexual behavior in this population, recreational drug use, and an increase in the incidence of sexually transmitted diseases.
- Transmission of drug-resistant virus continues to increase.

of infection from young MSM. Results from the Young Men's Survey found that heterosexual sex was prevalent among young MSM and that this group represents a possible "bridge" for transmitting HIV to women (Valleroy et al. 2004a). Young African American MSM who do not acknowledge their sexual identity are at high risk for HIV infection and represent a particular risk factor for transmission to the heterosexual population (Fitzpatrick et al. 2004; Millett 2004).

The number of pediatric AIDS cases diagnosed each year has declined dramatically since the introduction of effective antiretroviral interventions to reduce mother-to-child HIV transmission. In 1992, an estimated 952 total cases of pediatric cases were reported in the United States; in 2003, that number had dropped to 59 (CDC 2004). The results of an epidemiologic study of HIV in adolescents found that the large majority of adolescents with HIV were perinatally infected, suggesting that HIV prevalence in adolescents will likely increase due to improving survival (Liu et al. 2004).

Epidemiologic data indicate that those groups disproportionately affected by HIV infection also have less access to health care because of poverty and social disadvantage (CDC 2004). Socioeconomic factors that render populations vulnerable to HIV infection in include elevated rates of addiction and risk behaviors such as sharing needles, as well as stigmatization of homosexuality. Also, the threat of physical or emotional abuse may obstruct a person's willingness and ability to negotiate condom use (Wingood and DiClemente 1997).

Trends also indicate that the number of newly infected persons is on the rise among both MSM and heterosexuals (CDC 2003a; Fleming et al. 2002). Furthermore, many of those who are newly infected are unaware of their status (Fleming et al. 2002); nearly one-third of those who test positive do not return for their test results (CDC 2003b). This increase in HIV incidence rates is occurring in conjunction with a rise in sexually transmitted diseases (STDs). A retrospective study of adolescent use of U.S. emergency departments between 1992 and 1998 revealed that a large proportion of adolescents visited an emergency room for treatment of an STD (Beckmann et al. 2004). Increasing rates of syphilis are being reported from urban HIV clinics (Buchacz et al. 2004; Zweibel 2004); other data show an increase in gonorrhea cases among MSM and other groups in some areas of the country (Rietmeijer et al. 2003).

High rates of HIV risk behaviors are reported among young gay men (Jacobson et al. 2004; Valleroy et al. 2004b), with 41% reporting at least 1 episode of unprotected anal sex within the preceding 6 months (Valleroy et al. 2000). One study of 6 major metropolitan areas revealed a high incidence of HIV infection reported among young gay men (Table I.1-1) (CDC 2001). Since the introduction of highly active antiretroviral therapy (HAART), there has been an increase in reporting of risky sexual behavior among MSM, which appears to be related to length of time taking the medications, lower educational levels, and use of recreational drugs (Jacobson et al. 2004).

Table I.1-1. Increasing incidence of HIV infection among young gay men (CDC 2001).

	New infections each year [a]		Overall infections [b]	
Race/ethnicity	1994-1998	1998-2000	1994-1998	1998-2000
Black	4.0%	14.7%	14.1%	32.0%
Hispanic	1.8%	3.5%	6.9%	14.0%
White	2.4%	2.5%	3.3%	7.0%

Cities surveyed: Baltimore, Dallas, Los Angeles, Miami, New York, San Francisco, Seattle. Subjects were 15-22 years old (1994-1998; N = 3449) or 23-29 years old (1998-2000, N = 2942).

[a] Percentage of the population becoming infected with HIV each year; incidence.

[b] Overall percentage infected with HIV, regardless of when they became infected; prevalence.

Two multicenter surveys in newly diagnosed or recently infected persons with HIV indicated that resistant strains of HIV are being transmitted in the United States. In a 10-city 1997-2001 study of over 1000 treatment-naive individuals newly diagnosed with HIV, Weinstock and colleagues found that 8.3% had mutations associated with HIV drug resistance (Weinstock et al. 2004). Another 10-city North American study of 377 recently infected patients showed a rise in transmitted HIV drug resistance from 3.4% to 12.4% between 1995 and 2000 (Little et al. 2002). Both these studies utilized convenience samples from consenting individuals in participating centers and were not designed to represent the newly diagnosed or recently infected population of the country as a whole. A more recent study found a significant rise in the transmission of drug-resistant virus in New York City between 2003 and 2004 (Shet et al. 2005).

For newly infected patients, use of resistance testing before initiating antiretroviral therapy may influence the choice of antiretroviral agents. Although prospective clinical trials have not examined this, most recent guidelines for using resistance testing advocate its use in those newly infected (defined as infection within the last 12 months) as well as in some who are chronically infected and about to initiate therapy (DHHS 2004; Hirsch et al. 2003).

Determining the incidence and prevalence of HIV infection is complicated by the increasing HIV-1 genetic diversity occurring in the United States. A survey of African-born patients in selected Minnesota clinics showed that 90% were infected with HIV-1 non-B subtypes (Sides et al. 2004). The researchers did not find any evidence of non-B subtypes among U.S.-born persons. Although it is assumed that the U.S. epidemic is predominantly HIV-1 subtype B, the prevalence of other strains may be substantially higher in cities and states where a relatively greater proportion of HIV cases are individuals originating in countries where other strains predominate.

References

Beckmann KR, Melzer-Lange MD, Gorelick MH. Emergency department management of sexually transmitted infections in US adolescents: Results from the National Hospital Ambulatory Medical Care Survey. *Ann Emerg Med.* **2004**;43:333-338.

Buchacz K, Kellogg T, McFarland W, et al. Trends in primary and secondary syphilis and HIV seroincidence among men who have sex with men in San Francisco, 1998-2002. In: Program and abstracts of the 11th Conference on Retroviruses and Opportunistic Infections; February 8-11, **2004**; San Francisco, California. Abstract 88.

Centers for Disease Control and Prevention (CDC). HIV incidence among young men who have sex with men — seven U.S. cities, 1994-2000. *MMWR Morb Mortal Wkly Rep.* **2001**;50:440-444.

Centers for Disease Control and Prevention (CDC). Increases in HIV Diagnoses – 29 States, 1999-2002. MMWR. **2003a**;52:1145-1148. Available at: http://www.cdc.gov/mmwr/preview/mmwrhtml/mm5247a2.htm [accessed February 21, 2005].

Centers for Disease Control and Prevention (CDC). Advancing HIV Prevention: New Strategies for a Changing Epidemic—United States, 2003. MMWR. **2003b**;52:329-332. Available at: http://www.cdc.gov/mmwr/preview/mmwrhtml/mm5215a1.htm [accessed February 21, 2005].

Centers for Disease Control and Prevention (CDC). Cases of HIV infection and AIDS in the United States, 2003. HIV/AIDS Surveill Rep. **2004**;15. Available at: http://www.cdc.gov/hiv/stats/2003SurveillanceReport.pdf [accessed March 11, 2005].

Department of Health and Human Services (DHHS). Guidelines for the use of antiretroviral agents in HIV-1-infected adults and adolescents. October 29, **2004**. Available at: http://www.aidsinfo.nih.gov/guidelines [accessed February 21, 2005].

Fitzpatrick LK, Grant L, Eure C, et al. Investigation of HIV transmission among young black men who have sex with men (MSM) in North Carolina: Implications for prevention. In: Program and abstracts of the XV International AIDS Conference; July 11-16, **2004**; Bangkok, Thailand. Abstract C10746.

Fleming PL, Byers RH, Sweeney PA, Daniels D, Karon JM, Janssen RS. HIV prevalence in the United States, 2000. In: Program and abstracts of the 9th Conference on Retroviruses and Opportunistic Infections; February 24-28, **2002**; Seattle, Washington. Abstract 11.

Hall HI, Ling Q, Song R, McKenna MT. Recent trends in HIV diagnoses in the United States. In: Program and abstracts of the 11th Conference on Retroviruses and Opportunistic Infections; February 8-11, **2004**; San Francisco, California. Abstract 86.

Hirsch M, Brun-Vezinet F, Bonaventura C, et al. Antiretroviral drug resistance testing in adults infected with human immunodeficiency virus type 1: 2003 recommendations of an international AIDS society–USA panel. *Clin Infect Dis*. **2003**;37:113-128.

Jacobson LP, Ostrow D, Hylton J, Gore ME, Weisberg M, Silvestre A. Unsafe sexual behavior among homosexual men increases in the era of highly active antiretroviral therapy. In: Program and abstracts of the XV International AIDS Conference; July 11-16, **2004**; Bangkok, Thailand. Abstract 1090.

Little SJ, Holte, S, Routy JP, Daar ES, et al. Antiretroviral-drug resistance among patients recently infected with HIV. *N Engl J Med*. **2002**;347:385-394.

Liu KL, Peters V, Brooks A, et al. Epidemiology of adolescents living with HIV in New York City. In: Program and abstracts of the XV International AIDS Conference; July 11-16, **2004**; Bangkok, Thailand. Abstract 4769.

Manning SE, Ramaswamy C, Hajat A, et al. Estimation of HIV prevalence, risk factors, and testing frequency among sexually active men who have sex with men aged 18-64 years, New York City, 2001. In: Program and abstracts of the 11th Conference on Retroviruses and Opportunistic Infections; February 8-11, **2004**; San Francisco, California. Abstract 863.

Millett G. Men on the 'down low': more questions than answers. In: Program and abstracts of the 11th Conference on Retroviruses and Opportunistic Infections; February 8-11, **2004**; San Francisco, California. Abstract 83.

Rietmeijer CA, Patnaik JL, Judson FN, Douglas JM Jr. Increases in gonorrhea and sexual risk behaviors among men who have sex with men: A 12-year trend analysis at the Denver Metro Health Clinic. *Sex Transm Dis*. **2003**;30:562-567.

Shet A, Mohri H, Berry L, et al. Transmission of drug resistant HIV-1 in patients with acute and early HIV-1 infection in 2003 to 2004. In: Program and abstracts of the 12th Conference on Retroviruses and Opportunistic Infections, February 22-25, **2005**; Boston, Massachusetts. Abstract 289.

Sides T, Akinsete O, Henry K, et al. Substantial HIV-1 diversity in Minnesota (USA). In: Program and abstracts of the XV International AIDS Conference; July 11-16, **2004**. Bangkok, Thailand. Abstract 3427.

Valleroy LA, MacKellar D, Behel S, Secura G. The bridge for HIV transmission to women from 15- to 29-year-old men who have sex with men in 7 US cities. In: Program and abstracts of the XV International AIDS Conference; July 11-16, **2004a**; Bangkok, Thailand. Abstract 1367.

Valleroy LA, MacKellar DA, Behel S, Secura G, Mei JV. High HIV incidence among 23- to 29-year-old men who have sex with men in 6 U.S. cities. In: Program and abstracts of the XV International AIDS Conference; July 11-16, **2004b**; Bangkok, Thailand. Abstract 2071.

Valleroy LA, MacKellar DA, Karon JM, et al. HIV prevalence and associated risks in young men who have sex with men. Young Men's Survey Study Group. *JAMA*. **2000**;284:198-204.

Weinstock HS, Zaidi I, Heneine W, et al. The epidemiology of antiretroviral drug resistance among drug-naïve HIV-1-infected persons in 10 US cities. *J Infect Dis*. **2004**;189:2174-2180.

Wiewel EW, Bennani Y, Ramaswamy C, Sackoff JE, Torian LV. High prevalence and late diagnosis of HIV among Black men aged 40-54 in New York City. In: Program and abstracts of the XV International AIDS Conference; July 11-16, **2004**; Bangkok, Thailand. Abstract 3506.

Wingood GM, DiClemente RJ. The effects of an abusive primary partner on the condom use and sexual negotiation practices of African-American women. *Am J Public Health*. **1997**;87:1016-1018.

Zweibel M. Increasing rates of syphilis in an urban HIV clinic. In: Program and abstracts of the XV International AIDS Conference; July 11-16, **2004**; Bangkok, Thailand. Abstract 7389.

(RLO-2)

I.2. GLOBAL VIROLOGY

LEARNING OBJECTIVE: Discuss the global prevalence and geographic distribution of HIV-1 and HIV-2 infection, including HIV-1 subtypes (also known as clades), and recognize the impact that geographic site of HIV acquisition may have on HIV type and its implications for therapy.

Global estimates of HIV are staggering. The latest UNAIDS estimates are 4.9 million new cases in 2004 (range 4.3-6.4 million) and 39.4 million persons living with HIV/AIDS (range 35.9-44.3 million) as of midyear 2004 — the highest number ever (UNAIDS 2004a). (Note: The use of ranges in estimates of incidence and prevalence reflects the large variation in the quality of HIV surveillance systems among countries [Garcia-Calleja et al. 2004].) Approximately two-thirds (64%) of all cases are in sub-Saharan Africa, with this region also accounting for three-quarters (76%) of all women infected with HIV (UNAIDS 2004a). However, the number of HIV-infected persons is rising in every area of the world (Table I.2-1), with the sharpest increases seen in East Asia, Eastern Europe, and Central Asia, with these increases being driven mainly by new cases reported from China, Ukraine, India, and the Russian Federation.

The number of children (less than 15 years old) living with HIV is 2.2 million (range 2.0-2.6 million), with 640,000 newly infected in 2004 (UNAIDS 2004a). There are an estimated 10 million young people between the ages of 15 and 24 years living with HIV, mostly in sub-Saharan Africa (62%) and Asia (22%). This age group is the most vulnerable for infection, accounting for one-half of new HIV infections in 2004 (UNAIDS 2004b).

Table 1.2-1. Estimates of HIV/AIDS worldwide (UNAIDS 2004a).

	Adults and children living with HIV/AIDS	
Region	**2002**	**2004**
Sub-Saharan Africa	24.4 million	25.4 million
South and Southeast Asia	6.4 million	7.1 million
Latin America	1.5 million	1.7 million
Eastern Europe and Central Asia	1.0 million	1.4 million
East Asia	760,000	1.1 million
North America	970,000	1.0 million
Western and Central Europe	600,000	610,000
North Africa and Middle East	430,000	540,000
Caribbean	420,000	440,000
Oceania	28,000	35,000
TOTAL	**36.6 million**	**39.4 million**

The epidemics in Sub-Saharan Africa appear to be stabilizing, but the region of southern Africa still accounts for one-third of AIDS deaths worldwide (UNAIDS 2004a). In addition, AIDS has killed one or both parents of 12 million orphans in sub-Saharan Africa (UNAIDS 2004b), and this number is expected to rise to 18 million by the end of this decade. The

What's New

Prevalence of HIV infection continues to rise in all regions of the world, with the steepest increases now occurring in Eastern Europe and Asia. Adult and adolescent women now account for almost one-half of all HIV infections. Increasing genetic diversity in HIV subtypes is occurring.

Key Points

- An estimated 40 million people worldwide are infected with HIV, and the prevalence of HIV is increasing in all global regions, with women appearing to be at the greatest risk of infection.
- HIV occurs as types 1 and 2, with several groups and subtypes comprising HIV-1.
- Subtype B predominates in the Western Hemisphere and Western Europe, but other varieties and recombinant forms are more prevalent elsewhere. However, introduction of different subtypes and recombinant strains is occurring in the Western Hemisphere and Western Europe.
- Extrapolation of the HIV prevalence in Minnesota Africans and the proportion (98%) of non-B viruses found in this population to all U.S. Africans suggest that at least 4% of the annual 40,000 U.S. HIV cases may be non-B subtypes.

Caribbean has the second highest HIV prevalence in the world, and AIDS is the leading cause of death in adults ages 15 to 44 in this region (UNAIDS 2004a). Adult and adolescent women represent groups in which HIV prevalence is increasing, with almost one-half of all HIV cases now in women and girls. Areas in which the proportion of adult and adolescent women is growing include Eastern Europe, Asia, and Latin America.

Women are at greatest risk in areas where heterosexual transmission represents a major mode of transmission, such as Sub-Saharan Africa and the Caribbean. In Sub-Saharan Africa, young women are 3 to 6 times more likely to become infected than are men of the same ages (UNAIDS 2004a). In other regions of the world, HIV is mostly transmitted through injection-drug use and unprotected sex between men or with a commercial sex worker or a combination of these modes. However, in all global regions, a sizable proportion of men who have sex with men also have sex with women, and young injection-drug users are often sexually active. These two factors are affecting the increases of infection seen in heterosexual women and shifting the mode of transmission in areas like Latin America, Eastern Europe, and the Far East, where HIV infection has typically involved unprotected sex between men, injection-drug users, or commercial sex workers.

It is important to note that the epidemic in different geographic areas cannot be seen as limited to one risk group or mode of transmission (UNAIDS 2004b; Buve et al. 2001). The factors influencing the HIV epidemic globally are heterogenous and complex, especially in regions like sub-Saharan Africa. The prevalence of HIV is increasing in all regions of the world due not only to risky sexual behavior but also to factors that enhance HIV transmission, such as political and cultural barriers, migration, lack of male circumcision, and the rise of sexually transmitted diseases such as syphilis and herpes simplex virus type 2 infection (Celum 2004; Jin et al. 2004; Marcus et al. 2004; Reynolds et al. 2003; Buve et al. 2001).

The introduction of potent antiretroviral therapy around 1995 and 1996 interrupted the steady increase of 16% in AIDS mortality seen annually from 1987 through 1994, with a subsequent and dramatic decline in AIDS deaths from 1995 to 1997 in the United States (Minino and Smith 2001). AIDS epicenters in developing countries have not realized such progress given the lack of health services and access to antiretroviral therapy. Approximately only 1 out of 10 people needing antiretroviral treatment in low- and middle-income countries were receiving treatment in 2004 (WHO 2004).

Geographic Distribution of HIV Subtypes

HIV is categorized primarily as type 1 or type 2. HIV-1 may be more infectious and virulent than HIV-2. The majority of HIV-2 cases are found in West Africa, with few reported cases in the United States (CDC 1998).

HIV-1 strains fall under three genetically related groups, with group M being most common and groups O and N being relatively rare. Within group M are at least nine subtypes (also called clades): A through I (NIAID 2003).

Africa has the most diversity in HIV-1 strains. Subtype C is the most prevalent subtype in southern and eastern Africa, although subtypes A and D are most prominent in a focused central region of eastern Africa. West Africa harbors primarily recombinant forms: AG, plus a low prevalence of others. Central Africa, the putative home of the epidemic, contains a wide variety of rare subtypes and recombinants (IAVI 2003).

Subtype B is the predominant subtype in the Western Hemisphere, Australia, and Western Europe. The sole exception is in eastern regions of South America, where BF recombinants are also common. In Eastern Europe, subtypes A, B, and AB recombinant strains are the main subtypes. Asia possesses three different patterns: The Indian subcontinent has mostly subtype C; China has mainly B, C, and BC recombinants; and Southeast Asia has a mixture of subtype B and AE recombinant (IAVI 2003).

Subtype differences may be relevant to vaccine development, although this is not yet confirmed (NIAID 2003; Johnston and Flores 2001). Specifically, the global distribution of different subtypes of HIV-1 may have implications for vaccine development in that a single vaccine may be unable to provide cross-subtype immunity (NIAID 2003). Subtype variability may also influence how antiretroviral therapy is used. Although preliminary studies suggest that current antiretrovirals appear to be equally effective regardless of viral subtype, patterns of resistance may vary (Spira et al. 2003; Gomes et al. 2002). A recent study showed that discordant viral load results were obtained in persons with non-B subtypes (Hackett et al. 2004). There is scant information on the effect of antiretroviral therapy for HIV-2 infection. An in vitro study found that while the HIV-2 isolates tested were susceptible to the antiviral activities of nucleoside reverse transcriptase inhibitors (NRTIs) and most protease inhibitors (PIs), HIV-2 was highly resistant to nonnucleoside reverse transcriptase inhibitors (NNRTIs) (Witvrouw et al. 2004). Of the PIs, amprenavir showed diminished antiviral activity. Other studies of patients infected with HIV-2 receiving antiretroviral treatment have found mutations in HIV-2 reverse transcriptase and protease that are associated with HIV-1 drug resistance for each drug class, including enfuvirtide (Colson et al. 2005; Damond et al. 2005; Witvrouw et al. 2004; Rodés et al. 2000).

As HIV infection persists and becomes more prevalent globally, increasing genetic diversity in HIV subtypes is being reported (Aggarwal et al. 2004; Dos Santos et al. 2004; Hackett et al. 2004; Linka et al. 2004; Sides et al. 2004). Emigration and travel related to migrant work, tourism and military service are the likely causes for the emergence of new subtypes and recombinant strains. One study in the United States found a high proportion of non-B HIV in the African immigrant population, which if extrapolated to the entire country would represent 4% of the estimated 40,000 new HIV infections in 2004 (Sides et al. 2004). Once introduced, ongoing transmission of non-B subtypes in predominantly B-subtype regions can increase the amount of strain diversity (Aggarwal et al. 2004).

See also information on HIV variants in Objective I.13 on Testing Methods in this Update.

References

Aggarwal I, Smith M, Tatt I, et al. Evidence of onward transmission of HIV-1 non-B subtype strains in the UK. In: Program and abstracts of the XV International AIDS Conference; July 11-16, **2004**; Bangkok, Thailand. Abstract 1363.

Buve A, Carael M, Hayes RJ, et al. The multicentre study on factors determining the differential spread of HIV in four African cities: summary and conclusions. *AIDS*. **2001**;15(suppl 4):S127-S131.

Celum C. Herpes simplex and the global epidemiology of HIV. In: Program and abstracts of the 11th Conference on Retroviruses and Opportunistic Infections; February 8-11, **2004**; San Francisco, California. Abstract 142.

Centers for Disease Control and Prevention (CDC). Fact Sheet: Human Immunodeficiency Virus Type 2. **1998**. Available at: http://www.cdc.gov/hiv/pubs/facts/hiv2.htm [accessed February 21, 2005].

Colson P, Henry M, Tivoli N, et al. Polymorphism and drug-selected mutations in the reverse transcriptase gene of HIV-2 from patients living in southeastern France. *J Med Virol.* **2005**;75:381-390.

Damond F, Brun-Vezinet F, Matheron S, et al. Polymorphism of the human immunodeficiency virus type 2 (HIV-2) protease gene and selection of drug resistance mutations in HIV-2-infected patients treated with protease inhibitors. *J Clin Microbiol.* **2005**;43:484-487.

Dos Santos G, Ouka M, Cabie A, et al. Monitoring of HIV genetic diversity in Guadeloupe, Martinique and French Guiana emphasize the need for a regional surveillance network. In: Program and abstracts of the XV International AIDS Conference; July 11-16, **2004**; Bangkok, Thailand. Abstract 3445.

Garcia-Calleja JM, Zaniewski E, Ghys PD, Stanecki K, Walker N. A global analysis of trends in the quality of HIV sero-surveillance. *Sex Transm Infect.* **2004**;80(suppl 1):i25-i30.

Gomes P, Diogo I, Goncalves MF, et al. Different pathways to nelfinavir genotypic resistance in HIV-1 subtypes B and G. In: Program and abstracts of the 9th Conference on Retroviruses and Opportunistic Infections; February 24-28, **2002**; Seattle, Washington. Abstract 46.

Hackett Jr J, Holzmayer V, Swanson P, et al. Analysis of HIV-1 genetic diversity in London and its impact on the performance of viral load assays. In: Program and abstracts of the XV International AIDS Conference; July 11-16, **2004**; Bangkok, Thailand. Abstract 3419.

International AIDS Vaccine Initiative (IAVI). Global distribution of HIV-1 subtypes and recombinants. August **2003**. Available at: http://www.aegis.com/pubs/iavi/2003/HIV-clademap.pdf [accessed March 3, 2005].

Jin FY, Prestage G, Van de Ven P, et al. Prevalence, incidence and risk factors for HIV, syphilis, gonorrhoea and chlamydia in an HIV negative cohort of homosexual men. In: Program and abstracts of the XV International AIDS Conference; July 11-16, **2004**; Bangkok, Thailand. Abstract 7358.

Johnston MI, Flores J. Progress in HIV vaccine development. *Curr Opin Pharmacol.* **2001**;1:504-510.

Linka M, Bruckova M, Vandasova J, Reinis M, Stankova M. Study of HIV-1 subtypes identified in the Czech Republic. In: Program and abstracts of the XV International AIDS Conference; July 11-16, **2004**; Bangkok, Thailand. Abstract 3432.

Marcus U, Hamouda O, Voss L, Bremer V, Kollan C. Large increase of syphilis incidence among MSM in Germany since 2000 accompanied by only small increase of newly diagnosed HIV infections. In: Program and abstracts of the XV International AIDS Conference; July 11-16, **2004**; Bangkok. Abstract 7332.

Minino AM, Smith BL. Deaths: preliminary data for 2000. *Natl Vit Stat Rep.* **2001**;49:1-40.

National Institute on Allergies and Infectious Diseases (NIAID). Vaccines, Science. **2003**. Available at: http://www.niaid.nih.gov/daids/vaccine/science.htm [accessed February 21, 2005]

Reynolds SJ, Risbud AR, Shepherd ME, et al. Recent herpes simplex virus type 2 infection and the risk of human immunodeficiency virus type 1 acquisition in India. *J Infect Dis.* **2003**;187:1513-1521.

Rodés B, Holguin A, Soriano V, et al. Emergence of drug resistance mutations in human immunodeficiency virus type 2-infected subjects undergoing antiretroviral therapy. *J Clin Microbiol.* **2000**;38:1370-1374.

Sides T, Akinsete O, Henry K, et al. Substantial HIV-1 diversity in Minnesota (USA). In: Program and abstracts of the XV International AIDS Conference; July 11-16, **2004**; Bangkok, Thailand. Abstract 3427.

Spira S, Wainberg MA, Loemba H, Turner D, Brenner BG. Impact of clade diversity on HIV-1 virulence, antiretroviral drug sensitivity and drug resistance. *J Antimicrob Chemother.* **2003**;51:229-240.

United Nations Programme on HIV/AIDS (UNAIDS). AIDS epidemic update 2004. December **2004a**. Available at: http://www.unaids.org/wad2004/report.html [accessed February 21, 2005].

United Nations Programme on HIV/AIDS (UNAIDS). 2004 report on the global AIDS epidemic. **July 2004b**. Available at: http://www.unaids.org/bangkok2004/report.html [accessed February 21, 2005].

Witvrouw M, Pannecouque C, Switzer WM, Folks TM, De Clercq E, Heneine W. Susceptibility of HIV-2, SIV and SHIV to various anti-HIV-1 compounds: implications for treatment and postexposure prophylaxis. *Antivir Ther.* **2004**;9:57-65.

World Health Organization (WHO). Investing in a comprehensive health sector response to HIV/AIDS — Scaling up treatment and accelerating prevention: WHO HIV/AIDS Plan (January 2004-December 2005). Geneva: World Health Organization; **2004**. Available at www.wpro.who.int/pdf/rcm55/en/docs/RC55_INFDOC2.pdf [accessed January 5, 2005].

(RLO-3)

I.5. PREDICTIVE FACTORS FOR HIV DISEASE PROGRESSION

LEARNING OBJECTIVE: Demonstrate knowledge of the factors predictive of HIV disease progression, including host factors that can result in differences in progression and how to communicate this concept to patients.

The natural history of HIV infection is extremely heterogeneous across the human population. It is estimated that the average individual progresses from infection to symptomatic HIV disease over a period of 8 to 10 years (Biggar et al. 1990; Rutherford et al. 1990). However, approximately 10% of individuals will progress to AIDS during the first 4 years (Phair et al. 1992), whereas others remain asymptomatic, with high CD4 counts and low plasma HIV RNA levels, for more than 8 to 10 years (Ashton et al. 1998; Cao et al. 1995). There has been much interest in studying these so-called "rapid progressors" and "long-term nonprogressors" to determine markers that predict, and factors that are associated with, immunologic and clinical progression.

There are many viral factors that influence HIV disease progression. Similarly, host factors differ among individuals and influence both the acquisition of infection and disease progression once infection is established. Research is ongoing to determine the complex interactions that might be at work.

Host Factors Associated With HIV Disease Progression

Research has focused on the host factors that influence clinical HIV disease progression and that may in part explain the heterogeneity of HIV disease (Fauci 1996). These factors include variation in host immune responses, HLA type, and genetic markers, such as the 32-base pair deletion in the chemokine co-receptor CCR5 gene. All appear to have an influence on infection and/or disease progression. Many more genetic polymorphisms that have been identified are being investigated, and probably others remain to be discovered as well as their complex interactions that influence HIV infection and disease progression (Tang and Kaslow 2003).

Immune Responses and the Natural History of HIV Disease

There are many studies that have demonstrated a relationship between host immune responses and disease progression. In particular, studies have focused on cellular immune responses, focusing on the role that HIV-1-specific CD4+ and CD8+ T cells play in controlling HIV replication. Several analyses indicate a relationship among the development, magnitude, and breadth of cellular immune responses and the initial control of viral replication during primary infection (Gloster et al. 2004; Musey et al. 1997). The data are compatible with the hypothesis that preservation of a strong immune response is associated with being a long-term nonprogressor (Rosenberg et al. 1997). Although it is always difficult to prove cause and effect in cohort studies, recent data demonstrate a relationship between the development of mutations in epitopes targeted by immune responses and increasing plasma HIV RNA level, so called mutational escape of virus from immunologic control. These data provide additional evidence for a direct link between immune responses and viral replication (Oxenius et al. 2004).

What's New

There is growing but incomplete evidence that complex host and viral factors may influence HIV infectivity and disease progression. Among the host factors are the CCR5 co-receptor (both its variation in sequence and density on cells), human leukocyte antigen (HLA), natural killer cell killer immunoglobulin-like receptor (KIR), and APOBEC3F and APOBEC3G proteins. Viral co-infection factors may include the impact of GB virus C (GBV-C) on disease progression, although data are inconclusive at this point.

Key Points

- HIV disease progression is affected by both host and viral factors.
- Host factors, such as immune response, HLA type and genetic mutations of co-receptors, their ligands and others, may influence the likelihood of infection and/or disease progression.
- Viral factors affecting disease progression include virulence of virus type and, possibly, co-infection with other viruses, such as GBV-C (hepatitis G).
- Markers of disease progression are well established and include levels of HIV RNA and CD4+ T cells.

Genetic Factors Associated With Natural History of HIV Infection

There are increasing numbers of studies identifying genetic polymorphisms that influence both HIV-1 infection and the rate of disease progression. Most data correlate disease progression and HLA types, genetic variations in chemokine receptor genes, such as CCR5, their natural ligands, and various cytokines. This was reviewed recently by O'Brien and Nelson (2004).

HLA type and HIV disease

Human leukocyte antigen (HLA) on the surface of antigen-presenting and other cells display foreign rotein to provoke immune activity. Certain HLA types, most notably B27 and B57, have been associated with significantly slower disease progression in some studies (Migueles et al. 2000; Kaslow et al. 1996) but not all (Migueles et al. 2000). Alternatively, HLA-B*35 carriers appear to develop AIDS twice as rapidly as those without this HLA type (O'Brien and Nelson 2004; Carrington and O'Brien 2003; Gao et al. 2001). The reason for the association between disease progression and certain HLA haplotypes is under investigation and may relate to important differences in one's ability to make effective cellular immune responses against important virus epitopes (Migueles et al. 2000). Consistent with this hypothesis are recent data from the Swiss Cohort study demonstrating a relationship between select HLA types and differences in disease progression and host immune response (Scherer et al. 2004). As is true with many genetic mutations associated with alterations in the natural history of HIV disease, individual HLA haplotypes can be shown to predict disease course in populations but may not do so in a specific individual because of the simultaneous effect of many other factors. Therefore, on the basis of our knowledge, these select genetic markers cannot reliably be used to guide clinical decisions.

Co-receptors

HIV employs specific cellular receptors and co-receptors in order to enter the cell and initiate infection (Paxton et al. 1998; reviewed in Cohen et al. 1999). Although the CD4 molecule is the primary receptor for HIV, a secondary co-receptor is needed for infection to occur. The most important co-receptors are the chemokine receptors CCR5 and CXCR4. The chemokine receptors have important functions unrelated to HIV-1 and have natural ligands that play a role in host immune responses to a variety of pathogens (Lin et al. 2002; Paxton et al. 1998). Data indicate that CCR5 density may influence viral load and disease progression, with increasing density associated with accelerated disease progression (Reynes, et al. 2001) and modulation of the efficiency of viral replication (Lin et al. 2002). Of more interest are observations that genetic polymorphisms in this chemokine receptor gene and its promoter are associated with ability to become infected with HIV and disease progression.

Individuals who homozygous for the well-characterized 32 base pair deletion in the CCR5 gene do not express this co-receptor on the surface of their cells and are resistant to becoming infected with HIV-1 (Paxton et al. 1998). In rare circumstances, such individuals can be infected with HIV that uses another chemokine receptor, CXCR4, in which case rapid progression is likely to occur (Sheppard et al. 2002). Approximately 1% of individuals of northern and western European descent have this genetic mutation (Paxton et al. 1998). The mutation has not been identified in patients from Africa and Asia (Cohen et al. 1999). Although chemokine receptors have important functions, there are many different types with much crossover function among them, so the loss of the CCR5 receptor does not seem to cause any significant health problems.

Having only one abnormal gene for CCR5 is considerably more common than having two. Although those who are heterozygous for the CCR5 gene mutation are not protected from infection, they have a slower rate of disease progression to death by approximately 2 to 4 years (reviewed in Carrington et al. 2001). Genetic polymorphisms have also been seen in the CCR5 promoter (P1) that, when present in both genes, possibly increase CCR5 density on the surface of the cells and thus accelerate progression to AIDS (Martin et al. 1998). Mutations resulting in changes in another chemokine receptor, CCR2, are associated with a statistically significant reduction in the rate of disease progression (Carrington et al. 2001; Kostrikis et al. 1998). Once again, these effects are based on average survival and do not predict what will happen in a given individual.

Other genetic factors influencing disease progression

In addition to the above, other factors that may inhibit or promote HIV infectivity and disease progression are under investigation. Among these is the natural killer cell killer immunoglobulin-like receptor (KIR)—more specifically, the activating KIR allele KIR3DS1. One study demonstrated its delaying effect on progression to AIDS in an interaction with HLA-B Bw4-80Ile (Martin et al. 2002). Other factors recently reviewed are APOBEC3F and APOBEC3G, proteins that block HIV replication during reverse transcription. Their anti-HIV action is blocked by the viral Vif protein (Zheng et al. 2004), and alterations in these genes may influence the natural history of HIV disease (An et al. 2004).

Viral Factors Associated With HIV Disease Progression

The most commonly used viral markers of disease progression have been viral load (plasma HIV RNA levels) and assays of in vitro virulence and fitness. Studies of virulence have focused primarily on the ability of HIV to replicate to high levels in tissue culture systems, induce syncytia in peripheral blood mononuclear cells, and infect T-cell tumor lines. These viruses, described as "syncytium-inducing" (SI) strains, use the CXCR4 chemokine receptor and are referred to as "X4" viruses. These strains are seen in approximately 50% of individuals with AIDS.

In contrast, the majority of asymptomatic patients are initially infected by viruses that are non-syncytium-inducing (NSI) in vitro, infect monocytes/macrophages but not T-cell tumor lines, and use the CCR5 chemokine receptor; these are referred to as "R5" viruses (Berger 1998; Schuitemaker et al. 1992; Tersmette et al. 1988). The transition from NSI to SI virus is often associated with a precipitous decline in CD4 counts and presages clinical progression (Daar et al. 1995; Tersmette et al. 1989). Several studies have demonstrated that the presence of SI virus predicts disease progression (Koot et al. 1993) and, more recently, that the detection of X4 virus is also associated with more rapid CD4+ T cell decline and progression to AIDS (Daar et al. 2003).

HIV-1 fitness has also been proposed to be variable and to potentially influence the natural history of HIV disease. Measuring fitness is complex and has been reviewed by Bates et al. (2003). Several cross-sectional studies have shown relationships between various measures of viral fitness, plasma HIV RNA level, and stage of disease (Campbell et al. 2003; Quinones-Mateu et al. 2000). More recent data also show the relationship between viral fitness defined by reverse transcriptase- and protease-determined (*pol*) replication capacity and disease progression in newly and chronically infected individuals (Barbour et al. 2004; Daar et al. 2003). In fact, it has been proposed that changes in *pol* replication capacity associated with drug resistance mutations may influence disease progression in those failing antiretroviral therapy (Deeks et al. 2001). (Viral fitness is described in greater detail in Objective IV.28 on Viral Fitness and Replicative Capacity in this Update.)

In addition to specific properties of HIV-1, co-infection with other viruses may also alter the natural history of HIV-1 disease. Tillmann and colleagues (2001) reported that HIV-positive individuals who are co-infected with persistent GBV-C had slower HIV disease progression than individuals who were not co-infected. Williams and associates confirmed this finding, documenting improved survival for both those with GBV-C at 12 to 18 months after seroconversion and those evaluated at 5 to 6 years (Williams et al. 2004). In contrast, Bjorkman and colleagues (2004) found no correlation between GBV-C infection and disease outcome for those with asymptomatic infection but did see improved survival for the subset of patients who had symptomatic GBV-C. Both Williams and Bjorkman noted that the poorest prognosis was seen for those patients who experienced a loss of GBV-C viremia, which happened with more frequency during later follow-up (Bjorkman et al. 2004; Williams et al. 2004). GBV-C infection is not currently associated with any disease, and the mechanism by which GBV-C may render a protective effect on HIV disease progression is unclear.

Co-infection with other viruses, such as hepatitis C, may also affect HIV disease progression (see Objective III.42 on Hepatitis in this Update).

References

An P, Bleiber G, Duggal P, et al. APOBEC3G genetic variants and their influence on the progression to AIDS. *J Virol.* **2004**;78:11070-11076.

Ashton LJ, Carr A, Cunningham PH, et al. Predictors of progression in long-term nonprogressors. *AIDS Res Hum Retroviruses.* **1998**;14:117-122.

Barbour JD, Hecht FM, Wrin T, et al. Higher CD4+ T cell counts associated with low viral *pol* replication capacity among treatment-naive adults in early HIV-1 infection. *J Infect Dis.* **2004**;190:251-256.

Bates M, Wrin T, Huang W, et al. Practical applications of viral fitness in clinical practice. *Curr Opin Infect Dis.* **2003**;16:11-18.

Berger EA. HIV-1 phenotype classified by co-receptor usage [letter]. *Nature.* **1998**;291:240.

Biggar RJ, and the International Registry of Seroconverters. AIDS incubation in 1,891 HIV seroconverters from different exposure groups. *AIDS.* **1990**;4:1059-1066.

Bjorkman P, Flamholc L, Naucler A, et al. GB virus C during the natural course of HIV-1 infection: Viremia at diagnosis does not predict mortality. *AIDS.* **2004**;18:877-886.

Campbell TB, Schneider K, Wrin T, Petropoulos CJ, Connick E. Relationship between in vitro human immunodeficiency virus type 1 replication rate and virus load in plasma. *J Virol.* **2003**;77:12105-12112.

Cao Y, Qin L, Zhang L, Safrit J, Ho DD. Virologic and immunologic characterization of long-term survivors of human immunodeficiency virus type 1 infection. *N Engl J Med.* **1995**;332:201-208.

Carrington M, Nelson G, O'Brien SJ. Considering genetic profiles in functional studies of immune responsiveness to HIV-1. *Immunol Lett.* **2001**;79:131-140.

Carrington M, O'Brien SJ. The influence of *HLA* genotype on AIDS. *Annu Rev Med.* **2003**;54:535-551.

Cohen O, Weissman D, Fauci AS. The immunopathogenesis of HIV infection. In: Paul WE, ed. *Fundamental Immunology.* 4th ed. New York: Raven Press; **1999**:1455-1509.

Daar ES, Chernyavskiy T, Zhao JQ, Krogstad P, Chen ISY, Zack JA. Sequential determination of viral load and phenotype in human immunodeficiency virus type 1 infection. *AIDS Res Hum Retroviruses.* **1995**;11:3-9.

Daar ES, Kesler K, Lail A, et al. HIV co-receptor tropism (CRT)and replication capacity (RC) predict HIV progression. In: Program and abstracts of the 43rd Interscience Conference on Antimicrobial Agents and Chemotherapy; September 14-17, **2003**; Chicago, Illinois.

Deeks SG, Wrin T, Liegler T, et al. Virologic and immunologic consequences of discontinuing combination antiretroviral-drug therapy in HIV-infected patients with detectable viremia. *N Engl J Med.* **2001**;344:472-480.

Fauci AS. Host factors and pathogenesis of HIV-induced disease. *Nature.* **1996**;384:529-534.

Gao X, Nelson GW, Karacki P, et al. Effect of a single amino acid change in MHC class I molecules on the rate of progression to AIDS. *N Engl J Med.* **2001**;344:1668-1675.

Gloster SE, Newton P, Cornforth D, et al. Association of strong virus-specific CD4 T cell responses with efficient natural control of primary HIV-1 infection. *AIDS.* **2004**;18:749-755.

Kaslow R, Carrington M, Apple R, et al. Influence of combinations of major histocompatibility complex genes on the course of HIV-1 infection. *Nat Med.* **1996**;2:405-411.

Koot M, Keet IPM, Vos AHV, et al. Prognostic value of HIV-1 syncytium-inducing phenotype for rate of CD4+ cell depletion and progression to AIDS. *Ann Intern Med.* **1993**;118:681-688.

Kostrikis LG, Huang Y, Moore JP, et al. A chemokine receptor CCR2 allele delays HIV-1 disease progression and is associated with a *CCR5* promoter mutation. *Nat Med.* **1998**;4:350-353.

Lin, Y, Mettling C, Portales P, Reynes J, Clot J, Corbeau P. Cell surface CCR5 density determines the postentry efficiency of R5 HIV-1 infection. *Proc Natl Acad Sci U S A.* **2002**;99:15590-15595.

Martin MP, Dean M, Smith MW, et al. Genetic acceleration of AIDS progression by a promoter variant of CCR5. *Science.* **1998**;282:1907-1911.

Martin MP, Gao X, Lee J, et al. Epistatic interaction between *KIR3DS1* and *HLA-B* delays the progression to AIDS. *Nat Genetics.* **2002**;31:429-434.

Migueles SA, Sabbaghian MS, Schupert WL, et al. HLA B*5701 is highly associated with restriction of virus replication in a subgroup of HIV-infected long term nonprogressors. *Proc Natl Acad Sci U S A.* **2000**;97:2709-2714.

Musey L, Hughes J, Schacker T, et al. Cytotoxic-T-cell responses, viral load, and disease progression in early human immunodeficiency virus type 1 infection. *N Engl J Med.* **1997**;337:1267-1274.

O'Brien, SJ, Nelson, GW. Human genes that limit AIDS. *Nat Genetics.* **2004**;36:565-574.

Oxenius A, Price DA, Trkola A, et al. Loss of viral control in early HIV-1 infection is temporally associated with sequential escape from CD8+ T cell responses and decrease in HIV-1-specific CD4+ and CD8+ T cell frequencies. *J Infect Dis.* **2004**;190:713-721.

Paxton WA, Kang S, Koup RA. The HIV type 1 coreceptor CCR5 and its role in viral transmission and disease progression. *AIDS Res Hum Retroviruses.* **1998**;14(suppl 1):S89-S92.

Phair J, Jobson L, Detels R, et al. Acquired immune deficiency syndrome occurring within 5 years of infection with human immunodeficiency virus type-1: the Multicenter AIDS Cohort Study. *J Acquir Immune Defic Syndr.* **1992**;5:490-496.

Quinones-Mateu ME, Ball SC, Marozsan AJ, et al. A dual infection/competition assay shows a correlation between ex vivo human immunodeficiency virus type 1 fitness and disease progression. *J Virol.* **2000**;74:9222-9233.

Reynes J, Portales P, Segondy M, et al. CD4 T cell surface CCR5 density as a host factor in HIV-1 disease progression. *AIDS.* **2001**;15:1627-1634.

Rosenberg ES, Billingsley JM, Caliendo AM, et al. Vigorous HIV-1-specific CD4+ T cell responses associated with control of viremia. *Science.* **1997**;278:1447-1450.

Rutherford GW, Lifson AR, Hessol NA, et al. Course of HIV-1 infection in a cohort of homosexual and bisexual men: an 11 year follow-up study. *Br Med J.* **1990**;301:1183-1188.

Scherer A, Frater J, Oxenius A, et al. Quantifiable cytotoxic T lymphocyte responses and HLA-related risk of progression to AIDS. *Proc Natl Acad Sci U S A.* **2004**;101:12266-12270.

Schuitemaker H, Koot M, Kootstra NA, et al. Biological phenotype of human immunodeficiency virus type 1 clones at different stages of infection: progression of disease is associated with a shift from monocytotropic to T-cell-tropic virus populations. *J Virol.* **1992**;66:1354-1360.

Sheppard HW, Celum C, Michael NL, et al. HIV-1 infection in individuals with the CCR5-delta32/delta32 genotype: acquisition of syncytium-inducing virus at seroconversion. *J Acquir Immune Defic Syndr.* **2002**;29:307-313.

Tang J, Kaslow RA. The impact of host genetics on HIV infection and disease progression in the era of highly active antiretroviral therapy. *AIDS.* **2003**;17(suppl 4):S51-S60.

Tersmette M, De Goede R, Al BJM, et al. Differential syncytium-inducing capacity of HIV isolates: frequent detection of syncytium-inducing isolates in patients with AIDS and ARC. *J Virol.* **1988**;62:2026-2032.

Tersmette M, Gruters RA, de Wolf F, et al. Evidence for a role of virulent human immunodeficiency virus (HIV) variants in the pathogenesis of acquired immunodeficiency syndrome: studies on sequential HIV isolates. *J Virol.* **1989**;63:2118-2125.

Tillmann HL, Heiken H, Knapik-Botor A, et al. Infection with GB virus C and reduced mortality among HIV-infected patients. *N Engl J Med.* **2001**;345:715-724.

Williams CF, Klinzman D, Yamashita TE, et al. Persistent GB virus C infection and survival in HIV-infected men. *N Engl J Med*. **2004**;350:981-990.

Zheng Y, Irwin D, Kurosu T, et al. Human APOBEC3F is another host factor that blocks human immunodeficiency virus type 1 replication. *J Virol*. **2004**;78:6073-6076.

(RLO-4)

I.10. SUPERINFECTION

LEARNING OBJECTIVE: Discuss the data regarding HIV coinfection and superinfection/reinfection, and the implications for patient education/management.

Dual Infection

In one study of 31 female sex workers, blood samples showed that 19% were dually infected, although none showed evidence of superinfection. All dual infections were detected within 3 months of seroconversion, suggesting that occurrences were at or near the time of seroconversion (Grobler et al. 2004). In another study, a retrospective analysis of multiple cohorts identified 5 subjects who had been dually infected. Data suggest that all 5 progressed to AIDS more rapidly, with an AIDS-defining event occurring within 3 to 4 years and with the average time for CD4 counts to drop below 200 cells/mm^3 being less than 3.1 years (Gottlieb et al. 2004).

Superinfection

Animal data and the presence of circulating recombinant viruses throughout the world have long supported the possibility of superinfection; however, it has been difficult to prove that this phenomenon actually occurs in humans (Sharpe et al. 1997; McCutchan et al. 1996; Robertson et al. 1995). One of the first cases of probable HIV superinfection in humans was published by Jost and colleagues (2002). They described a person, followed from the time of seroconversion with a type AE strain of HIV, who was subsequently found to be infected with a subtype B strain after a new sexual exposure in Brazil. Given the comprehensive documentation of the patient's medical history in the case report, the authors concluded that this new strain emerged as a result of HIV superinfection. Although this provides strong evidence that superinfection can occur, it does not definitively prove it given the absence of documentation that the new subtype B virus matched that of the new contact.

Another reasonably convincing case of HIV superinfection was reported by investigators in Boston, where a person treated at the time of primary infection was able to control the virus after stopping therapy for a prolonged period of time, only to later experience viral rebound. Phylogenetic evidence strongly supported the conclusion that the person rebounded with a virus different from that with which he was initially infected. Using highly sensitive molecular techniques, the second virus was not detected before viral rebound. Once again, the potential source of the second virus was not available for evaluation. This study was also notable because HIV-specific immune responses in this subject were thoroughly characterized. In fact, he had strong responses to both the first and the second viruses, suggesting that despite preexisting immunity to the second virus he appears to have been superinfected (Altfeld et al. 2002).

In addition to these studies, other case reports also suggest that superinfection occurs (Koelsch et al. 2003; Ramos et al. 2002). Thus far, the evidence in these cases relies primarily on phylogenetic data showing that the second virus is distinct from the first. In addition, these cases were unable to identify the second virus at an earlier time point. A mathematical model examined the possibility that superinfection occurrences, even if rare, could account

What's New

Documented cases of superinfection remain rare and are limited to small case reports or case series, usually in subjects followed from the time of suspected superinfection. Among the limited cases identified, superinfection has not been fully documented among chronically infected individuals. Cases of dual infection have been documented with higher levels of frequency.

Key Points

- Dual infection, meaning infection with two HIV strains at or close to the time of seroconversion, has been documented.
- Infection with a second strain after initial infection has occurred (i.e., superinfection), although the frequency is unknown.
- Phylogenetic studies that show a high prevalence of circulating recombinant strains suggest that infection with more than one HIV-1 strain can occur and may be more common than is currently reported.
- HIV health care providers should counsel their patients about the risk of superinfection, possibly with a virus that could be drug-resistant or poorly handled by their immune system.

for a high level of recombinant infections (Gross et al. 2004). In the model, 20% of HIV-1 infections were calculated to be recombinant infections in a scenario in which superinfection susceptibility was limited to a 30-day period, post initial infection. This finding was consistent with rates of recombinant virus seen in some sub-Saharan African settings.

Several studies have attempted to define the frequency with which HIV superinfection occurs. One group of investigators reported that dual infection was present in 5% of recently infected injection-drug users, with one of these cases likely to be a result of superinfection. Follow-up data in this same study (median of 14.5 months) identified two additional cases of superinfection among chronically infected clients, as determined from a review of 5 of 156 cases that demonstrated an unexpected 1-$\log_{10}$ increase in plasma HIV RNA that was not associated with treatment change (Yerly et al. 2004). Another study assessed the frequency of superinfection among those followed from the time of primary HIV infection. This phylogenetic study included 78 individuals who were newly HIV-infected and who deferred therapy for at least 6 months. In this study, it was reported that 3 (3.8%) individuals became superinfected (Smith et al. 2004). Moreover, superinfection in these 3 individuals was associated with an increase in plasma HIV RNA level (mean 1.6 $\log_{10}$ copies/mL) and a decline in CD4+ T cells (mean 132 cells/mm^3).

The above cases mostly demonstrate that superinfection can occur during early HIV infection. Other groups have attempted to define the frequency with which superinfection occurs in those with chronic HIV infection. Gonzales and colleagues (2003) failed to detect any cases of superinfection from 718 person samples. Tsui and associates (2004) likewise failed to document superinfection from among a sample of 37 injection-drug users. Finally, Grant and associates (2004) also failed to document superinfection from a prospective study of 19 seroconcordant couples with years of high-risk exposure. The investigators involved in the latter two studies postulated that the absence of superinfection in chronically infected individuals might be attributable to the new strain's inability to compete, given the existing immune responses or as a result of competitive pressure from existing viruses. Alternatively, these findings could be a result of technical difficulties in identifying dual infection in coinfected individuals, or other limitations of the study designs.

However, Chohan and colleagues (2005) recently reported a relatively high frequency of intersubtype superinfection among a cohort of 20 chronically infected women in Mombasa, Kenya, who continued to engage in high-risk heterosexual activity. Superinfection with subtype A virus was detected in 3 of the 20 women who initially were infected with non-subtype A viruses; these new infections occurred from 101 to 591 days after initial infections (Overbaugh 2005). Based on these results, Overbaugh posited that among high-risk individuals, persons with a high level of initial virus can be infected with a new virus subtype; that both viruses can coexist for years; and that superinfection may actually occur at a rate approaching the rate of first infections.

Several additional studies are under way to further define the significance of these findings and the frequency of superinfection (HISIS-Network 2004; CAPS-UCSF 2002). Nevertheless, on the basis of the evidence described above, health care providers must be aware of the possibility of superinfection and dual infection when counseling HIV-infected individuals regarding their sexual and needle-sharing practices. In fact, these individuals should be counseled to adhere to safe sexual and injection practices to avoid HIV superinfection as well as infection with other blood-borne or sexually transmitted organisms.

References

Altfeld M, Allen T, Yu X, et al. HIV-1 superinfection despite broad CD8+ T-cell responses containing replication of the primary virus. *Nature.* **2002**;420:434-439.

Center for AIDS Prevention Studies—University of California San Francisco (CAPS-UCSF). HIV superinfection among HIV seroconcordant couples. **2002**. Available at: http://www.caps.ucsf.edu/portfolio/index2002.html [accessed December 28, 2004].

Chohan B, Lavreys L, Rainwater S, et al. The biology of HIV-1 transmission and re-infection. In: Program and abstracts from the 12th Conference on Retroviruses and Opportunistic Infections, February 22-25, **2005**; Boston, Massachusetts. Abstract 66.

Gonzales MJ, Delwart E, Rhee SY, et al. Lack of detectable human immunodeficiency virus type 1 superinfection during 1072 person-years of observation. *J Infect Dis.* **2003**;188:397-405.

Gottlieb GS, Nickle DC, Jensen MA, et al. Dual HIV-1 infection associated with rapid disease progression. *Lancet.* **2004**;363:619-622.

Grant RM, McConnell JJ, Herring B, et al. No superinfection among seroconcordant couples after well-defined exposure. In: Program and abstracts of the XV International AIDS Conference; July 11-16, **2004**; Bangkok, Thailand. Abstract ThPeA6949.

Grobler J, Gray CM, Rademeyer C, et al. Incidence of HIV-1 dual infection and its association with increased viral load set point in a cohort of HIV-1 subtype C-infected female sex workers. *J Infect Dis.* **2004**;190:1355-1359.

Gross KL, Porco TC, Grant RM. HIV-1 superinfection and viral diversity. *AIDS.* **2004**;18:1513-1520.

HISIS-Network. HIV Superinfection Study and Vaccine Preparation Project. Copyright by Abteilung Für Infektions-Und Tropenmedizin; **2004**. Available at http://www.tropinst.med.uni-muenchen.de/ag/hivaids/hisis-brochure.htm [accessed December 28, 2004].

Jost S, Bernard M-C, Kaiser L, et al. A patient with HIV-1 superinfection. *N Engl J Med.* **2002**;347:731-736.

Koelsch KK, Smith DM, Little SJ, et al. Clade B HIV-1 superinfection with wild-type virus after primary infection with drug-resistant clade B virus. *AIDS.* **2003**;17:F11-F16.

McCutchan FE, Salminen MO, Carr JK, Burke DS. HIV-1 genetic diversity. *AIDS.* **1996**;10(suppl 3):S13-S20.

Overbaugh J. The biology of HIV-1 transmission and re-infection. Presented at the 12th Conference on Retroviruses and Opportunistic Infections, February 22-25, **2005**; Boston, Massachusetts. Plenary session 20. Available at http://www.retroconference.org/2005/Pages/webcasts.htm [accessed March 10, 2005].

Ramos A, Hu DJ, Nguyen L, et al. Intersubtype human immunodeficiency virus type 1 superinfection following seroconversion to primary infection in two injection drug users. *J Virol.* **2002**;76:7444-7452.

Robertson DL, Hahn BH, Sharp PM. Recombination in AIDS viruses. *J Mol Evol.* **1995**;40:249-259.

Sharpe SA, Whatmore AM, Hall GA, Cranage MP. Macaques infected with attenuated simian immunodeficiency virus resist superinfection with virulence-revertant virus. *J Gen Virol.* **1997**;78:1923-1927.

Smith DM, Wong JK, Hightower GK, et al. Incidence of HIV superinfection following primary infection. *JAMA.* **2004**;292:1177-1178.

Tsui R, Herring BL, Barbour JD, et al. Human immunodeficiency virus type 1 superinfection was not detected following 215 years of injection drug user exposure. *J Virol.* **2004**;78:94-103.

Yerly S, Jost S, Monnat M, et al. HIV-1 co/super-infection in intravenous drug users. *AIDS.* **2004**;18:1413-1421.

(RLO-5)

I.13. TESTING METHODS

LEARNING OBJECTIVE: Describe the benefits, limitations, appropriate use, interpretation, and confirmation of available testing methods for HIV-1 and its various subtypes (also referred to as clades) and for HIV-2.

Screening for HIV with antibody testing allows for the diagnosis of infection and entry into care. It also represents the opportunity to counsel individuals on ways to prevent transmission to others. When evaluating an individual for evidence of HIV infection, antibody assays are in most cases the diagnostic test of choice. Multiple types of HIV antibody tests are now available. The standard protocol for all of these tests is to detect the presence of HIV antibodies using the screening enzyme immunoassay (EIA), with positive results subsequently confirmed with the Western blot test or immunofluorescence assay (IFA) (see Interpreting HIV Antibody Tests, below) (Mylonakis et al. 2000; CDC 1989).

The molecular heterogeneity found in HIV results in differing sensitivities of various tests. This includes tests for serologic evidence of infection (antibody tests) and molecular diagnostic tests that detect plasma HIV RNA (viral load assays).

The classification of HIV variants begins by type: HIV-1 predominates in the United States, whereas HIV-2 is highly endemic to western Africa with only occasional cases identified in the United States (CDC 1995a). HIV-1 is further classified into group M, the predominant group throughout the world, and the less common groups N and O. Within group M there are a variety of subtypes, including subtype B (which predominates in the Americas, Western Europe, and Australia); subtype E (which predominates in Southeast Asia); and subtype C (in southern Africa, Ethiopia, and India) (Osmanov et al. 2002). Moreover, recombination has been demonstrated between viruses of different subtypes (Eshleman et al. 2002; Holguin et al. 2002; Magiorkinis et al. 2002). (See also Objective I.2 on Global Virology in this Update.)

Types of HIV Antibody Tests

In the past, HIV antibody tests were serum-based only. Newer tests have been developed to help clinicians more easily test for HIV. These include rapid blood tests (which provide results during the course of a clinic visit) and tests that use oral fluid or urine, thus not requiring a blood draw or finger-stick from the person being tested. Urine-based tests are sensitive and specific but less so than comparable serum-based EIAs (Oelemann et al. 2002; Granade et al. 1998). Oral-based tests are of comparable accuracy (OraQuick 2003).

In recent years, the U.S. Food and Drug Administration (FDA) has approved a number of rapid antibody tests (FDA 2005). These tests have comparable accuracy with other EIAs and are able to identify the presence of HIV-1 antibodies within about 20 minutes (CDC 2002). Like other HIV tests, they also require confirmation by Western blot testing. Some of these rapid tests can be performed as a "point-of-care" test at such places as HIV counseling centers and public clinics (FDA 2002). The benefit of rapid testing is that

What's New

Within the past few years, oral and rapid HIV tests have been introduced, providing potential opportunities to expand testing activities and overcome such barriers as client resistance to serum-based tests and clinic visits. On the screening and test verification front, it may be possible to use RNA testing of pooled antibody-negative serum specimens to detect acute HIV infection cases.

Key Points

- HIV infection may be diagnosed with a number of antibody assays that use serum, urine or oral fluids.
- The gold standard for antibody testing is the enzyme immunoassay (EIA) with confirmation by Western blot.
- Antibody assays cannot be used to diagnose HIV infection in newborns. Instead, other assays, such as an HIV RNA (RT-PCR) or viral culture are required.
- Rapid test kits take only minutes, rather than days, to return a result.
- Indeterminate HIV test results should prompt examination of patient risk factors and appropriate follow-up.
- Most EIA tests are reactive to HIV-1, and some identify HIV-2 as well.
- Many current assays may miss rarer forms of HIV-1, including non-group M virus, and may be less sensitive for the detection of some group M, non-subtype B virus. The two most recently approved EIAs detect group O.
- Current viral load assays are only able to quantify HIV-1 and vary in their ability to measure subtypes that are less prevalent in the United States.

individuals tested in these settings using standard assays often do not return to receive their results (FDA 2002; Reynolds et al. 2002).

Among the approved rapid tests, two are approved for point-of-care. They include OraQuick ADVANCE (approved June 2004; can be used with finger-stick, whole blood, oral fluid, or plasma and has an indication for HIV-1 and -2 screening) and UniGold Recombigen (approved December 2003). Other tests, which are not approved for point-of-care, include Reveal (approved April 2003; can be used only with serum/plasma; screens for HIV-1), and Multispot (approved November 2004; can be used for both HIV-1 and HIV-2) (FDA 2005).

A federal initiative, Advancing HIV Prevention: New Strategies for a Changing Epidemic, seeks to reduce barriers to early diagnosis by improving access to medical care (CDC 2003). This initiative focuses on providing HIV testing to as many potentially infected individuals as possible. It is hoped that rapid testing may enhance the success of this effort. The efficacy of rapid testing was documented in the Mother Infant Rapid Intervention at Delivery (MIRIAD) study to diagnose women in labor whose HIV status is not in their medical records. In the study, 4849 women accepted rapid testing, and sensitivity and specificity of rapid test results were comparable to the EIA (Bulterys et al. 2004).

A recent advance in HIV serologic technology is the development of assays that estimate the duration of infection in a person found to be antibody-positive. This "less-sensitive EIA," also referred to as the "detuned assay," can be used to classify infection as either recent or long-standing in those found to be antibody-positive by standard assays. This tool remains investigational and has been modified several times since its introduction. Although the assay is not suitable for clinical use, it has been successfully employed in epidemiologic studies to estimate HIV incidence rates (Kothe et al. 2003; Rawal et al. 2003; Parekh et al. 2001; Janssen et al. 1998).

Interpreting HIV Antibody Tests

The Western blot should only be used for individuals who are positive on EIA or rapid test because it is not uncommon for a Western blot to detect a cross-reacting antibody to a single HIV protein.

There are other circumstances that require special consideration. For example, if an HIV antibody EIA test is negative, it is possible that the person may have recently been infected but has not yet seroconverted. In this case, CDC recommends that follow-up after an exposure include periodic testing for at least 6 months and, after a documented definite exposure, at 6 weeks, 12 weeks and 6 months (CDC 2001c).

Currently there are no recommendations for follow-up of patients who are positive on EIA and negative Western blot. All persons with indeterminate Western blot should have follow-up testing (CDC 2001b). In subjects with a positive EIA and a negative or indeterminate Western blot, a risk assessment should establish the likelihood of recent infection. All sexually active persons, as well as those who inject drugs, are theoretically at risk. Evidence of symptoms consistent with acute seroconversion should be sought. If the indeterminate results are a consequence of an emerging humoral immune response, the Western blot should become positive in the coming weeks. In the case of a reactive rapid HIV test, CDC emphasizes that results must be confirmed with a Western blot or IFA. This confirmation should be done even if a later EIA is nonreactive. If the confirmatory test provides negative or indeterminate results, CDC further recommends conducting follow-up testing 4 weeks after the first reactive rapid HIV test result (CDC 2004).

An indeterminate finding in a low-risk individual usually represents a false-positive result; such individuals are very unlikely to be in the seroconversion process (Jackson et al. 1990). If recent exposure is possible, follow-up testing should be performed to rule out new infection in EIA-positive patients who are Western blot-indeterminate. Even patients without recent exposure will usually require retesting for reassurance.

Individuals who may have been infected by a partner from overseas, where different strains may be endemic, should be evaluated for the possibility of infection with HIV-2 or uncommon groups of HIV-1, such as group O. FDA-licensed assays are capable of detecting such infections (Koch et al. 2001; Nkengasong et al. 1999). No qualitative DNA polymerase chain reaction (PCR) tests (or RNA, for that matter) are available for diagnostic use in the United States.

Although further investigation is needed, several studies have explored, with success, the use of pooling of serum specimens from those undergoing routine HIV antibody testing. The purpose here is to detect HIV RNA by PCR in infected persons who are in the process of developing antibodies, a situation in which the diagnosis might be missed through EIA testing alone. In one study, over 8000 individuals who tested HIV antibody-negative had their serum pooled for PCR assays, which resulted in the identification of 5 positive specimens. It should be noted that 2 of these subjects were found to be antibody-positive on the Abbott EIA and 1 proved to be a false positive (Pilcher et al. 2002). In another study, Stramer and colleagues (2004) reported results from the American Red Cross pooled nucleic acid amplification detection of both HIV and HCV from 37 million blood donors who were antibody-negative for these pathogens. They calculated that this technology helped to prevent approximately 5 HIV-1 and 56 HCV transfusion-associated infections annually.

Testing in Newborns

Standard antibody assays are not useful for diagnosing HIV infection in children younger than 18 months. This is because infants born to HIV-infected mothers acquire maternal antibodies and thus test antibody-positive for up to 18 months after birth, even if they are not infected. Therefore, diagnosis of HIV infection in newborns requires the use of other assays. A positive virologic test (i.e., detection of HIV by culture, DNA PCR or RNA assays) indicates possible HIV infection and should be confirmed by a repeat virologic test on a second specimen as soon as possible after the results of the first test become available. Diagnostic testing should be performed within 48 hours of birth, at age 1 to 2 months and at age 3 to 6 months. Additional testing at age 14 days might allow for early detection of infection; however, HIV infection can be diagnosed definitively in most HIV-infected infants by 1 month of age and in almost all HIV-infected infants by 6 months of age. HIV infection can be reasonably excluded in non-breast-fed infants with two or more negative virologic tests performed after 1 month of age, with one of the tests performed after 4 months of age. HIV. Non-infection can be definitively confirmed by documenting loss of HIV antibody in children who have had previously negative HIV DNA PCR tests as early as 12 months of age but in most by 15 to 18 months of age (CDC 1995b).

Antibody Testing for HIV-1 and HIV-2

The HIV antibody EIAs used in the United States are designed to detect antibodies either to HIV-1, to both HIV-1 and HIV-2, or to HIV-2 (FDA 2005). Although considerable serologic cross-reaction occurs between HIV-1 and HIV-2, HIV-2 infection may be negative or indeterminate on standard HIV-1 Western blot (CDC 1992). Therefore, an HIV-2 Western blot should be performed in patients with a positive HIV-1/2 EIA and a negative or indeterminate HIV-1 Western blot, if HIV-2 infection is suspected on the basis of epidemiologic information (CDC 1992).

Quantitative Assays for HIV-1 RNA

There are three commercially available assays that reliably quantitate HIV-1 RNA in plasma. They are: (1) the reverse transcriptase polymerase chain reaction (RT-PCR) assay Amplicor (Roche Diagnostics; Basel, Switzerland); (2) the branched chain DNA (bDNA) assay Versant (Bayer Diagnostics; Tarrytown, NY); and (3) the nucleic acid sequence-based amplification (NASBA) assay (bioMérieux, The Netherlands). Currently available RNA assays detect most HIV-1 subtypes (Peter and Sevall 2004).] HIV-2 RNA viral load tests are not commercially available (CDC 2001a). Hence, HIV-2 disease currently must be managed without the benefit of viral load measures.

References

Bulterys M, Jamieson DJ, O'Sullivan MJ et al. Rapid HIV-1 testing during labor: A multicenter study. *JAMA.* **2004**;292:219-223.

Centers for Disease Control and Prevention (CDC). Interpretation and use of the Western blot assay for serodiagnosis of human immunodeficiency virus type 1 infections. *MMWR Morb Mortal Wkly Rep.* **1989**;38:1-7.

Centers for Disease Control and Prevention (CDC). Testing for antibodies to human immunodeficiency virus type 2 in United States. *MMWR Morb Mortal Wkly Rep.* **1992**;41(RR-12):1-9.

Centers for Disease Control and Prevention (CDC). Update: HIV-2 infection among blood and plasma donors—United States, June 1992-June 1995. *MMWR Morb Mortal Wkly Rep.* **1995a**;44:603-606.

Centers for Disease Control and Prevention (CDC). 1995 Revised guidelines for prophylaxis against Pneumocystis carinii pneumonia for children infected with or perinatally exposed to human immunodeficiency virus. *MMWR Morb Mortal Wkly Rep.* **1995b**;44(RR-4):1-11.

Centers for Disease Control and Prevention (CDC). Guidelines for laboratory test result reporting of human immunodeficiency virus type 1 ribonucleic acid determination: recommendations from a CDC working group. *MMWR Morb Mortal Wkly Rep.* **2001a**;50(RR-20):2-12.

Centers for Disease Control and Prevention (CDC). Revised guidelines for HIV counseling, testing, and referral and revised recommendations for HIV screening of pregnant women. *MMWR Morbid Mortal Wkly Rep.* **2001b**;50(RR-19):1-86.

Centers for Disease Control and Prevention (CDC). Updated U.S. Public Health Services guidelines for management of occupational exposures to HBV, HCV and HIV and recommendations for postexposure prophylaxis. *MMWR Morb Mortal Wkly Rep.* **2001c**;50(RR-11):1-42.

Centers for Disease Control and Prevention (CDC). Notice to readers: Approval of a new rapid test for HIV antibody. *MMWR Morb Mortal Wkly Rep.* **2002**;51:1051-1052.

Centers for Disease Control and Prevention (CDC). Advancing HIV prevention: New strategies for a changing epidemic—United States, 2003. *MMWR Morb Mortal Wkly Rep.* **2003**;52:329-332.

Centers for Disease Control and Prevention (CDC). Protocols for confirmation of reactive rapid HIV tests. *MMWR Morb Mortal Wkly Rep.* **2004**;53:221-222.

Eshleman SH, Gonzales MJ, Becker-Pergola G, et al. Identification of Ugandan HIV Type 1 variants with unique patterns of recombination in pol involving subtypes A and D. *AIDS Res Hum Retroviruses.* **2002**;18:507-511.

Food and Drug Administration (FDA). FDA approves new rapid HIV test kit [press release]. U.S. Food and Drug Administration; November 7, **2002**.

Food and Drug Administration (FDA). Licensed/approved HIV, HTLV and hepatitis tests. Updated January 10, **2005**. Available at: http://www.fda.gov/cber/products/testkits.htm [accessed February 4, 2005].

Granade TC, Phillips SK, Parekh B, et al. Detection of antibodies to human immunodeficiency virus type 1 in oral fluids: a large-scale evaluation of immunoassay performance. *Clin Diagn Lab Immunol.* **1998**;5:171-175.

Holguin A, Alvarez A, Soriano V. HIV-1 Subtype J recombinant viruses in Spain. *AIDS Res Hum Retroviruses.* **2002**;18:523-529.

Jackson JB, MacDonald KL, Cadwell J, et al. Absence of HIV infection in blood donors with indeterminate western blot tests for antibody to HIV-1. *N Engl J Med.* **1990**;322:217-222.

Jaffe HW, Schochetman G. Group O human immunodeficiency virus-1 infections. *Infect Dis Clin North Am.* **1998**;12:39-46.

Janssen RS, Satten GA, Stramer SL, et al. New testing strategy to detect early HIV-1 infection for use in incidence estimates and for clinical and prevention purposes. *JAMA.* **1998**;280:42-48.

Koch WH, Sullivan PS, Roberts C, et al. Evaluation of United States-licensed human immunodeficiency virus immunoassays for detection of group M viral variants. *J Clin Microbiol.* **2001**;39:1017-1020.

Kothe D, Byers RH, Caudill P, et al. Performance characteristics of a new less sensitive HIV-1 enzyme immunoassay for use in estimating HIV seroincidence. *J Acquir Immune Defic Syndr.* **2003**;33:625-634.

Magiorkinis G, Paraskevis D, Magiorkinis E, Vandamme AM, Hatzakis A. Reanalysis of the HIV-1 circulating recombinant form A/E (CRF01 AE): evidence of A/E/G recombination. *J Acquir Immune Defic Syndr.* **2002**;30:124-129.

Mylonakis E, Paliou M, Lally M, Flanigan TP, Rich JD. Laboratory testing for infection with the human immunodeficiency virus: established and novel approaches [review]. *Am J Med.* **2000**;109:568-576.

Nkengasong JN, Maurice C, Koblavi S, et al. Evaluation of HIV serial and parallel serologic testing algorithms in Abidjan, Cote d'Ivoire. *AIDS.* **1999**;13:109-117.

Oelemann WMR, Lowndes CM, Veríssimo da Costa GC, et al. Diagnostic detection of human immunodeficiency virus type 1 antibodies in urine: a Brazilian study. *J Clin Microbiol.* **2002**;40:881-885.

OraQuick (rapid HIV-1 antibody est) [package insert]. Bethlehem, PA: OraSure Technologies, October **2003**.

Osmanov S, Pattou C, Walker N, et al. Estimated global distribution and regional spread of HIV-1 genetic subtypes in the year 2000. *J Acquir Immune Defic Syndr.* **2002**;29:184-190.

Parekh BS, Pau C, Kennedy MS, et al. Assessment of antibody assays for identifying and distinguishing recent from long-term HIV type 1 infection. *AIDS Res Hum Retroviruses.* **2001**;17:137-146.

Peter JB, Sevall JS. Molecular-based methods for quantifying HIV viral load. *AIDS Patient Care STDs.* **2004**;18:75-79.

Pilcher CD, McPherson JT, Leone PA, et al. Real-time, universal screening for acute HIV infection in a routine HIV counseling and testing population. *JAMA.* **2002**;288:216-221.

Rawal BD, Degula A, Lebedeva L, et al. Development of a new less-sensitive enzyme immunoassay for detection of early HIV-1 infection. *J Acquir Immune Defic Syndr.* **2003**;33:349-355.

Reynolds SJ, Ndongala LM, Luo CC, et al. Evaluation of a rapid test for the detection of antibodies to human immunodeficiency virus type 1 and 2 in the setting of multiple transmitted viral subtypes. *Int J STD AIDS.* **2002**;13:171-173.

Stramer SL Glynn SA, Kleinman SH, et al. Detection of HIV-1 and HCV infections among antibody-negative blood donors by nucleic acid-amplification testing. *N Engl J Med.* **2004**;351;760-768.

Working Group on Antiretroviral Therapy and Medical Management of HIV-Infected Children. Guidelines for the use of antiretroviral agents in pediatric HIV infection. November 30, **2004**. Available at: http://aidsinfo.nih.gov/guidelines/pediatric/PED_113004.pdf [accessed December 15, 2004].

APPROACH TO THE PATIENT WITH HIV

This section covers the most recent information developments in the medical evaluation and counseling of a patient with HIV infection.

Upon completion of this section, clinicians should be able to evaluate large-joint pain in light of increasing incidence of osteopenia and osteonecrosis in patients with HIV disease; discuss the evidence supporting anal and genital tract dysplasia screening; identify appropriate HIV and STD risk assessment and risk-reduction counseling; describe current research on preventive HIV vaccines; and discuss legal issues related to confidentiality and HIV in light of the Health Insurance Portability and Accountability Act (HIPAA) provisions.

At-a-glance

What's New - Overview

Those with acute HIV infection may be highly infectious, and efforts should focus on early diagnosis, use of HIV RNA testing, and prevention counseling. In established infection, the incidence of bone fractures may increase with the growing age of the HIV-infected population.

(RLO-6)

II.11. LARGE-JOINT PAIN, OSTEOPOROSIS, AND BONE FRACTURES

LEARNING OBJECTIVE: Discuss the evaluation of large-joint pain and the increased incidence of age-related diseases, such as osteoporosis, in HIV-infected patients.

The evaluation of large-joint pain, particularly hip pain, in HIV-infected patients differs little from that in the general population. However, patients with one sexually transmitted disease may also have another, and Reiter's syndrome and gonococcal arthritis should therefore be higher on the differential diagnosis than for the general population (as reviewed in Solinger 2003).

Clinicians should be aware of recent reports of unexpectedly high rates of osteoporosis in HIV-infected patients (Tebas et al. 2000) as well as an increased risk for fragility fractures (McComsey et al. 2004) and osteonecrosis (avascular necrosis [AVN]) of joints (Miller et al. 2002; Keruly et al. 2001) in HIV-infected patients.

Osteonecrosis most commonly affects the hip joint; however, other parts of the body, such as the shoulder, wrist, knee and ankle, can also be affected (Powderly 2001). Cohort studies suggest that a small proportion of patients may have asymptomatic osteonecrosis, but routine screening of asymptomatic patients is not currently recommended (Powderly 2001). Bilateral disease is common, so both hips should be assessed in patients who present with pain in one hip. A standard x-ray of both hips may be normal (Miller et al. 2002), in which case CT or MRI of the pelvis should be performed, which can establish the diagnosis (Powderly 2001).

Studies have shown that a significant percentage of HIV-infected patients with AVN possess one or more traditional AVN risk factors, including corticosteroid use, hyperlipidemia, hypercoagulability, alcoholism and smoking (Gutierrez et al. 2002; Ries et al. 2002), so diagnosis should include an assessment for these. However, because the same studies have shown that 14% to 57% of HIV-infected patients with AVN have no traditional risk factors, the absence of these should not preclude an appropriate work-up for the condition. Two studies have shown that the use of megestrol acetate (Megace) is correlated to AVN in HIV-infected patients (Gutierrez et al. 2002; Koller et al. 2000), so past or present use of this drug could be considered another risk factor for the condition.

The cause of AVN in HIV-infected patients is currently unknown. There has been speculation that the condition may be a result of HIV infection itself or a side effect of combination antiretroviral therapy or of specific antiretroviral classes or agents, although to date AVN has not been associated with a specific antiretroviral regimen (CDC 2002). It has been postulated that the various hypercoagulable states that often accompany HIV infection may be the cause of AVN of bone in HIV disease (Scribner et al. 2000). (For more on AVN, see Objective III.52 on Skeletal and Rheumatologic Disorders, and IV.50 on Bone Complications, in the AAHIVM 2003 Study Guide.)

Since the early 1990s, HIV has increasingly become a disease of older persons (CDC 1998). From 1990 to 2001, a fivefold increase was seen in the incidence of HIV infection in people

What's New

Rising gonorrhea rates may increase the incidence of gonococcal arthritis. Tenofovir and abacavir use are associated with reduced bone mineral density, although no increase in fracture rate has been reported. As HIV infection becomes a disease of the elderly, the incidence of fractures due to osteoporosis may increase.

Key Points

- Reiter's syndrome, gonococcal arthritis, other reactive arthritides and septic arthritis should be higher on the differential diagnosis of large-joint pain for HIV-infected patients than for the general population.
- Increasing incidence of osteonecrosis has recently been reported among HIV-infected patients.
- The most common presentation of osteonecrosis is hip pain, and bilateral disease is common; its cause is currently unknown.
- High rates of osteoporosis in HIV-infected individuals is occurring because of the increased incidence of HIV infection among people aged 50 years and older.
- Low bone mineral density is common among HIV-infected patients and is a risk factor for nontraumatic fractures, often in patients without osteoporosis or osteopenia.

over 50 years of age (as reviewed in Mack and Ory 2003), which has led to an increase in the incidence of age-related diseases, such as osteoporosis, within the HIV-infected population. Additionally, reductions in bone mineral density (BMD) have been associated with antiretroviral therapies, such as tenofovir and abacavir (Anastos and Hessol 2004; Gallant et al. 2004). Low BMD is a risk factor for osteoporosis and nontraumatic fractures, although nontraumatic fractures also occur in HIV-infected patients without osteoporosis or osteopenia (McComsey et al. 2004). The pathogenesis of osteopenia and osteoporosis in HIV-infected patients is more closely associated with traditional risk factors and advanced HIV infection than with HIV treatment (Mondy et al. 2003).

A review of 49 cases of fractures among HIV-infected patients in nine HIV clinics found that 57% of fractures were not due to trauma, while the remaining 43% were due to minor trauma (McComsey et al. 2004). The median age of patients was 45 years (range 25-75 years), 76% were male, the majority (96%) were receiving antiretroviral therapy at the time of fracture, 48% were smokers, and 14% had a history of steroid use, although only 4% were receiving chronic steroid therapy at the time of the fracture. The median duration of HIV infection in this population was 6 years. According to lumbar spine and hip t-scores in 10 patients with DEXA scans, at least 50% of patients did not meet the criteria for osteopenia or osteoporosis. Most fractures were to vertebrae (45%) or lower extremities (31%), followed by ribs (8%), upper extremities (6%), clavicle (4%), and combinations of vertebrae and foot, femur, or pelvis (2% each). After an average 10-month follow-up, 9 patients experienced another fracture, 7 of which were to new sites. These results suggest that more screening for fractures is indicated in HIV-infected patients.

A study comparing 184 HIV-infected (~50% receiving HAART) and 88 HIV-negative women found significantly lower BMD associated with HIV infection (6%-8%; $P < .03$); BMD was similar in HIV-infected women receiving and not receiving HAART (Anastos and Hessol 2004). However, only 1.8% of HIV-infected women with low BMD met the t-score criteria for osteoporosis (less than -2.5). A significantly higher prevalence of osteopenia/osteoporosis at any body site was found in HIV-infected women compared with HIV-negative women ($P = .03$). Abacavir use was associated with low BMD. White race, relatively lower body mass index, and self-reported postmenopausal status were independently associated with lower BMD. Therefore, the study concluded that women with HIV infection might have an increased risk for bone fracture.

References

Anastos K, Hessol N. The association of bone mineral density with HIV infection and antiretroviral treatment in women. In: Program and abstracts of the 11th Conference on Retroviruses and Opportunistic Infections; February 8-11, **2004**; San Francisco, California. Abstract 744.

Centers for Disease Control and Prevention (CDC). AIDS among persons aged greater than 50 years—United States, 1991-1996. *MMWR Morbid Mortal Wkly Rep*. **1998**, 47:21-27.

Centers for Disease Control and Prevention (CDC). Guidelines for using antiretroviral agents among HIV-infected adults and adolescents. *MMWR Morbid Mortal Wkly Rep*. **2002**;51(RR-7).

Gallant JE, Staszewski S, Pozniak AL, et al. Efficacy and safety of tenofovir DF vs stavudine in combination therapy in antiretroviral-naive patients: a 3-year randomized trial. *JAMA*. **2004**;292:191-201.

Gutierrez F, Padilla S, Ortega E, et al. Avascular necrosis of the bone in HIV-infected patients: incidence and associated factors. *AIDS*. **2002**;16:481-482.

Keruly JC, Chaisson RE, Moore RD. Increasing incidence of avascular necrosis of the hip in HIV-infected patients. *J Acquire Immun Defic Syndr*. **2001**;28:101-102.

Koller E, Mann M, Malozowski S, Bacsanyi J, Gibert C. Aseptic necrosis in HIV seropositive patients: a possible etiologic role for megestrol acetate. *AIDS Patient Care STDs*. **2000**;14:405-410.

Mack KA, Ory MG. AIDS and older Americans at the end of the twentieth century. *J Acquir Immune Defic Syndr.* **2003**;33(suppl 2):S68-S75.

McComsey G, Huang J, Woolley I, et al. Fragility fractures in HIV-infected subjects, an area for improvement. In: Program and abstracts of the 11th Conference on Retroviruses and Opportunistic Infections; February 8-11, **2004**; San Francisco, California. Abstract 743.

Miller KD, Masur H, Jones EC, et al. High prevalence of osteonecrosis of the femoral head in HIV-infected adults. *Ann Intern Med.* **2002**;137:17-25.

Mondy K, Yarasheski K, Powderly WG, et al. Longitudinal evolution of bone mineral density and bone markers in human immunodeficiency virus-infected individuals. *Clin Infect Dis*. **2003**;36:482-490.

Powderly WG. Bone disorders in HIV-infected patients. Medscape General Medicine. **2001**;3(1). Available at: http://www.medscape.com/viewarticle/403863 [accessed February 12, 2005].

Ries MD, Barcohana B, Davidson A, Jergesen HE, Paiement GD. Association between human immunodeficiency virus and osteonecrosis of the femoral head. *J Arthroplasty.* **2002**;17:135-139.

Scribner AN, Troia-Cancio PV, Cox BA, et al. Osteonecrosis in HIV: a case-control study. *J Acquir Immun Defic Syndr.* **2000**;25:19-25.

Solinger AM. Rheumatic manifestations of human immunodeficiency virus. *Curr Rheumatol Rep*. **2003**;5:205-209.

Tebas P, Powderly WG, Claxton S, et al. Accelerated bone mineral loss in HIV-infected patients receiving potent antiretroviral therapy. *AIDS*. **2000**;14:F63-F67.

(RLO-7)

II.20. PAP SMEARS

LEARNING OBJECTIVE: Discuss the recommended frequency and specimen collection technique, and cite indications for specialist referral for colposcopy or high-resolution anoscopy or biopsy, for the following: (a) genital tract Pap smears in HIV-infected women; (b) anal Pap smears in HIV-infected men and women.

Cervical Dysplasia and Cancer

Infection with human papillomavirus (HPV) is responsible for the transformation of cervical epithelial cells into precancerous and cancerous tissue. Although there are many types of HPV, certain high-risk types have been associated with the development of highly abnormal cells and cervical cancer, notably HPV-16 and HPV-18 (Munoz et al. 2003).

The prognosis of cervical cancer is worse in HIV-infected women than in HIV-negative women (Einstein and Kadish 2004; Maiman 1998). Immunologic studies by researchers at the University of Milan have found weakened cellular immunity in the mucosal tissues of HIV-infected women coinfected with HPV compared with monoinfected women with HIV or HPV (Maffeis et al. 2004). Coinfection with HIV and HPV may synergistically weaken cellular immunity in mucosal tissues, allowing the growth of HPV-infected cells.

As previously mentioned, HPV-16 and -18 are associated with an increased risk of cervical cancer in HIV-negative women. These two types of HPV are the focus of development efforts to create a vaccine to prevent the development of HPV-related complications (Harper et al. 2004). Whether these vaccines will be effective in HIV-infected women has not been formally studied. However, data on the types of HPV associated with cervical dysplasia in HIV-infected women (Luque et al. 2004) suggest the possibility that these vaccines may not be as effective in this population.

Luque and colleagues (2004) prospectively assessed and monitored 229 HIV-infected women for up to 7 years at 6-month intervals using Pap smears and cervicovaginal lavage. They found that the commonly detected strains of HPV included HPV-56 (18%), HPV-53 (12%) and HPV-16 (8%). Moreover, among women with abnormal Pap smear results, many types of HPV were common. In the same study, there were 16 women with high-grade lesions: 3 were in women with HPV-58, 3 were in women with HPV-52, and 2 were in women with HPV-16. All in all, although having HPV-16 or -18 was significantly associated with an increased risk for an abnormal Pap smear, the presence of other high-risk HPV types was also associated with the development of abnormal Pap smear results. The findings by Luque and colleagues suggest the possibility that vaccines for the prevention or modification of HPV-related disease in HIV-infected women may need to contain additional epitopes from several high-risk types of HPV, not just HPV-16 and -18.

Although HAART has improved or restored immunity to many infections seen in HIV/AIDS, immunity to HPV does not appear to be restored. In a study assessing the impact of HAART in 146 treatment-naive HIV-infected women, Squires and colleagues (2004) found that, at baseline, abnormal Pap smear results were more likely in women who were white than

What's New

Regular screening with high-resolution anoscopy confirmation of anal Pap smear results (for oncogenic types) is needed. Risk factors for anal cancer include male-male sex, CD4 count over 200 cells/mm^3 and age of over 34 years. Risk factors for human papillomavirus (HPV)-related anal dysplasia in HIV-infected women include smoking, presence of oncogenic HPV subtypes, and CD4 count under 500 cells/mm^3. In addition to HPV-16 or -18, other high-risk HPV types were also associated with the development of abnormal cervical Pap smears in HIV-infected women, having implications for HPV vaccine development to prevent cervical cancer.

Key Points

- Abnormal cervical Pap smears are associated with behavioral and gynecologic factors but not overall immune status.
- HPV infection in HIV/HPV-coinfected women is associated with altered mucosal immunity and, in particular, with the activation of proinflammatory cytokines and an impairment of cell-mediated immunity.
- There are several HPV types in the pathogenesis of serious HPV disease in HIV-infected women, having implications for HPV vaccine development.
- The use of HAART appears to have had little impact on the prevalence of high-risk HPV-related anal dysplasia; therefore, anal dysplasia screening in all HIV-infected men and women is needed.
- HPV genotypes and the level of HPV E6 transcripts correlated with severity of anal pathology in HIV-infected men.

Key Points (cont.)

- Persons with HIV infection are at increased risk for anorectal cancer compared with the general population. Recently, anorectal cancer was associated with male-male sex, older age, and more advanced HIV disease.
- High prevalence of anal squamous intraepithelial lesions (SIL), including high-grade SIL, and anal HPV infection in HIV-infected men who have sex with men (MSM) occur despite immune restoration under HAART.
- Risk factors for HPV-related anal dysplasia in HIV-infected women include smoking, the presence of oncogenic HPV subtypes and CD4 count below 500 cells/mm^3.
- If any anal Pap smear shows atypical squamous cells of undetermined significance (ASCUS) or SIL, refer to a specialist for anoscopy and biopsy.
- Perform anal Pap smears on a yearly basis, increasing to every 6 months after detecting any neoplasm.

black or Hispanic and who previously had abnormal Pap smears or gynecologic surgery. Current smoking was also marginally associated with abnormal Pap smears in this study. However, immune status was not associated with abnormal Pap results.

The U.S. Public Health Service recommends a complete gynecologic evaluation with Pap smear as part of the initial evaluation for all HIV-infected women (CDC 2002a,b). The Pap smear should be obtained twice in the first year of diagnosis and, if normal, annually thereafter (CDC 2002a,b; Abulanach and Anderson 2001). More frequent Pap smears should be considered in women with a previous abnormal Pap smear, those with symptomatic HIV infection or significant immunosuppression, and those infected with HPV and after treatment for cervical dysplasia (ACOG 1995).

Abnormalities are seen in a high percentage of HIV-infected women: 30% to 60% have abnormal cytology, and 15% to 40% have dysplasia, as much as 10 times the prevalence observed in noninfected women (Maiman 1998). Current recommendations therefore vary with the clinical status of the patient (Table II.20-1).

Table II.20-1. Suggested frequency of pap smears in HIV-infected women.

Clinical scenario	Screening frequency
Normal Pap	Annually
Symptomatic HIV infection or CD4 count under 200 cells/mm^3	Every 6 months, x 2; if both Paps are normal, then screen annually; if either Pap is abnormal, then screen every 6 months until normal
ASCUS/LSIL (evaluated and monitored without treatment)	Every 4-6 months
Following treatment of preinvasive lesions	Every 3-4 months during first year, then every 6 months

ASCUS, atypical squamous cells of undetermined significance ; LSIL, low-grade squamous intraepithelial lesion.

Adapted from CDC 2002a; Abulanach and Anderson 2001.

A single Pap smear may be associated with a false-negative rate of 10% to 25%, which is the same as in noninfected women (Abulanach and Anderson 2001). (For more details on cervical dysplasia, see Objectives III.14 and III.15 on Human Papillomavirus and Cervical Dysplasia in the AAHIVM 2003 Study Guide.)

Anal Dysplasia and Cancer

Screening for anal dysplasia is not yet standard practice. There is, however, mounting evidence to support the use of routine anal Pap smears in male and female HIV-infected patients. One study found that HIV-infected male intravenous-drug users (IVDUs) in France were at increased risk for anal HPV even though they did not report practicing anal intercourse (Piketty et al. 2003), but no similar study has been reported in male IVDUs in the United States. U.S. surveys have found that the rates of anal HPV infection, anal intraepithelial neoplasia (AIN) and anal cancer are elevated overall in men and women with HIV (Chin-Hong and Palefsky 2002; Frisch et al. 2000).

Anal Pap smears involve cell collection and examination techniques similar to those used for cervical screening. The cytology rating system also mirrors that of cervical Pap smears. If Pap screening reveals abnormal findings, patients should be referred to a specialist or surgeon for high-resolution anoscopy (similar to colposcopy) and biopsy (Chin-Hong and Palefsky 2002). Treatment is given on detection of high-grade lesions (AIN II or III) or cancer.

A study screening 417 HIV-infected men who have sex with men (MSM), by Lee and colleagues (2004), followed up 163 abnormal anal Pap smear results with high-resolution anoscopy and biopsies. The study revealed that 8% had severe dysplasia and 4% had carcinoma. Although anal Pap smears are highly sensitive, this study shows the value of confirmatory techniques even in the case of normal Pap smears.

In another screening program, Mahony and colleagues (2004) found that 57% of more than 200 HIV-infected men with a history of anal-receptive intercourse had dysplasia. Multiple types of HPV were found in 92% of patients, and in 88%, strains of HPV associated with a high risk of oncogenesis were found (HPV-16, -18, -31, -52, and -53). In the same study, levels of the HPV peptide E6 were more frequently found in biopsies from high-grade lesions in those with HPV-16. This was generally not the case for HPV-18 and HPV-31. However, levels of the combined total E6 levels from these three oncogenic types were greater in high-grade lesions than mildly abnormal or normal tissue. Because of this finding, the study team suggested that further study is needed to assess the potential for using E6 levels as a biomarker of HPV disease progression.

Anal dysplasia can progress to invasive cancer, but this occurs only in a small number of cases (Klencke and Palefsky 2003). Sullivan and colleagues (2004) sought to assess factors associated with the development of anorectal cancer in HIV-infected people. Using data collected between 1992 and 2002 on 58,039 subjects, they found 150 documented cases of anorectal cancer. Of these, 92% were male, and 79% acquired HIV infection through male-male sex. The team calculated that the risk of anorectal cancer increased with age, particularly in those over the age of 34 years (the risk was even higher among those 45 years or older). Also, having less than 200 CD4 cells/mm^3 was another risk factor.

Separately, at least two studies have found that the use of HAART appears to have little impact on the prevalence of high-risk HPV infection in heterosexuals and MSM (Piketty et al. 2004; Wilkin et al. 2004). These findings again underscore the need for regular screening in HIV-infected men for anal dysplasia and cancer.

Treatment options for anal cancer in HIV-infected people are similar (chemotherapy, radiation) to those in HIV-negative people (Klencke et al. 2003). However, the tolerability of these therapies in HIV-infected patients appears to be worse (Klencke et al. 2003). There is an urgent need for prospective clinical studies and, consequently, for treatment guidelines for anal cancer in HIV-infected people.

The development of anal lesions and invasive cancer generally occurs at the level of the transformation zone, the area where the stratified squamous epithelium of the anus meets the columnar epithelium of the rectum. Anal cytology, i.e., Pap smears, can detect the presence of abnormal cells that may be at risk for progression to cancer if untreated.

Sensitivity appears to be similar to that of cervical Pap smears. In this setting, however, finding low-grade squamous intraepithelial lesions (LSIL) or atypical squamous cells of undetermined significance (ASCUS) does not reliably predict the true lesion grade found on anoscopy and biopsy (Mathews et al. 2004; Chin-Hong and Palefsky 2002). In these cases, histologic examination frequently detects AIN (Mathews et al. 2004; Chin-Hong and Palefsky 2002).

Anal Pap smears are performed as follows (Martins 2001): A moistened Dacron swab is inserted 1-1.5 inches into the anal canal and rotated firmly as it is slowly withdrawn in a tight spiral motion. The transformation zone is located approximately 1 inch from the anal verge, and both rectal columnar and anal squamous cells must be obtained to have an adequate specimen. The sampling process should take 15 to 20 seconds. Evaluation using liquid-based media may be the easiest method, with the swab vigorously shaken in the fixative, followed by centrifugation and the cells spread as a monolayer. Abnormalities on anal cytology should be further evaluated with anoscopy and biopsy (Chin-Hong and Palefsky 2002).

There are no universally accepted guidelines for anal Pap smear screening. The suggested approach for HIV-infected women and men closely resembles recommendations for cervical cytologic screening (Martins 2001):

1. Perform anal Pap at time of initial diagnosis and, if normal, repeat in 6 months.

2. If the first two Pap smears are normal, repeat annually; consider more frequent screening with CD4 count below 500 cells/mm^3.

3. If any Pap shows ASCUS or SIL, refer for anoscopy and biopsy.

Chin-Hong and Palefsky (2002) recommended slightly less rigorous monitoring (see algorithm below). Their recommendations arose from cost-effectiveness modeling based on MSM (Goldie et al. 1999). In this model, semiannual screening provided little or no additional benefit over annual or biannual screening. Providers should consider a similar Pap smear schedule for HIV-infected women and heterosexual males although there are no data on the cost-effectiveness of screening in these populations (Chin-Hong and Palefsky 2002).

Although the prevalence of anal cytologic abnormalities in HIV-infected women and heterosexual male IVDUs is high, it is lower than that observed in MSM (Hillemanns et al. 1996; Piketty et al. 2003). Factors such as smoking, the presence of oncogenic HPV subtypes and having fewer than 500 CD4 cells/mm^3 placed HIV-infected women at increased risk for HPV-related anal dysplasia (Durante et al. 2003).

Little is known about the rate of anal dysplasia in non-IVDU heterosexual men, a comparatively small group. One large study of HPV-related malignancy looked at the records of 309,365 men and women drawn from local U.S. AIDS registries. Male heterosexuals without drug use made up only 3% of the total (Frisch et al. 2000). The study could find no additional risk of anal cancer in such men.

Figure II.20-1. Protocol for screening anal intraepithelial neoplasia (AIN).

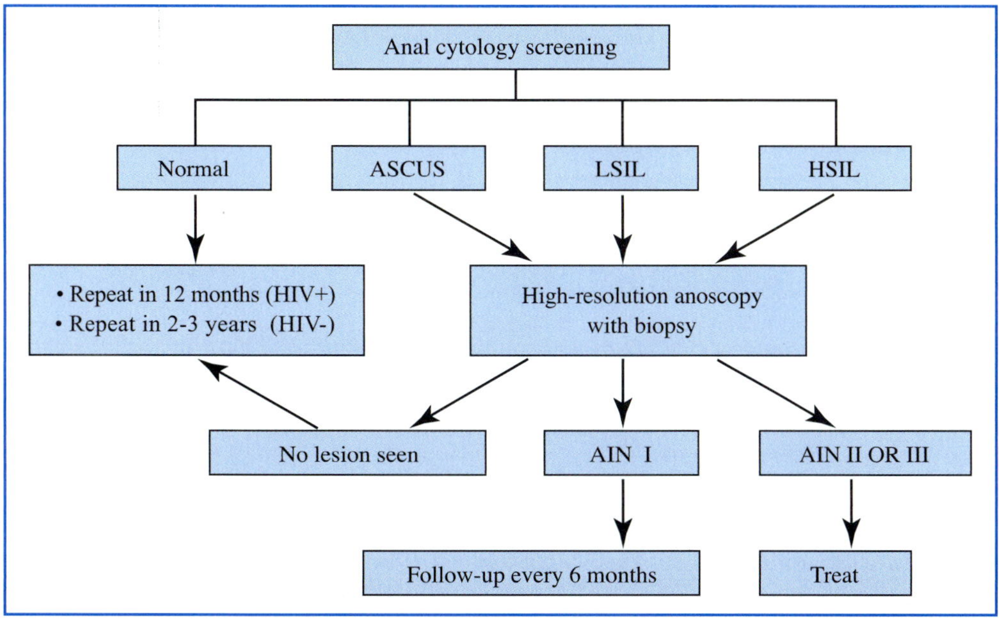

ASCUS, atypical squamous cells of indeterminate significance; HSIL, high-grade squamous intraepithelial lesions; LSIL, low-grade squamous intraepithelial lesions.

Reprinted with permission from University of Chicago Press. Source: Chin-Hong PV, Palefsky JM. Natural history and clinical management of anal human papillomavirus disease in men and women infected with human immunodeficiency virus. Clin Infect Dis. 2002;35:1127-1134.

Screening for anal dysplasia is not yet standard practice; however, there is growing evidence supporting the use of routine anal Pap smears in certain patients (Palefsky 2000). The technique is similar to that used for cervical screening. If anal Pap screening is not available, or if Pap screening reveals abnormal findings, these patients should be referred to a specialist or surgeon for high-resolution anoscopy and biopsy and subsequent treatment of high-grade lesions or cancer (Palefsky 2000).

References

Abulanach S, Anderson J. Gynecologic problems. In: Anderson JR, ed. *A Guide to the Clinical Care of Women With HIV.* Rockville, Md: U.S. Department of Health and Human Services, Health Resources Services Administration, HIV/AIDS Bureau; **2001**:149-196. Available at: http://hab.hrsa.gov/publications/womencare.htm [accessed December 2001].

American College of Obstetricians and Gynecologists (ACOG). *Recommendations on Frequency of Pap Test Screening*. Committee Opinion No. 152. Washington, DC, March **1995**.

Centers for Disease Control and Prevention (CDC). Guidelines for preventing opportunistic infections among HIV-infected persons — 2002 recommendations of the U.S. Public Health Service and the Infectious Diseases Society of America. *MMWR Morb Mortal Wkly Rep*. **2002a**;51(RR-8).

Centers for Disease Control and Prevention (CDC). Sexually transmitted diseases treatment guidelines 2002. *MMWR Morb Mortal Wkly Rep*. **2002b**:51(RR-6).

Chin-Hong PV, Palefsky JM. Natural history and clinical management of anal human papillomavirus disease in men and women infected with human immunodeficiency virus. *Clin Infect Dis*. **2002**;35:1127-1134.

Durante AJ, Williams AB, Da Costa M, Darragh TM, Khoshnood K, Palefsky JM. Incidence of anal cytological abnormalities in a cohort of human immunodeficiency virus-infected women. *Cancer Epidemiol Biomarkers Prev*. **2003**;12:638-642.

Einstein MH, Kadish AS. Anogenital neoplasia in AIDS. *Curr Opin Oncol.* **2004**;16:455-462.

Frisch M, Biggar RJ, Goedert JJ. Human papillomavirus-associated cancers in patients with human immunodeficiency virus infection and acquired immunodeficiency syndrome. *J Natl Cancer Inst.* **2000**;92:1500-1510.

Goldie SJ, Kuntz KM, Weinstein MC, Freedberg KA, Welton ML, Palefsky JM. The clinical effectiveness and cost-effectiveness of screening for anal squamous intraepithelial lesions in homosexual and bisexual HIV-positive men. *JAMA.* **1999**;281:1822-1829.

Harper DM, Franco EL, Wheeler C, et al. Efficacy of a bivalent L1 virus-like particle vaccine in prevention of infection with human papillomavirus types 16 and 18 in young women: a randomised controlled trial. *Lancet.* **2004**;364:1757-1765.

Hillemanns P, Ellerbrock TV, McPhillips S, Dole P, et al. Prevalence of anal human papillomavirus infection and anal cytologic abnormalities in HIV-seropositive women. *AIDS.* **1996**;10:1641-1647.

Klencke BJ, Palefsky JM. Anal cancer: an HIV-associated cancer. *Hematol Oncol Clin North Am.* **2003**;17:859-872.

Lee A, Young T, Hanks D, Ung R, Stansell J. The evaluation of anal dysplasia with anal cytology (PAP) followed by high resolution anoscopy (HRA) and biopsy in HIV-infected men. In: Program and abstracts of the XV International Conference on AIDS; July 11-16, **2004**; Bangkok, Thailand. Abstract ThOrB1407.

Luque AE, Messing S, Rose RC, Reichman RC. Prevalence of human papillomavirus (HPV) genotypes in HIV-infected women. In: Program and abstracts of the XV International Conference on AIDS; July 11-16, **2004**; Bangkok, Thailand. Abstract MoPeB3323.

Maffeis G, Agarossi A, Trabattoni D, et al. Mucosal immunity in the natural history of HPV in HIV-seropositive women. In: Program and abstracts of the 11th Conference on Retroviruses and Opportunistic Infections; February 8-11, **2004**; San Francisco, California. Abstract 776.

Mahony J, Salit IE, Chong S, et al. Screening for anal dysplasia: correlation of HPV genotypes and E6 transcripts with anal pathology. In: Program and abstracts of the XV International Conference on AIDS; July 11-16, **2004**; Bangkok, Thailand. Abstract MoPeB3131.

Maiman M. Management of cervical neoplasia in human immunodeficiency virus-infected women. *J Natl Cancer Inst Monogr.* **1998**;23:43-49.

Martins CR. HPV-induced anal dysplasia: what do we know and what can we do about it? *Hopkins HIV Report.* **2001**;13:3-5, 16.

Mathews C, Sitapati A, Caperna J, Barber R, Go EY. Measurement characteristics of anal cytology, histopathology, and colposcopic visual impression in an anal dysplasia screening program. In: Program and abstracts of the 11th Conference on Retroviruses and Opportunistic Infections; February 8-11, **2004**; San Francisco, California. Abstract 775.

Munoz N, Bosch FX, de Sanjose S, et al. Epidemiologic classification of human papillomavirus types associated with cervical cancer. *N Engl J Med.* **2003**;348:518-527.

Palefsky JM. Human papillomavirus-related tumors. *AIDS.* **2000**;14(suppl 3):S189-S195.

Piketty C, Darragh TM, Da Costa M, et al. High prevalence of anal human papillomavirus infection and anal cancer precursors among HIV-infected persons in the absence of anal intercourse. *Ann Intern Med.* **2003**;138:453-459.

Piketty C, Darragh TM, Heard I, et al. High prevalence of anal squamous intraepithelial lesions in HIV-positive men despite the use of highly active antiretroviral therapy. *Sex Transm Dis.* **2004**;31:96-99.

Squires KE, Nyangweso PM, Brown D, et al. Prevalence of human papilloma virus (HPV) DNA in women who are antiretroviral-naïve and initiating highly active antiretroviral therapy (HAART): baseline (BL) analysis of A5029. In: Program and abstracts of the XV International Conference on AIDS; July 11-16, **2004**; Bangkok, Thailand. Abstract ThPeA6952.

Sullivan PS, Juhasz M, Brooks J, Wolfe M, and The Adult/Adolescent Spectrum of HIV Disease Study Group. Incidence and associations of anorectal cancers in persons with HIV infection. In: Program and abstracts of the 11th Conference on Retroviruses and Opportunistic Infections; February 8-11, **2004**; San Francisco, California. Abstract 777.

Wilkin TJ, Palmer S, Brudney KF, Chiasson MA, Wright TC. Anal intraepithelial neoplasia in heterosexual and homosexual HIV-positive men with access to antiretroviral therapy. *J Infect Dis.* **2004**;190:1685-1691.

(RLO-8)

II.27. HIV TRANSMISSION RISK ASSESSMENT AND RISK-REDUCTION COUNSELING

LEARNING OBJECTIVE: Describe appropriate and comprehensive HIV and STD risk assessment and risk reduction/behavioral intervention counseling for patients, in accordance with current CDC guidelines, with special attention to "prevention for positives" (HIV-infected patients) and high-risk groups of HIV-infected patients; and identify where to find information and materials to assist in these HIV prevention efforts.

HIV infection is most commonly acquired from exposure to body fluids infected with HIV: blood, semen, vaginal fluids or breast milk. A sexually active adult is most likely to come into contact with HIV-infected body fluids by sexual contact; the second most likely way is by injecting intravenous drugs with previously used needles. Because the sexual drive is an integral part of being human, the need for health care professionals to discuss sexual practices with patients is crucial. Appropriate counseling for injection-drug users is discussed in Objective II.25 on Injection Drug Abuse and Objective II.54 on Drug Abuse in HIV+ Patients in the AAHIVM 2003 Study Guide.

Recent studies have found that a core group of HIV-infected patients have frequent unprotected sex. Some of these persons harbor drug-resistant HIV and need to be a particular focus of counseling (Chin-Hong et al. 2004; Kozal et al. 2004).

Trends also indicate that the number of new HIV infections is on the rise among men who have sex with men (MSM), Hispanics and non-Hispanic whites (CDC 2003a). Furthermore, many of those with new infections are unaware of their status (Fleming et al. 2002); nearly one-third of those who test positive do not return for their test results (CDC 2003b). In light of these developments, CDC is focusing efforts on both finding those with HIV infection and directing prevention efforts toward them. This initiative comprises four strategies:

- Make HIV testing part of routine medical care by all providers
- Implement new models, such as rapid HIV tests, for quicker HIV diagnosis outside medical settings (e.g., correctional facilities; testing partners of HIV-infected persons)
- Incorporate HIV prevention into the regular medical care of HIV-infected persons including testing all of their sexual partners
- Reduce perinatal infection by promoting routine screening of all pregnant women and all infants whose mothers were not screened

Sexual Risk Behaviors

Among sexual practices, two are noted as being particularly high risk: receptive vaginal or anal intercourse without the use of condoms. Insertive intercourse may also be associated with HIV acquisition, as may oral sex (for more details, see Objective I.6 on Modes [of transmission] in the AAHIVM 2003 Study Guide). HIV can also be transmitted from an HIV-infected mother to her child, either during pregnancy or labor or through breast-feeding (for more details, see Objective II.26 on Breast-Feeding in the AAHIVM 2003 Study Guide).

What's New

The continuing rise in the incidence of STDs among HIV-infected men who have sex with men (MSM) indicates persisting unsafe sex practices. Those with acute HIV infection may be highly infectious and efforts should focus on early diagnosis, use of HIV RNA testing and prevention counseling.

Key Points

- Health care professionals must discuss HIV transmission and sexual practices with patients and be aware that people may be reluctant to disclose sexual behavior.
- Health care professionals should ask simple, open-ended questions to assess patients' understanding of HIV transmission.
- Recent studies have found that a small group of HIV-infected patients have frequent unprotected sex. Some members of this group have drug-resistant virus.
- Recent increases in the incidence of syphilis and other STDs among HIV-infected MSM indicate that safer sex messages are not being followed as well as in the past.
- Complete sexual abstinence is the only infallible way to prevent transmission of STDs.
- Correctly used condoms, male or female, are an effective barrier against most STDs.
- The presence of genital ulcers may increase the susceptibility of HIV transmission.
- Knowledge that antiretroviral therapy is effective and sometimes results in undetectable levels of HIV may reinforce patients' beliefs that unprotected sex may be safe.

Key Points (cont.)

- Viral load levels peak during the first month after infection. This argues in favor of adding HIV RNA screening to the battery of routine diagnostic tests performed for patients presenting with any viral syndrome.
- CDC recommends that all providers incorporate HIV testing into their routine medical care.
- CDC recommends that clinicians screen for HIV transmission risk behaviors and STDs, and deliver brief behavioral interventions, as a routine and continuing part of medical care of all HIV-infected patients.
- Rapid tests for HIV can facilitate testing and counseling in primary care practices.

Questions to assess patients' understanding of HIV transmission should be simple and designed to avoid overly technical terms whenever possible. Questions should be open-ended, encouraging a patient to give more than a simple "yes" or "no" answer. Questions that might be asked of HIV-infected patients in order to examine their knowledge of the routes of HIV transmission include the following:

- "Can you please tell me three ways in which a person can become infected with HIV?"
- "How can you avoid becoming infected with STDs?"
- "If a medicine reduces the amount of virus so much that it can't be found in a person's bloodstream, can that person still infect someone else?"

STD Incidence

Misconceptions about HIV transmission and treatments contribute to behavioral trends that increase the risk of HIV transmission (CDC et al. 2003c). Increased incidences of STDs, such as syphilis and chlamydia, serve as biological markers of these trends. Although syphilis rates fell 90% between 1990 and 2000 (CDC 2003), the number of reported primary and secondary syphilis cases rose by 12.4% from 2001 to 2002, with the rate of infections in men 3.5 times higher than that in women (CDC 2003e).

The incidence of STDs is increasing at a disproportionate rate among MSM (CDC 2003d). A study in the United Kingdom of bacterial STD incidence among HIV-infected MSM, heterosexual HIV-infected men and HIV-negative MSM found that the incidence of gonorrhea, chlamydia and syphilis was significantly higher in the HIV-infected MSM cohort than in the HIV-negative MSM cohort and the HIV-infected heterosexual cohort (Fisher et al. 2003).

Infectiousness and Acute Infection

Recent data from Pilcher and colleagues (2004a) in North Carolina have found that viral loads peak approximately 4 weeks after acute HIV infection, and that semen concentrations of HIV rise in parallel with blood levels. Thus, the time span between acute HIV infection and development of measurable antibodies represents a period of high infectiousness, which increases in the presence of an STD.

The significance for risk reduction is obvious: Few people are tested early after acute infection; fewer than 1000 individuals (of the roughly 60 million HIV-infected worldwide) have been diagnosed within the first month of infection (Pilcher et al. 2004b). In large part, this is because symptoms of acute HIV infection, present in 50% to 90% of newly infected persons, are nonspecific and can resemble a number of other viral syndromes including influenza and mononucleosis, among others (Schacker et al. 1996; Tindall et al. 1988). In a cohort of 29 patients with primary HIV infection, Weintrob and colleagues (2003) found that more than half were seen in an acute care setting at least 3 times before being diagnosed with HIV infection.

Thus, incorporating HIV-RNA testing as a part of a diagnostic work-up of any acute viral syndrome could uncover early, acute infection. Early diagnosis could enhance response to treatment, but by detecting infection in those who otherwise would be unaware of their HIV status and counseling them about safer sex practices and common misconceptions outlined subsequently, it may also reduce transmission rates (Pilcher et al. 2004b).

Important Misconceptions

Common misconceptions contributing to increased risk-taking sexual behaviors include beliefs that antiretroviral treatments have changed HIV/AIDS from a life-threatening disease to a chronic, manageable one; that postexposure prophylaxis with antiretrovirals is effective in preventing HIV transmission; that antiretroviral-induced low viral loads eliminate the risk of HIV transmission; and that HIV-infected individuals can safely have unprotected sex with HIV-infected sex partners without the risk of superinfection (CDC et al. 2003c). Clinicians should be aware of these misconceptions and provide accurate information to their patients, especially in areas where the STD rates are highest and with patients at the greatest risk, i.e., people of color, MSM, people with STDs, women, young people (aged 13-24 years) and injection-drug users (CDC 2001).

As with all other STDs, complete sexual abstinence is the only infallible method to prevent transmission of HIV. However, a commitment to abstinence is not necessarily held. One recent NIH-sponsored survey followed 15,000 youths aged 12 to 24 years, of whom over 3000 reported taking a "virginity pledge" at one time or another (Bearman and Brückner 2004). Of the 940 who were most committed to their pledge (to observe abstinence until marriage), 88% admitted to eventually breaking that pledge. Overall, pledgers' STD rates were similar to those who had never pledged. Factors associated with virginity pledgers' unexpectedly high STD rate were lower perception of risk, less STD testing and treatment and less use of condoms during sex.

Monogamy between two partners can also significantly reduce the risk of transmission. However, sexually active adults should understand their risks for contracting STDs and HIV, even when engaged in a monogamous relationship. Condoms, when used properly, remain the most effective barrier against transmission of HIV and most other STDs for individuals who choose not to remain abstinent and who are not in a monogamous relationship with an uninfected partner. Improper use of condoms, however, can significantly reduce their effectiveness. Of note, MSM have increasingly used "serosorting," or intercourse preferentially among HIV-infected individuals (McConnell and Grant 2004) to reinforce the effect of condoms. Despite a continued high overall level of unprotected sex, there is a declining rate of unprotected sex between HIV-negative and HIV-infected MSM partners (Truong et al. 2004).

Condoms

Most condoms are made of very thin latex, are inexpensive and their use is associated with few adverse effects. For individuals with an allergy to latex, polyurethane condoms are available. Standard condoms are made to fit over the penis and down the shaft entirely. Some of the most important guidelines to proper condom use are outlined below.

- No oil-based lubricants should be used with latex condoms, because the latex in the condom can be degraded by contact with oil and may tear. Also, nonoxynol-9 should not be used because it irritates mucosal tissue, making HIV transmission more likely.
- The condom should be rolled down to the very base of the shaft of the penis before insertion into the vagina or rectum of the partner. The outside of the condom should also be lubricated before insertion if the condom was not prelubricated.

- After ejaculation, the base of the condom should be held tightly and removed carefully to avoid leaking of ejaculate into or onto the partner.

Polyurethane "female" condoms are also available. Rather than fitting over the penis, and thus requiring the male partner's cooperation, the female condom is built to fit inside the vagina, with rubber rings to hold it in place. This may enable women to protect themselves when their male partners are unwilling to use a traditional condom. The "female" condom has proven relatively effective when used correctly (Beksinska et al. 2001; Farr et al. 1994) but can be more expensive and more difficult to use (Artz et al. 2002; Sakondhavat et al. 2001). Some studies have suggested that these condoms can be safely washed in bleach and reused up to eight times (Beksinska et al. 2001; Smith et al. 2001), but thus far the World Health Organization does not recommend reuse (WHO 2002). Furthermore, when compared with the "male" condom, users have disliked the "female" condom, finding it awkward and inconvenient to insert and unpleasant during sex (Kulczycki et al. 2004). Additional educational interventions are needed to introduce women to the female condom; this can be accomplished through health care providers in a culturally sensitive and appropriate way (Hoffman et al. 2004; Van Devanter et al. 2002).

Avoiding sexual intercourse during periods of genital or anal ulceration may decrease the risk of acquiring or transmitting other STDs, including HIV infection (Torian et al. 1995). One study suggested that the presence of genital ulcers may increase the infectiousness of HIV (Morse 1999). Among seronegative individuals, the presence of genital ulcers may increase susceptibility both because mucosal integrity is interrupted and because target cells for HIV infection, such as activated lymphocytes, are recruited in high numbers to the ulcerated area (reviewed in Cohen 1998).

Studies have been mixed regarding whether screening and treating high-risk populations for genital ulcer disease and urethritis reduces HIV transmission. However, active screening and treatment of STDs among sexually active adults does reduce morbidity in general (Tovanabutra et al. 2002; Chakraborty et al. 2001; Gray et al. 2001).

References

Artz L, Demand M, Pulley L, Posner SF, Macaluso M. Predictors of difficulty inserting the female condom. *Contraception*. **2002**;65:151-157.

Bearman P, Brückner H. The relationship between virginity pledges in adolescence and STD acquisition in young adulthood. Presented at the 2004 National STD Prevention Conference. Philadelphia. March 8-11, **2004**. Available at: http://www.sociology.columbia.edu/people/faculty/bearman/papers/std_prevention.pdf. [accessed February 16, 2005].

Beksinska ME, Rees HV, Dickson-Tetteh KE, Mqoqi N, Kleinschmidt I, McIntyre JA. Structural integrity of the female condom after multiple uses, washing, drying, and re-lubrication. *Contraception*. **2001**;63:33-36.

Centers for Disease Control and Prevention (CDC). HIV prevention strategic plan through 2005. **2001**. Available at: http://www.cdc.gov/hiv/pubs/prev-strat-plan.pdf [accessed December 20, 2003].

Centers for Disease Control and Prevention (CDC). Increases in HIV diagnoses – 29 States, 1999-2002. *MMWR Morbid Mortal Wkly Rpt*. **2003a**;52:1145-1148.

Centers for Disease Control and Prevention (CDC). Advancing HIV prevention: New strategies for a changing epidemic—United States, 2003. *MMWR Morbid Mortal Wkly Rpt*. **2003b**;52:329-332.

Centers for Disease Control and Prevention (CDC), Health Resources and Services Administration, National Institutes of Health, HIV Medicine Association of the Infectious Diseases Society of America. Incorporating HIV prevention into the medical care of persons living with HIV. *MMWR Recomm Rep.* **2003c**;52(RR-12):1-24.

Centers for Disease Control and Prevention (CDC). *National STD Surveillance Report 2003.* **2003d**. Available at: http://www.cdc.gov/std/stats/ [accessed December 20, 2003].

Centers for Disease Control and Prevention (CDC). Primary and secondary syphilis – United States, 2002. *MMWR Morbid Mortal Wkly Rpt.* **2003e**;52:1117-1120.

Chakraborty H, Sen PK, Helms RW, et al. Viral burden in genital secretions determines male-to-female sexual transmission of HIV-1: a probabilistic empiric model. *AIDS.* **2001**;15:621-627.

Chin-Hong PV, Deeks S, Liegler T, et al. High risk sexual behavior in HIV-infected adults with genotypically proven antiretroviral resistance. In: Program and abstracts of the 11th Conference on Retroviruses and Opportunistic Infections; February 8-11, **2004**; San Francisco, California. Abstract 845.

Cohen MS. Sexually transmitted diseases enhance HIV transmission: No longer a hypothesis. *Lancet.* **1998**;351(suppl 3):5-7.

Farr G, Gabelnick H, Sturgen K, Dorflinger L. Contraceptive efficacy and acceptability of the female condom. *Am J Public Health.* **1994**;84:1960-1964.

Fisher M, Barrett S, Sabin C, Williams D, Dean G. Increasing bacterial sexually transmitted infections (STIs) in HIV positive men who have sex with men (MSM). In: Program and abstracts from the 2nd International AIDS Society Conference on HIV Pathogenesis and Treatment; July 13-16, **2003**; Paris, France. Abstract 998.

Fleming PL, Byers RH, Sweeney PA, et al. HIV prevalence in the United States, 2000. In: Program and abstracts of the 9th Conference on Retroviruses and Opportunistic Infections; February 24-28, **2002**; Seattle, Washington. Abstract 11.

Gray RH, Wawer MJ, Brookmeyer R, et al. Probability of HIV-1 transmission per coital act in monogamous, heterosexual, HIV-1-discordant couples in Rakai, Uganda. *Lancet.* **2001**;357:1149-1153.

Hoffman S, Mantell J, Exner T, Stein Z. The future of the female condom. *Int Fam Plan Perspec.* **2004**;30:139-145.

Kozal M, Amico R, Chiarella J, et al. In: Program and abstracts of the 11th Conference on Retroviruses and Opportunistic Infections; February 8-11, **2004**; San Francisco. Abstract 35LB.

Kulczycki A, Kim D, Duerr A, et al. The acceptability of the female and male condom: A randomized crossover trial. *Perspect Sex Reprod Health.* **2004**;36:114-119.

McConnell J, Grant R. Sorting out serosorting with sexual network methods. In: Program and abstracts of the 11th Conference on Retroviruses and Opportunistic Infections; February 8-11, **2004**; San Francisco. Abstract 41.

Morse SA. Etiology of genital ulcer disease and its relationship to HIV infection. *Sex Transm Dis.* **1999**;26:63-65.

Pilcher CD, Tien HC, Eron JJ, et al. Brief but efficient: Acute HIV infection and the sexual transmission of HIV. *J Infect Dis.* **2004a**;189:1785-1792.

Pilcher CD, Eron JJ, Galvin S, et al. Acute HIV revisited: New opportunities for treatment and prevention. *J Clin Invest.* **2004b**;113:937-945.

Sakondhavat C, Weeravatrakul Y, Benette T, et al. Consumer preference study of the female condom in a sexually active population at risk of contracting AIDS. *J Med Assoc Thai.* **2001**;84:973-981.

Schacker T, Collier AC, Hughes J, et al. Clinical and epidemiologic features of primary HIV infection. *Ann Intern Med.* **1996**;125:257-264.

Smith JB, Nkhama G, Trottier DA. Female condom reuse in Lusaka, Zambia: Evidence from 12 cases. *J Urban Health.* **2001**;78:638-646.

Tindall B, Barker S, Donovan B, et al. Characterization of the acute clinical illness associated with human immunodeficiency virus infection. *Arch Intern Med.* **1988**;148:945-949.

Torian L, Weisfuse I, Makki H, et al. Increasing HIV-1 seroprevalence associated with genital ulcer disease, New York City, 1990-1992. *AIDS.* **1995**;9:177-181.

Tovanabutra S, Robison V, Wongtrakul J, et al. Male viral load and heterosexual transmission of HIV-1 subtype E in northern Thailand. *J Acquir Immune Defic Syndr.* **2002**;29:275-283.

Truong HM, McFarland W, Kellogg T, Dilley J. Increases in "serosorting" may prevent further expansion of the HIV epidemic among MSM in San Francisco. In: Program and abstracts of the 11th Conference on Retroviruses and Opportunistic Infections; February 8-11, **2004**; San Francisco, California. Abstract 843.

Van Devanter N, Gonzales V, Merzel C, Parikh NS, Celantano D, Greenberg J. Effects of an STD/AIDS behavioral intervention on women's use of the female condom. *Am J Public Health.* **2002**;92:109-115.

Weintrob AC, Giner J, Menezes P, et al. Infrequent diagnosis of primary human immunodeficiency virus infection. *Arch Intern Med.* **2003**;163:2097-2100.

WHO Information Update: Considerations regarding reuse of the female condom (July **2002**). Available at: http://www.who.int/reproductive-health/rtis/docs/reuse_FC2.pdf [accessed March 10, 2005).

(RLO-9)

II.36. PREVENTIVE HIV VACCINE RESEARCH

LEARNING OBJECTIVE: Discuss current research on the development of vaccines to prevent HIV infection.

Government and private institutions have for some years been searching for a preventive HIV vaccine. In March 2005, a search of ClinicalTrials.gov, a central database sponsored by the National Institutes of Health, found 88 early-stage HIV preventive vaccine studies worldwide that are completed or are under way, sponsored by the National Institutes of Health, other U.S. federal agencies and the pharmaceutical industry (NIH 2005). Of these, 14 studies are either currently recruiting or not yet recruiting volunteers. Despite this substantial number of early-phase studies, only two vaccines have advanced to a phase III trial.

Obstacles to the development of a preventive vaccine include the global genetic diversity of HIV subtypes, the replication and mutagenesis rates of HIV, the rapid establishment of a latent reservoir following infection and the general absence of neutralizing antibodies elicited by the vaccines tested. Protective immunity from other vaccines occurs because of effective antibody responses that clear virus, after infection has occurred. Correlates of protective immunity against HIV remain to be identified. Additionally, the generation of antibodies (e.g., IgA) at mucosal surfaces by candidate vaccines has not been rigorously assessed. The life cycle of HIV is complex and rapid (see Objective I.4 on Viral Replication in the AAHIVM 2003 Study Guide) and involves constant mutation. A vaccine developed against one strain of HIV may not prevent infection by a different strain (Letvin 2002). Recent reports claim cases of HIV superinfection of an individual with a second strain of HIV, after already having sustained chronic HIV infection from a prior source (see Objective I.10 on Superinfection in this Update), and cases of infection despite a good CD8-specific T-cell response against the infecting strain (Fidler et al. 2003) cast doubt on the possibility of ever producing a vaccine that could fully protect against infection. Even if an appropriate vaccine candidate emerges, the generation of significant immune responses will likely require the use of appropriate adjuvants, although this aspect has not been fully studied to date.

Early attempts to develop HIV vaccines used gp120, an HIV glycoprotein, to induce neutralizing antibody, but they were unsuccessful (McMichael et al. 2002). Since 1999, more than 600 people have enrolled in ongoing preventive vaccine trials using two primary vaccine candidates that target the cellular immune system; a plasmid-based (naked DNA) vaccine and a modified adenovirus-5 (Ad5; modified common cold virus) vector vaccine (Kahn 2003). Both candidates carry the HIV-*gag* gene (Kahn 2003). The research program also includes variations of these two models, such as improved vectors, multigene vaccines and novel prime-boost combinations (Kahn 2003).

Early study results with the DNA vaccine include low immunogenicity in volunteers following four vaccinations given at intervals up to 26 weeks (Kahn 2003). The Ad5 vaccine study results showed responses in about 60% of volunteers at 8 and 30 weeks; however, in people with preexisting immunity to the vector there was a blunted response (Kahn 2003). Several approaches to improving responses of these investigational vaccines are being

What's New

Despite best efforts by scientists worldwide, development of preventive vaccines remains difficult, with disappointing results.

Key Points

- Clinical trials of potential AIDS vaccines are in progress.
- Current vaccine clinical trial data indicate that a preventive HIV vaccine is unlikely to be available in the near future.
- New investigational vaccine strategies include use of a priming vaccine followed by a boosting vaccine using an alternative antigen or delivery system.

investigated, including the use of higher Ad5 doses, different adenovirus serotypes and combining Ad5 with a DNA prime (Kahn 2003). An international study designed to track the epidemiology of preexisting neutralizing antibodies to Ad5 showed an international prevalence of anti-Ad5 neutralizing antibodies of 91.6%, much higher than the 61.2% in subjects in the United States (Mast et al. 2004); this finding highlights some of the difficulties of vaccine development for diverse global populations.

Additional phase I vaccine research reported favorable preclinical data in primates of a combination of the canarypox-based HIV vaccine (ALVAC vCP205) with the Ad5 vaccine, and the results enabled progression of phase I trial plans in healthy volunteers. The phase I trial entails vaccination with an ALVAC boost in volunteers who have previously been vaccinated with Ad5 (Kahn 2003). Another primate study evaluated two poxvirus-based, trivalent simian immunodeficiency virus (SIV) vaccines (MVA-SIV, ALVAC-SIV or ALVAC vector) to assess the ability of neonatal vaccination to provide protection against later oral SIV exposure (Marthas et al. 2004). In all, 10 of 15 vaccinated macaques were protected from infection after 20 weeks of daily, oral SIV inoculation, whereas all 5 unvaccinated controls were infected.

There is growing conviction that even if a wholly preventive HIV vaccine may not be possible, an AIDS vaccine that at least slows disease progression may be plausible (for further details, see Objective IV.55 on Therapeutic HIV Vaccines the AAHIVM 2003 Study Guide).

Phase III Trials

Two potential vaccines to prevent HIV infection have reached phase III clinical trials. The first is a phase III trial of a preventive HIV vaccine (bivalent rgp120/HIV-1 vaccine) that was ongoing in North America and Europe, with 5109 men who have sex with men and 309 women at heterosexual risk of HIV infection. Retention after two years was high (89%). The most common adverse effect was pain at the site of injection. Education has been effective in preventing trial-related social harms (e.g., mild disturbances in personal relationships) (Harro et al. 2002). The trial ended in late 2002, and results announced in February 2003 described this vaccine as safe but not effective in reducing HIV infection within the entire study population. A post-hoc subgroup analysis found a statistically significant increase in protection in a relatively small number of patients in African American and Asian subgroups. The increase in protection seen in these subgroups was accompanied by relatively higher levels of vaccine-induced neutralizing antibodies (rgp120 Vaccine Study Group 2005); however, this finding remains controversial. Further studies would be required to determine whether this subgroup protection is a truly significant result or just an artifact of this study. More recent data support the initial overall disappointing results (Chan et al. 2004).

Another trial, with bivalent B[MN]/E[A244] rgp120, enrolled 2545 intravenous-drug users in Thailand. Overall immunization compliance was 98%, with 97% receiving the fourth dose (Choopanya et al. 2002). The primary endpoint was prevention of HIV infection, and the secondary endpoints were related to delayed progression of HIV disease in participants who were vaccinated but later became infected with HIV (VaxGen 2003). Preliminary results reported in July 2004 indicated that the vaccine candidate was not effective for the primary or secondary endpoints. The annualized incidence of HIV infection among vaccinated participants was 3.1% (Choopanya et al. 2004).

References

Chan KJ, Lampinen TM, Logue K, et al. HIV incidence among AIDSVAX® B/B vaccine trial participants in Montreal, Toronto and Vancouver. In: Program and abstracts of the XV International AIDS Conference; July 11-16, **2004**; Bangkok, Thailand. Abstract ThOrC1432.

Choopanya K, Tappero J, Pitisuttithum P, et al. Ongoing follow-up of injecting drug users (IDUs) in the AIDSVAXreg;B/E vaccine efficacy trial in Bangkok, Thailand. In: Program and abstracts of the XIV International AIDS Conference; July 7-12, **2002**; Barcelona, Spain. Abstract WeOrD1300.

Choopanya K, Tappero JW, Pitisuttithum P, et al. Preliminary results of a phase III HIV vaccine efficacy trial among injecting drug users in Thailand. In: Program and abstracts of the XV International AIDS Conference; July 11-16, **2004**; Bangkok, Thailand. Abstract ThOrA1427.

Fidler S, Pinheiro S, Nicholson C, et al. Pre-existing HIV-specific CD8+ CTL fail to prevent HIV infection in an HIV sero-discordant couple. In: Program and abstracts from the 10th conference on retroviruses and Opportunistic Infections; February 10-14, **2003**; Boston, Massachusetts. Abstract 506.

Harro C, Judson F, Brown S, et al. Conduct of the first phase III efficacy trial of a preventive HIV-1 vaccine (AIDSVAXreg; B/B) in North America and Europe. In: Program and abstracts of the XIV International AIDS Conference; July 7-12, **2002**; Barcelona, Spain. Abstract WeOrD1299.

Kahn P. Update on Merck's AIDS Vaccine Program. IAVI Report. **2003**;7(1):3-4, 17, 19. Available at: http://www.iavireport.org/Issues/0403/2003FebAprIR.pdf [accessed February 16, 2005].

Letvin NL. Strategies for an HIV vaccine. *J Clin Invest*. **2002**;110:15-27.

Marthas ML Van Rompay KKA, Lawson JR, et al. Neonatal poxvirus-based vaccines provide long-term, protection of macaques against oral SIV exposure. In: Program and abstracts of the XV International AIDS Conference; July 11-16, **2004**; Bangkok, Thailand. Abstract ThPeA6997.

Mast TC, Gupta S, Nikas A, et al. International epidemiology of human pre-existing anti-adenovirus Type-5 (Ad5) neutralizing antibodies in areas representative of potential HIV vaccine trial sites. In: Program and abstracts of the XV International AIDS Conference; July 11-16, **2004**; Bangkok, Thailand. Abstract ThPeC7432.

McMichael A, Mwau M, Hanke T. Design and tests of an HIV vaccine. *Br Med Bull*. **2002**;62:87-98.

National Institutes of Health (NIH). Clinical trials database. Search term: HIV prevention vaccine. Available at: http://clinicaltrials.gov/ct/action/GetStudy [accessed March 10, 2005].

The rgp120 HIV Vaccine Study Group. Placebo-Controlled Phase 3 Trial of a Recombinant Glycoprotein 120 Vaccine to Prevent HIV-1 Infection. *J Infect Dis*. **2005**;191:654-665.

VaxGen. VaxGen Announces results of its phase III HIV vaccine trial in Thailand: Vaccine fails to meet endpoints. November 12, **2003**. Available at: http://www.vaxgen.com [accessed February 13, 2005].

(RLO-10)

II.83. CONFIDENTIALITY

LEARNING OBJECTIVE: Discuss legal issues related to confidentiality and HIV, including health information protected under HIPAA's Privacy Rule and HIPAA's impact on communicating a patient's personal health information.

The rationale for confidentiality in the medical setting is that an effective physician-patient relationship is based upon trust and strict confidentiality regarding the patient's medical information. Almost all would agree that keeping patient information confidential has particular importance when the patient is infected with HIV. HIV-infected patients may choose to keep their status private in order to avoid the significant emotional, social and financial stigmatization, isolation and loss that many HIV-infected persons encounter when their status becomes known. Therefore, every physician should seek to respect the privacy of his or her patients, including persons living with HIV, and respect their wish not to have intimate and personal information about themselves made available to others.

The Hippocratic Oath and other ethical guidelines instruct physicians that information gained through the physician–patient relationship is confidential. Confidentiality requirements are also underscored by various state laws and federal provisions. The Health Insurance Portability and Accountability Act of 1996 (HIPAA) has implications for nearly all health care providers and facilities, including federally funded facilities that provide substance abuse treatment services (SAMHSA 2004).

In general, both state and federal confidentiality requirements address the following areas:

- **Handling of medical information.** State laws require patient consent for releasing information to all or only certain requestors (AMA 2004). HIPAA oversees transmission of information within the current interrelated healthcare system for purposes of treatment, payment or other health care functions. It oversees multiple providers and payers and the electronic information shared between them.
- **Procedures for handling exceptional situations.** State laws typically provide for disclosure of information for public health purposes, such as the "duty to warn" an individual facing imminent harm from a patient. Assaults and communicable diseases are reportable and may be legally mandated (AMA 2004). Physician–patient confidentiality is not absolute under the law of most states. The courts and legislators in many states have attempted to strike a balance between competing rights: those of patients to confidentiality and those of others to information about the significant dangers they may face (see Objective II.82 on Issues in Nondisclosure in the AAHIVM 2003 Study Guide). It seems reasonable that the patient's right to privacy should be breached only when it is necessary to avoid imminent and serious harm. If the chance of contracting HIV from contact with the patient is remote (e.g., a household contact), then the right to confidentiality should be considered paramount. However, if the chance of contracting HIV is high (e.g., a sexual contact), then the duty to warn may take precedence.

What's New

In addition to the Privacy Rule, HIPAA regulations call for Security Standards: Clinicians must enact administrative, physical and technical safeguards that will protect information that the clinician collects, maintains, uses and transmits. The compliance date for the Security Standards is April 21, 2005, with a 1-year extension for small health plans.

Key Points

- Multiple reasons for strict confidentiality exist in the medical setting, including maintaining effective clinician-patient relationships.
- Various state and federal regulations govern confidentiality of medical information. Noncompliance carries the risk of civil and/or criminal penalties.
- Federal provisions governing confidentiality were established in the Health Insurance Portability and Accountability Act of 1996 (HIPAA). The Act defines which health entities are covered, what kind of medical information is covered, how information can be used and requirements for notifying patients. The deadline for compliance with the HIPAA Privacy Rule was April 14, 2003.
- The HIPAA Security Standards dictate that "administrative, physical, and technical" safeguards must be in place to protect confidential information and its transmission and storage. Healthcare providers must comply with the HIPAA Security Standards by April 21, 2005, with a 1-year extension for small health plans.
- Available resources may assist clinicians in complying with HIPAA and other confidentiality provisions.

- **Penalties.** Physicians treating HIV-infected patients must seek to balance these legal and ethical obligations. There is no guarantee that the balance struck by the physician will be the same one struck by a court should the matter end up being the subject of litigation. Almost one-half of the states have provisions for revoking a physician's medical license or other disciplinary action when confidential patient information is inappropriately or unlawfully disclosed. HIPAA also contains penalty provisions. When in doubt, the physician should consult an attorney before taking any action or making any disclosure without consent.

HIPAA

Boyle and colleagues (2003) describe HIPAA regulations on privacy and disclosure of medical information (i.e., the "Privacy Rule"). HIPAA places the burden on health care providers and others who have access to confidential medical information to keep it private and protected, outlining who must comply, what information is protected and what providers must do to comply. Similar state laws take precedence if they are more stringent than HIPAA.

The Privacy Rule definition of who must comply (a detailed outline of "covered entities") covers most clinicians and health plans because it essentially applies to anyone who bills electronically. "Protected health information" (PHI), likewise, is broadly defined (i.e., medical records and other identifying information). Covered entities had to be in compliance with the Privacy Rule by April 14, 2003.

The Privacy Rule also stipulates, in great detail, how information may be used and disclosed. Key examples of allowed uses include release of information to the patient in question. In fact, patients must have access to their medical records along with information about who has been granted access to it. Information can also be used in treatment and payment. HIPAA also contains provisions for special circumstances under which medical information can be released, such as the "duty to warn" provisions cited previously.

Patient consent must be obtained for most disclosures of medical information. Covered entities are also required to provide patients with a written "Notice of Privacy Practices" that clearly explains the provider's privacy policy—and must document that their patients received it (Boyle et al. 2003). More generally, physicians must institute reasonable measures to prevent incidental disclosure of patient information. Such reasonable measures include steps to make sure that unauthorized persons cannot wander into record rooms or access computer databases—or overhear names during in-person or telephone communications. However, HIPAA is not intended to impede customary communications, nor does it require protection against any conceivable incidental disclosure, such as when a visitor glimpses patient names on a sign-in sheet (DHHS OCR 2003).

In addition to the Privacy Rule, HIPAA also requires clinicians and health plans to protect the security of patients' medical information that is stored or transmitted electronically (the "Security Standards"). The Security Standards call for all covered entities to enact administrative, physical and technical safeguards for electronic data (DHHS 2003).

Examples of such safeguards in an office setting are policies that limit access to database software to those who require it (physical safeguard), sanctions for employees who violate the Standards (administrative safeguard) and the maintenance of electronic "audit logs" on computer systems that are equipped to access PHI (technical safeguard).

The compliance date for the Security Standards is April 21, 2005. Small health plans have an additional year to comply with the rules.

Ideas for Compliance

Clinicians should establish compliance provisions, not only to fulfill HIPAA requirements, but also to be prepared to handle confidentiality in a responsible manner. Among the methods used is the securing of written informed consent from patients (required by HIPAA for certain situations) and formulation of clear procedures for handling patient information (e.g., secure storage, definitions of what information is protected, with whom it can be shared, strategies for handling special circumstances). Other options include designating a privacy officer who would be knowledgeable about the details of HIPAA and providing staff training on confidentiality (Boyle et al. 2003).

For handling situations in which a "duty to warn" another individual arises, such as a sex partner or injection-drug-using partner of the patient, clinicians can seek assistance. Most local or state health departments have partner notification programs that do this work.

Web-Based Resources

There are a number of Internet resources that may assist clinicians in complying with HIPAA and other confidentiality provisions. The Web site of the American Medical Association (AMA), available at http://www.ama-assn.org/go/hipaa, contains a number of sections related to HIPAA and complying with its provisions, including a frequently asked questions page, sample documents, links to other online resources for HIPAA information and compliance, and a complaint form for alerting the AMA to health plans and other payers that are not in compliance with the HIPAA electronic transaction standards.

In addition, the Web site of the US Department of Health and Human Services Office of Civil Rights (DHHS OCR) contains HIPAA information for both clinicians and patients, including fact sheets, sample documents and educational materials. This Web site is accessible at http://www.hhs.gov/ocr/hipaa/.

Finally, clinicians may consult the Centers for Medicare & Medicaid Services (CMS) online at http://www.cms.hhs.gov/hipaa/ to download standards and educational materials. The CMS Web site also lists educational events related to HIPAA implementation, including satellite broadcasts and teleconferences.

References

American Medical Association (AMA). Patient confidentiality. **2004**. Available at: http://www.ama-assn.org/ama/pub/category/4610.html [accessed February 19, 2005].

Boyle B, Bradley T, Bradley H. Health Insurance Portability and Accountability Act of 1996 ("HIPAA"): new national medical privacy standards. *AIDS Reader.* **2003**;13:261-266.

Department of Health and Human Services (DHHS). 45 CFR Parts 160, 162, and 164. Health insurance reform: Security Standards; final rule. *Federal Register.* **2003**;68:8333-8381.

Department of Health and Human Services Office for Civil Rights (DHHS OCR). Incidental uses and disclosures. Revised April 3, **2003**. Available at: http://www.hhs.gov/ocr/hipaa/guidelines/incidentalud.pdf [accessed February 19, 2005].

Substance Abuse and Mental Health Services Administration (SAMHSA). The confidentiality of alcohol and drug abuse patient records regulation and the HIPAA privacy rule: Implications for alcohol and substance abuse programs. June **2004**. Available at: http://www.hipaa.samhsa.gov/download2/SAMHSAHIPAAComparisonClearedPDFVersion.pdf [accessed February 19, 2005].

CLINICAL MANIFESTATIONS OF HIV INFECTION AND ASSOCIATED CONDITIONS

This section covers the most recent information developments in clinical manifestations of chronic HIV infection, including the various opportunistic infections seen in AIDS, and other HIV-related illnesses and comorbidities that are frequently encountered when caring for patients with HIV infection.

Upon completion of this section, clinicians should be able to describe when to initiate and discontinue prophylaxis for opportunistic infections; and identify what is needed to diagnose and treat methicillin-resistant *Staphylococcus aureus* (MRSA), eosinophilic folliculitis (EF), NASH, hepatitis B, hepatitis C and syphilis.

At-a-glance

What's New – Overview

The incidence of syphilis is still rising among MSM, and the threat of MRSA in patients with HIV is receiving increased attention, as is an outbreak of proctitis induced by lymphogranuloma venereum. A third nucleoside analog, entecavir, is now approved for hepatitis B, and pegylated interferon alfa-2a has received an additional indication for HCV/HIV coinfection.

(RLO-11)

III.8. OPPORTUNISTIC INFECTION PROPHYLAXIS

LEARNING OBJECTIVE: List the recommended prophylactic regimens for *Pneumocystis jiroveci* pneumonia (PCP), *Mycobacterium avium* complex (MAC), fungal infections, toxoplasmosis and herpesvirus infections (including cytomegalovirus [CMV]), citing the guidelines for initiation of prophylaxis (including co-trimoxazole desensitization) and discontinuation of prophylaxis.

Pneumocystis jiroveci Pneumonia (PCP)

Primary prophylaxis

Initiate if the patient has a CD4 count below 200 cells/mm^3 or a history of oropharyngeal candidiasis, or a history of other AIDS-defining opportunistic infections at a higher CD4 count. The preferred regimen is one double-strength tablet of trimethoprim/sulfamethoxazole (co-trimoxazole, TMP-SMX; Bactrim or Septra) administered once daily or three times weekly. One single-strength tablet daily is also effective and may be better tolerated.

In case of intolerance, rechallenge the patient with a lower dose or employ a desensitization protocol of gradual dose escalation (Tables III.8-1 and III.8-2). A study comparing desensitization (n = 34) and rechallenge (n = 25) to TMP-SMX treatment in HIV-infected patients receiving prophylaxis for PCP found comparable effectiveness between treatment strategies (Bonfanti et al. 2000). Desensitization protocols for TMP-SMX hypersensitivity in HIV-infected patients have had mixed success. Nguyen and colleagues (1995) achieved a 60% (27/45 subjects) success rate using graduated oral suspension doses of TMP-SMX administered over 36 hours. Patients who tolerated this regimen were switched to a daily regimen of oral tablets or intravenous formulation. The long-term outcomes of TMP-SMX desensitization were studied retrospectively in 22 patients (Gluckstein and Ruskin 1995). Of the 81% of patients successfully desensitized, 3 discontinued TMP-SMX treatment within 2 weeks due to fever and/or rash and three experienced transient rashes 1 week post desensitization but were able to continue treatment. No patient in either study was hospitalized for adverse reactions (Gluckstein and Ruskin 1995; Nguyen et al. 1995).

Alternative but possibly less effective regimens include dapsone alone (100 mg once daily) or dapsone (50 mg once daily) plus pyrimethamine (50 mg once weekly) plus leucovorin (25 mg once weekly). Aerosolized pentamidine administered with a Respirgard II nebulizer is another option but is less effective than TMP-SMX.

Secondary prophylaxis

Use the same regimens as above to prevent reoccurrence after an episode of PCP.

Discontinuation

Both primary and secondary prophylaxis for *Pneumocystis jiroveci* (formerly *P. carinii*) pneumonia may be discontinued in adults and adolescents who have responded to combination antiretroviral therapy with an increase in CD4 count above 200 cells/mm^3 for at least 3 months. However, continuing primary prophylaxis until the first observed CD4 count above 300 cells/mm^3 may further decrease the risk of PCP cases and be more cost-effective, especially in patients who began prophylaxis at lower CD4 counts and are in late-stage HIV disease (Goldie et al. 2002). PCP prophylaxis may also be safely discontinued in children with prolonged CD4+ T cell normalization (16 weeks or longer; CD4+ T cells over 25% for patients age 2 to 6 years; over 20% for patients older than 6 years) (Dankner et al. 2004).

What's New

Co-trimoxazole (trimethoprim/sulfamethoxazole; TMP-SMX) desensitization may be an effective treatment strategy for patients with a history of hypersensitivity to TMP-SMX requiring prophylaxis for PCP. Patients with sustained immunologic improvement due to antiretroviral therapy may be successfully discontinued from antifungal maintenance therapy for histoplasmosis.

Key Points

- It is generally safe to discontinue primary and secondary prophylaxis for opportunistic infections when CD4 counts rebound to protective levels as a result of successful combination antiretroviral therapy.
- Current guidelines from the U.S. Public Health Service on primary and secondary prophylaxis for opportunistic infections (CDC 2002) are briefly described. For full details, see http://www.cdc.gov/mmwr/PDF/rr/rr5108.pdf or http://www.cdc.gov/mmwr/preview/mmwrhtml/rr5108a1.htm.

Table III.8-1. Slow co-trimoxazole (TMP-SMX) desensitization.

Day	Dilution[1]
1	1:1,000,000
2	1:1000,000
3	1:10,000
4	1:1,000
5	1:100
6	1:10
7	1:1
8	Standard suspension[2]
≥ 9	1 double-strength tablet daily

Adapted with permission from Bartlett and Gallant (2004).

[1] Serial dilutions of oral suspension formulation containing 40 mg TMP and 200 mg SMX/5 mL. Treatment is administered four times daily for 7 days in doses of 1, 2, 4 and 8 mL.

[2] 8 mg TMP and 40 mg SMX per mL

Table III.8-2. Rapid co-trimoxazole (TMP-SMX) desensitization.

Hour	Dose (TMP-SMX)	Dilution
0	0.004/0.02 mg	1:10,000 (5 mL)
1	0.04/0.2 mg	1:1,000 (5 mL)
2	0.4/2.0 mg	1:100 (5 mL)
3	4/20 mg	1:10 (5 mL)
4	40/200 mg	(5 mL)
5	160/800 mg	1 double-strength tablet

Adapted with permission from Gluckstein and Ruskin (1995) and from Bartlett and Gallant (2004).

Mycobacterium avium Complex (MAC)

Primary prophylaxis

Initiate primary prophylaxis in patients with CD4 counts below 50 cells/mm^3. Clarithromycin (500 mg twice daily) and azithromycin (1200 mg once weekly), which also help to prevent respiratory infections, are the preferred agents. Rifabutin (300 mg once daily) is an alternative for those intolerant to clarithromycin and azithromycin. Note that rifabutin reduces the blood levels of a large number of drugs, including protease inhibitors and nonnucleoside reverse transcriptase inhibitors. The presence of active disseminated MAC or tuberculosis should be excluded before commencing prophylaxis to prevent the selection of drug-resistant disease.

Secondary prophylaxis

Once therapy has been commenced it should be continued indefinitely, or until the CD4 count has risen to a point when MAC prophylaxis can be safely discontinued. The recommended treatment regimen is either clarithromycin (500 mg twice daily) or azithromycin (500 mg once daily) plus ethambutol (15 mg/kg once daily), with or without rifabutin (300 mg once daily).

Discontinuation

Primary prophylaxis may be discontinued in adults and adolescents who have responded to combination antiretroviral therapy with an increase in CD4 count above 100 cells/mm^3 for at least 3 consecutive months. Patients with a history of MAC are at low risk for recurrence if they have been treated with a macrolide-based regimen for at least 12 months without MAC symptoms and have responded to combination antiretroviral therapy with an increase in CD4 count above 100 cells/mm^3 (Aberg et al. 2003). Secondary prophylaxis should be resumed if the patient's CD4 count declines again to below 100 cells/mm^3. MAC prophylaxis may also be safely discontinued in children with prolonged CD4+ T cell normalization (16 weeks or longer; CD4 cells over 25% for patients 2 to 6 years of age; over 20% for patients older than 6 years) (Dankner et al. 2004).

Fungal Infections

Candidiasis

The effectiveness of therapy for acute disease, low mortality rate, drug interactions and cost, as well as the risk of developing drug-resistant Candida, discourages routine prophylaxis. However, the use of fluconazole or itraconazole solution may be considered to prevent frequent or severe recurrences or oropharyngeal or vulvovaginal candidiasis, and oral fluconazole (100-200 mg daily) may be appropriate to prevent recurrent esophageal candidiasis in patients with CD4 counts below 100 cells/mm^3. Resistance can develop to azoles with long-term use (CDC 2002).

For infections not responding to fluconazole therapy, options include increasing the oral dose of fluconazole (up to 800 mg/day); switching to another azole, either itraconazole 200 mg/day or voriconazole 200 mg/day; or switching to intravenous therapy with amphotericin B 0.3-0.7 mg/kg/day or caspofungin 70 mg for Day 1, then 50 mg/day (Bartlett and Gallant 2004).

Cryptococcosis

Primary prophylaxis is not recommended. Although fluconazole and itraconazole reduce the incidence of cryptococcosis, the rarity of the disease as well as drug toxicity, resistance and cost issues discourage their use. If used, fluconazole at 100 to 200 mg once daily is appropriate for patients with CD4 counts below 50 cells/mm^3.

Fluconazole (200 mg once daily) is effective as secondary prophylaxis; itraconazole is a less effective alternative. Secondary prophylaxis should continue for life, or until the patient is asymptomatic and has responded to combination antiretroviral therapy with an increase in CD4 count above 100 to 200 cells/mm^3 for at least 6 months. Even then, recurrences are possible. Some specialists would not discontinue prophylaxis until the cerebrospinal fluid is culture-negative for Cryptococcus, although others do not agree that this is necessary.

Coccidioidomycosis

There is no routine primary prophylaxis. Secondary prophylaxis consists of fluconazole (400 mg once daily) or itraconazole (200 mg twice daily). There are insufficient data to allow a recommendation on discontinuing secondary prophylaxis (although this may be possible in patients with combination antiretroviral therapy-induced CD4 count rebounds above 200 cells/mm^3).

Histoplasmosis

There is no routine primary prophylaxis. Itraconazole might be used in patients with CD4 counts below 100 cells/mm^3 who are occupationally exposed or live in areas of very high incidence. For secondary prophylaxis, itraconazole is used at 200 mg once daily. In a recent study, itraconazole maintenance therapy was discontinued in 32 HIV-infected patients previously treated for disseminated histoplasmosis who received maintenance therapy for over 12 months (Goldman et al. 2004). After a median follow-up time of 24 months, no evidence of relapse was found in any patient. The success of itraconazole maintenance discontinuation may be due to the sustained immunologic improvement of patients throughout the study resulting from antiretroviral therapy (median CD4 counts increased from 289 to 338 cells/mm^3, and the proportion of patients with HIV-1 RNA levels below 50 copies/mL increased from 59% to 81%). At present, there are insufficient data to allow a recommendation on stopping secondary prophylaxis.

Toxoplasmic encephalitis

Primary prophylaxis. *Toxoplasma* antibody-positive patients with CD4 counts below 100 cells/mm^3 should receive primary prophylaxis with one double-strength TMP-SMX tablet/day (Bartlett and Gallant 2004).

Secondary prophylaxis. The combination of oral doses of pyrimethamine (25-50 mg/day) plus leucovorin (5-10 mg/day) plus sulfadiazine (500-750 mg q6h) is highly effective in preventing recurrence, and it also prevents PCP (Bartlett and Gallant 2004; CDC 2002). An alternative is substituting sulfadiazine with clindamycin (300 mg q6-8h), which is not effective against PCP. Pyrimethamine and leucovorin plus atovaquone, clarithromycin, dapsone or azithromycin is another alternative for patients who cannot tolerate sulfadiazine or clindamycin. Atovaquone may also be taken alone.

Discontinuation. Primary prophylaxis may be discontinued in patients who have responded to combination antiretroviral therapy with an increase in CD4 count above 200 cells/mm^3 for at least 3 consecutive months. There are insufficient data to support a definitive recommendation on stopping secondary prophylaxis; however, this may be considered in asymptomatic patients with combination antiretroviral therapy-induced increases in CD4 count above 200 cells/mm^3 for at least 6 months consecutively. Recurrences have been reported after secondary prophylaxis has been stopped. Some experts recommend that a new MRI scan of the brain be evaluated before deciding whether to cease secondary prophylaxis.

Herpes Viruses

Cytomegalovirus (CMV)

The most important means of preventing severe CMV retinitis is careful monitoring for early symptoms in patients with low CD4 counts. Primary prophylaxis with valganciclovir may be considered in patients with CD4 counts below 50 cells/mm^3, but this is not routinely prescribed because of its toxicities, cost and uncertain benefits. It might be considered in a patient with a very low CD4 count and refractory HIV while awaiting the availability of new antiretroviral agents for salvage.

Systemic regimens for chronic secondary prophylaxis that have been evaluated in randomized, controlled clinical trials include valganciclovir, the oral prodrug of ganciclovir, (900 mg/day), ganciclovir given intravenously (5-6 mg/kg 5-7 days/week) or orally (1000 mg three times daily), intravenous foscarnet (90-120 mg/kg/day), and intravenous cidofovir (5 mg/kg every other week) (Bartlett and Gallant 2004; CDC 2002). Sustained-release ganciclovir intraocular implants or intravitreous fomivirsen injections are additional options for local secondary prophylaxis for CMV retinitis. A combination of intraocular and systemic therapy provides more complete protection than either alone.

Multiple studies have found that adults and adolescents can safely discontinue secondary prophylaxis for CMV retinitis if they have had combination antiretroviral therapy-induced increases in CD4 count above 100 to 150 cells/mm^3 for longer than 6 months.

Herpes simplex virus

Neither primary nor secondary prophylaxis is required. Persons with frequent severe recurrences may take daily suppressive doses of oral acyclovir (400 mg twice daily), famciclovir (125-250 mg twice daily) or valacyclovir (500 mg twice daily or 1 g once daily). However, cases of acyclovir-, famciclovir-, valacyclovir- and penciclovir-resistant herpes simplex in immunocompromised patients have been reported (Sarisky et al. 2003; Kopp et al. 2002). Kopp and colleagues reported a case study of an HIV-infected patient who failed valacyclovir treatment (1500 mg/day) but was successfully treated with intravenous cidofovir (5 mg/kg) once weekly at semimonthly intervals. The patient was 95% healed after three treatment cycles (Kopp et al. 2002). Penciclovir-resistant herpes simplex virus isolates were found in patients with a variety of immunocompromising conditions (e.g., HIV/AIDS and septicemia) (Sarisky et al. 2003).

Varicella-zoster virus (VZV)

VZV antibody-negative patients who report close contact with a person who has chickenpox or shingles should receive VZV immunoglobulin as soon as possible. The chicken pox vaccine, which contains live attenuated virus, should be administered only to HIV-infected children who have normal CD4 counts. There are few data to support the use of the vaccine in HIV-infected adults or the use of prophylactic acyclovir.

References

Aberg JA, Williams PL, Liu T, et al. A study of discontinuing maintenance therapy in human immunodeficiency virus-infected subjects with disseminated Mycobacterium avium complex: AIDS Clinical Trial Group 393 Study team. *J Infect Dis.* **2003**;187:1046-1052. [Erratum: J Infect Dis. 2003;187:1346.]

Bartlett JG, Gallant JE. *Medical Management of HIV Infection*, 2004 ed. Baltimore, Md: Johns Hopkins Medicine; **2004**.

Bonfanti P, Pusterla L, Parazzini F, et al. The effectiveness of desensitization versus rechallenge treatment in HIV-positive patients with previous hypersensitivity to TMP-SMX: a randomized multicentric study. *Biomed Pharmacother.* **2000**;54:45-49.

Centers for Disease Control and Prevention (CDC). Guidelines for preventing opportunistic infections among HIV-infected persons—2002 recommendations of the U.S. Public Health Service and the Infectious Diseases Society of America. *MMWR Morbid Mortal Wkly Rep.* **2002**;51(RR-8).

Dankner W, Nachman S, Hughes W, et al. An observational study of the rate of opportunistic infections events in HIV-infected children who have demonstrated immunologic reconstitution and who have discontinued prophylaxis. In: Program and abstracts of the 11th Conference on Retroviruses and Opportunistic Infections; February 8-11, **2004**; San Francisco, California. Abstract 931.

Gluckstein D, Ruskin J. Rapid oral desensitization to trimethoprim-sulfamethoxazole (TMP-SMZ): Use in prophylaxis for *Pneumocystis carinii* pneumonia in patients with AIDS who were previously intolerant to TMP-SMZ. *Clin Infect Dis.* **1995**;20:849-853.

Goldie SJ, Kaplan JE, Losina E, et al. Prophylaxis for human immunodeficiency virus-related *Pneumocystis carinii* pneumonia: Using simulation modeling to inform clinical guidelines. *Arch Intern Med.* **2002**;162:921-928.

Goldman M, Zackin R, Fichtenbaum CJ, et al. Safety of discontinuation of maintenance therapy for disseminated histoplasmosis after immunologic response to antiretroviral therapy. *Clin Infect Dis.* **2004**;38:1485-1489.

Kopp T, Geusau A, Reiger A, Stingl G. Successful treatment of an aciclovir-resistant herpes simplex type 2 infection with cidofovir in an AIDS patient. *Br J Dermatol.* **2002**;147:134-138.

Nguyen M-T, Weiss PJ, Wallace MR. Two-day oral desensitization to trimethoprim-sulfamethoxazole in HIV-infected patients. *AIDS.* **1995**;9:572-575.

Sarisky RT, Bacon TH, Boon RJ, et al. Profiling penciclovir susceptibility and prevalence of resistance of herpes simplex virus isolates across eleven clinical trials. *Arch Virol.* **2003**;148:1757-1769.

(RLO-12)

III.18DF. DERMATOLOGIC PRESENTATION AND TREATMENT

LEARNING OBJECTIVE: Describe the presentation and therapy for common dermatoses seen in HIV-infected patients: (d) bacterial, including methicillin-resistant *Staphylococcus aureus* (MRSA); (f) other (eosinophilic folliculitis [EF]).

What's New

This objective contains further information on the MRSA epidemic: epidemiology, clinical presentation, treatment/management. It also examines the diagnosis and management of *Demodex*-associated EF.

Key Points

- High incidence of MRSA has been reported in men who have sex with men and among prison inmates.
- Eruptions of eosinophilic folliculitis — associated with *Demodex* mite infestation — have arisen in persons whose CD4 counts are rebounding after initiating HAART.

See Objective III.18 on Dermatologic Complications: Presentation and Treatment in the AAHIVM 2003 Study Guide for complete review of other bacterial infections of the skin.

Methicillin-Resistant *Staphylococcus aureus*

Staphylococcus aureus is a common cause of soft tissue infections, and is found normally on the skin of up to 20% of healthy people (Garthwaite et al. 2003). Methicillin-resistant *S. aureus* (MRSA) infections have become common in hospitalized patients, and recently, significant recurrent outbreaks have been reported among men who have sex with men and prison inmates (CDC 2003). One study of a retrospective HIV-infected cohort found that the incidence of clinically significant MRSA events increased more than 6 times from 2000 to 2003 (Mathews et al. 2005). The authors suggested that the increased prevalence was due to a direct effect that HIV has on defenses against staphylococcal infections.

Outside hospital settings, MRSA is usually transmitted through skin-to-skin contact or perhaps contact with fomites via a contaminated surface or towels, clothing, or soap (Rimland and Brooks 2004). Community-acquired MRSA strains have antibiotic resistance patterns different from those of hospital-acquired MRSA strains (Said-Salim et al. 2003). As a result, there is a growing trend in the infectious disease field to reclassify MRSA as community- or hospital-acquired MRSA. Reports suggest that there is an increase in the number of community-acquired MRSA infections among HIV-infected men who have sex with men. In fact, the majority of skin or soft tissue infections at many HIV clinics can be attributed to MRSA acquired from either skin to skin or skin to fomite contact outside of hospitals (Rieg et al. 2005).

MRSA-related dermatosis may present in any of a number of forms, including cellulitis, impetigo, folliculitis, furunculosis, carbuncle, abscess or infected laceration (Garthwaite et al. 2003). In addition, other inflammatory dermatoses flare when staphylococcal infection occurs, including eczemas, seborrheic dermatitis and psoriasis. Treating the underlying staph infection may lead to improvement of the coexistent dermatosis. Accurately detecting the staph infection is therefore critical. Microbiological culture of skin lesions should be obtained in symptomatic cases to guide the antibiotic therapy. These cultures are particularly useful when managing recurrent or persistent skin infection, in the presence of antibiotic failure and/or with advanced or aggressive infections. When no symptoms are present, culture of MRSA colonization is usually not necessary (Garthwaite et al. 2003).

Initial treatment recommendations include incision, drainage and local lesion care. Simple skin infections that have a low index of suspicion for bacteremia can often be treated with oral antibiotics depending on the susceptibility of the isolate (Rimland and Brooks 2004). The predominant strains in recent MRSA outbreaks have been susceptible to trimethoprim/

sulfamethoxazole (TMP/SMX; co-trimoxazole), clindamycin, gentamicin, rifampin and vancomycin (Jones et al. 2003; CDC 2001). MRSA often exhibits a lack of susceptibility to erythromycin, with inducible clindamycin resistance (Rimland and Brooks 2004). Dual antibiotic therapy (i.e., TMP/SMX plus rifampin) is sometimes administered (Garthwaite et al. 2003). Careful consideration must be given to all of the other drugs a patient might be taking because of the interaction between rifampin and some other HIV-related drugs. The affected drugs include some protease inhibitors, some non-nucleoside reverse transcriptase inhibitors (NNRTIs) and fluconazole (Diflucan 2004). New guidelines state that rifampin may be used in patients who are receiving nucleoside or nucleotide analogue reverse transcriptase inhibitors along with either ritonavir as their only protease inhibitor or with the NNRTI efavirenz (CDC 2004). Linezolid is a newer antimicrobial that is bacteriocidal for MRSA at oral doses of 600 mg twice daily. However, there is a risk of thrombocytopenia if used for longer than 2 weeks (reviewed in Lundstrom and Sobel 2004).

Where there are recurrent MRSA skin infections in an individual or among a group of people in contact with each other, decolonization protocols are sometimes invoked (Rimland and Brooks 2004). Careful hygiene, including frequent hand washing, is an often overlooked yet important part of preventing infection. Other measures include chlorhexidine body washes and avoidance of shared towels and clothing. Nasal decolonization of MRSA using topical 2% mupirocin (Bactroban) can be very effective (Walker et al. 2003). However, there have been increasing reports of mupirocin resistance (Walker et al. 2003). Another possible decolonization is TMP/SMX plus rifampin (Rimland and Brooks 2004).

Demodex-Associated Eosinophilic Folliculitis

The *Demodex folliculorum* mite has long been considered one of the many factors inducing HIV-associated eosinophilic folliculitis (EF) (Ellis and Scheinfeld 2004).

Several recent studies indicate that this mite is the source of an inflammatory folliculitis related to immune reconstitution. It occurs within the first few days, weeks or months after beginning highly active antiretroviral therapy (HAART) (Delfos et al. 2004; Aquilina et al. 2002; Bouscarat et al. 2000). Both the clinical presentation and response to treatment vary substantially among patients. Most commonly, there are lesions on the face and/or upper trunk (Delfos et al. 2004; Aquilina et al. 2002; Bouscarat et al. 2000); pruritus may (Delfos et al. 2004; Bouscarat et al. 2000) or may not (Aquilina et al. 2002) be present. In some cases, there are coalescing lesions (Aquilina et al. 2002) unlike the discrete follicular papules commonly seen with EF in HIV-infected patients (Ellis and Scheinfeld 2004).

Therapies that have proved effective in at least some patients include topical corticosteroid cream (betamethasone dipropionate 0.05%) (Bouscarat et al. 2000) and topical metronidazole (Metrocream) (Delfos et al. 2004). Oral ivermectin (Stromectol) is a possibility in patients who have failed topical remedies (Delfos et al. 2004; Aquilina et al. 2002). To prevent recurrence, it is followed by either topical permethrin cream (Nix) (Aquilina et al. 2002) or topical metronidazole (Delfos et al. 2004). It will be important for clinicians to watch for suspect skin changes in the period following HAART initiation, and to differentiate such problems from antiretroviral drug side effects. For additional information on this form of folliculitis, including a more detailed description of the clinical presentation as well as important warnings about possible drug interactions with ivermectin, see Objective IV.51 on Immune Reconstitution Inflammatory Syndrome in this Update.

References

Aquilina C, Viraben R, Sire S. Ivermectin-responsive *Demodex* infestation during human immunodeficiency virus infection: a case report and literature review. *Dermatology*. **2002**;205:394-397.

Bouscarat F, Maubec E, Matheron S, Descamps V. Immune recovery inflammatory folliculitis. *AIDS*. **2000**;14:617-618.

Centers for Disease Control and Prevention (CDC). Methicillin-resistant *Staphylococcus aureus* skin or soft tissue infections in a state prison—Mississippi, 2000. *MMWR Morb Mortal Weekly Rep*. **2001**;50:919-922.

Centers for Disease Control and Prevention (CDC). Outbreaks of community-associated methicillin-resistant Staphylococcus aureus skin infections — Los Angeles County, California, 2002-2003. *MMWR Morb Mortal Wkly Rep*. **2003**;52:88.

Centers for Disease Control and Prevention (CDC). Updated guidelines for the use of rifamycins for the treatment of tuberculosis among HIV-infected patients taking protease inhibitors or nonnucleoside reverse transcriptase inhibitors. January 20, **2004**. Available at: http://www.cdc.gov/nchstp/tb/tb_hiv_drugs/toc.htm [accessed February 19, 2005].

Delfos NM, Collen AFS, Kroon FP. Demodex folliculitis: a skin manifestation of immune reconstitution disease. *AIDS*. **2004**;18:701-702.

Diflucan (fluconazole) [prescribing information]. New York, NY. Pfizer, Inc. August **2004**.

Ellis E, Scheinfeld N. Eosinophilic pustular folliculitis: a comprehensive review of treatment options. *Am J Clin Dermatol*. **2004**;5:189-197.

Garthwaite T, Fielding J. Fact sheet for health care providers: Community-associated methicillin-resistant Staphylococcus aureus skin infections. Los Angeles, Calif: Los Angeles County Department of Health Services, March 20, **2003**. Available at: http://lapublichealth.org/acd/docs/CAMRSA_ProviderFactSheet.pdf [accessed February 19, 2005].

Jones ME, Karlowsky JA, Draghi DC, et al. Epidemiology and antibiotic susceptibility of bacteria causing skin and soft tissue infections in the USA and Europe: a guide to appropriate antimicrobial therapy. Int J Antimicrob Agents. **2003**;22:406-419.

Lundstrom TS, Sobel JD. Antibiotics for gram-positive bacterial infections: vancomycin, quinupristin-dalfopristin, linezolid, and daptomycin. *Infect Dis Clin North Am*. **2004**;18:651-668.

Mathews C, Torriani F, Miller L, et al. Incidence of and risk factors for clinically significant MRSA infection in a cohort of HIV-infected adults: relation to severity of HIV disease. In: Program and abstracts of the 12th Conference on Retroviruses and Opportunistic Infections; February 22-25, **2005**; Boston, Abstract 142.

Rieg G, Daar E, Witt M, Guerrero M, Miller L. Community-acquired methicillin-resistant staphylococcus aureus colonization among HIV-infected men who have sex with men: a point prevalence survey. In: Program and abstracts of the 12th Conference on Retroviruses and Opportunistic Infections; February 22-25, **2005**; Boston, Abstract 877.

Rimland D, Brooks J. Antiretroviral Rounds: A patient with painful skin nodules. *AIDS Clinical Care*. **2004**;16:82.

Said-Salim B, Mathema B, Kreiswirth BN. Community-acquired methicillin-resistant Staphylococcus aureus: An emerging pathogen. *Infect Control Hosp Epidemiol*. **2003**;24:451-455.

Walker ES, Vasquez JE, Dula R, Bullock H, Sarubbi FA. Mupirocin-resistant, methicillin-resistant Staphylococcus aureus: Does mupirocin remain effective? *Infect Control Hosp Epidemiol*. **2003**;24:342-346.

(RLO-13)

III.42ABC. HEPATITIS

LEARNING OBJECTIVE: Discuss the following aspects of hepatitis in HIV-infected patients:

- **(a) clinical presentation, diagnosis and treatment of nonalcoholic steatohepatitis (NASH);**
- **(b) clinical presentation, diagnosis, treatment and treatment complications of hepatitis B;**
- **(c) clinical presentation, diagnosis, treatment and treatment complications of hepatitis C.**

An elevation of liver-associated enzymes is commonly seen among HIV-infected patients, usually as a hepatocellular pattern of enzyme elevation (increased alanine aminotransferase [ALT] and aspartate aminotransferase [AST]). The most common causes of hepatitis are viral pathogens and the effects of medication. Although the most prevalent causes of viral hepatitis include hepatitis B and hepatitis C, atypical viral pathogens may also cause hepatocellular necrosis in patients with AIDS, including hepatitis A virus (HAV), cytomegalovirus (CMV) and herpes simplex virus (HSV), among others.

NASH

NASH, or nonalcoholic steatohepatitis, is a type of fatty liver disease that develops in the absence of alcohol abuse (Medina et al. 2004; Neuschwander-Tetri and Caldwell 2003). It can lead to progressive fibrosis, cirrhosis and end-stage liver disease (Brunt 2004). In NASH, fatty infiltration of hepatic cells causes varying degrees of inflammation and fibrosis (Medina et al. 2004). The exact etiology is unclear, but in HIV disease, metabolic syndromes such as hyperlipidemia or insulin resistance or diabetes that are potentially HAART-related may be important factors (Pol et al. 2004). Although NASH can occur in patients without classic risk factors (Yu and Keefe 2002), in the general population, obesity, type 2 diabetes, hyperlipidemia (Neuschwander-Tetri and Caldwell 2003; Yu and Keeffe 2002) and insulin resistance leading to the accumulation of hepatocellular fat are common factors (Medina et al. 2004). This last link may be especially important in HIV patients who have acquired insulin resistance as a result of long-term exposure to certain antiretroviral agents, such as stavudine or protease inhibitors. Hyperlipidemia is also common in HIV-infected patients, especially in those on protease inhibitors. In addition, there are several factors known to be present in HIV disease, including oxidative stress, elevated levels of tumor necrosis factor-alpha, and, especially in patients on nucleoside analog drugs, mitochondrial dysfunction. These are thought to cause hepatocellular injury in the steatotic liver that may lead to disease progression and establishment of NASH (Medina et al. 2004; Neuschwander-Tetri and Caldwell 2003).

Clinical presentation of NASH may vary from completely asymptomatic to nonspecific symptoms such as fatigue, weakness, malaise and, less commonly, vague right upper quadrant pain and/or abdominal distention (Yu and Keeffe 2002). Severe pain is rare. The typical signs of acute liver failure such as jaundice are also missing unless cirrhosis has developed. Physical exam may show acanthosis nigricans (Neuschwander-Tetri and Caldwell 2003), a dark pigmentation under the armpits and neck typically seen in insulin

What's New

Either adefovir or the similar drug tenofovir can yield effective HBV suppression even with lamivudine-resistant virus. A third nucleoside analog, entecavir, is now approved for hepatitis B, and pegylated interferon alfa-2a has received an additional indication for HCV/HIV coinfection. Recent studies indicate that of the currently available drugs, pegylated interferon combined with ribavirin provides the highest level of effectiveness against hepatitis C. Temporary eye problems, including cataracts, decreased color vision and cotton wool spots, have been reported to occur in a significant percentage of those HIV/HCV-coinfected patients given pegylated interferon with ribavirin. A potential alternative to liver biopsy for patients either unwilling or unable to undergo this procedure has emerged in the form of blood tests that use several different hepatic inflammatory markers in order to approximate hepatic inflammation and fibrosis. NASH (nonalcoholic steatohepatitis) should be considered in the differential diagnosis of unexplained fatty liver in an HIV-infected patient.

Key Points

- Nonalcoholic steatohepatitis should be considered in the diagnosis of unexplained fatty liver because of the associated factors common to both HIV and NASH.
- Available antiviral agents with significant activity against HBV include the nucleoside/nucleotide analogs lamivudine, tenofovir and emtricitabine.
- Emergence of lamivudine-resistant HBV is very common in patients taking this drug.

Key Points (cont.)

- Interferon alfa is used to treat hepatitis C; with the availability of the new oral agents for hepatitis B, interferon is rarely used for this indication.
- Treatment responses to interferon alfa are lower in persons with HIV coinfection.
- HBV and HCV viral load monitoring has greatly improved evaluation of patients' response to treatment.
- The introduction of pegylated interferon has improved response to treatment in HIV/HCV-coinfected patients.
- New blood test markers of hepatic inflammation and/or fibrosis may be an option if liver biopsy is difficult or undesired.

resistance. After years of NASH, there is an increased risk of cirrhosis, with the typical associated signs of compensated or decompensated liver disease, and hepatocellular carcinoma (Yu and Keeffe 2002).

Laboratory abnormalities, including liver enzymes, are generally thought to be insensitive and incapable of confirming the diagnosis or staging the extent of fibrosis with NASH (Neuschwander-Tetri and Caldwell 2003). Serum aminotransferase levels may be normal in some patients with NASH (Yu and Keeffe 2002). Others may exhibit ALT increases (more so than AST in early stages), and elevated gamma-glutamyl transferase (GGT) (Neuschwander-Tetri and Caldwell 2003). In later stages, as NASH progresses to cirrhosis, AST levels may become higher than ALT levels (Neuschwander-Tetri and Caldwell 2003; Yu and Keeffe 2002). Diagnosis is ultimately accomplished through liver biopsy and exclusion of other causes of fatty liver such as alcohol, medications, and viral, autoimmune or genetic diseases (Yu and Keefe 2002). The morphologic changes on liver biopsy that establish a diagnosis of NASH are similar to those seen with alcoholic hepatitis. These include hepatocellular fat accumulation, evidence of cell injury and lobular inflammation, and, in some cases, progressive fibrosis (Brunt 2004; Yu and Keeffe 2002).

Treatment of NASH in the general population is controversial, and there are no trials showing effective treatments for HIV-infected patients with NASH. In general, it is thought that treatment should include weight loss via diet and exercise when obesity is present (Neuschwander-Tetri and Caldwell 2003; Yu and Keefe 2002). Various medications are under investigation in non-HIV populations, including insulin-sensitizing agents such as metformin (Glucophage) (Marchesini et al. 2001), pioglitazone (Actos) (Promrat et al. 2004) and rosiglitazone (Avandia) (Neuschwander-Tetri et al. 2003); anti-TNF-alpha agents such as pentoxifylline (Trental) (Satapathy et al. 2004); antioxidants (Harrison et al. 2003); and the weight-reduction medication orlistat (Xenical) (Harrison et al. 2003a). Although there is no clear link between HIV and NASH, hypertriglyceridemia, insulin resistance and diabetes are associated with both diseases, and therefore NASH should be considered in the differential diagnosis of unexplained fatty liver in an HIV-infected patient.

Hepatitis B

Hepatitis B virus (HBV) infection is a serious viral infection that is common worldwide. When it causes chronic hepatitis, it may lead to cirrhosis or hepatocellular carcinoma. Because both HBV and HIV share the epidemiologic risks of sexual contact (homosexual or heterosexual), injection-drug use and (in the past) use of blood products, up to 90% of HIV-infected patients have serologic markers of past HBV infection (Rodriguez-Mendez et al. 2000), and about 10% are chronic carriers (Ockenga et al. 1997).

Coinfection complications

Coinfection with HIV negatively affects hepatitis B infection. First, it decreases the chance for clearing hepatitis during acute infection. Second, it accelerates the progression of liver disease in those with chronic hepatitis B (Thio 2004).

The immune response plays a key role in viral clearance as well as the hepatic damage associated with HBV infection (Gilson et al. 1997). The risk for chronic HBV infection is increased in HIV-infected patients if infection with HIV preceded acquisition of HBV (Sinicco et al. 1997; Hadler et al. 1991), but is unchanged if HBV infection preceded HIV infection (Sinicco et al. 1997). HIV-induced immunosuppression also amplifies the risk of reactivation of quiescent HBV (Waite et al. 1988; Gilson et al. 1997), a rarity in the immunocompetent patient.

Decreased anti-HBV immune surveillance also results in heightened HBV replication (Ockenga et al. 1997) manifested by higher levels of HBV DNA (Colin et al. 1999; Goldin et al. 1990), increased HBV e antigen (HBeAg) titer (Goldin et al. 1990) and a lower rate of spontaneous HBeAg seroconversion (Gilson et al. 1997). Although immunocompromised HIV-infected patients exhibit lower transaminase levels and less histologic damage (Colin et al. 1999; Goldin et al. 1990), it is clear that the coinfected have an increased risk for cirrhosis and mortality (Thio 2004). In one large study, men with HIV/HBV coinfection had a mortality rate from liver disease of 14.2 per 1000 person-years, compared with a rate of 0.8 in those with HBV alone and 1.7 in those with HIV alone (Thio et al. 2002). In these men, there was a trend toward more severe liver disease in those with lower CD4 counts.

Immune reconstitution that accompanies initiation of combination antiretroviral therapy may result in a severe exacerbation of HBV hepatitis (Manegold et al. 2001) and can be responsible for death from liver failure (Martin-Carbonero et al. 2001). Stopping a lamivudine-containing combination antiretroviral therapy regimen can have a similar effect (Bellini et al. 2003). The Swiss HIV Cohort Study examined the records of patients with HIV-HBV coinfection who terminated lamivudine temporarily or permanently. Two out of 66 such terminations resulted in fulminant hepatitis, 6 in grade 4 liver function elevations and 2 in grade 2 elevations. There were no fatalities.

Symptoms and signs

HBV infection can be associated with a constellation of symptoms and signs that result from hepatic inflammation. Acute hepatitis is seen in approximately 25% of patients and can present as an acute illness characterized by the abrupt onset of malaise, fever, anorexia, nausea, headache and abdominal pain. Jaundice may be seen and may be accompanied by dark urine and acholic stools. Diagnosis of patients at this stage of disease necessitates serologies because viral hepatitis cannot be distinguished from hepatitis due to medications and toxins such as alcohol.

During the acute symptomatic phase of disease, which typically occurs 1 to 6 months after exposure, the patient's serum becomes positive for HBV surface antigen (HBsAg), HBV DNA and HBeAg. During this phase, there is a concomitant rise in transaminases (5-20x upper limit of normal [ULN]) and a moderate rise in alkaline phosphatase (2-10x ULN). If the patient clears the virus, the HBV DNA, HBsAg and HBeAg will become undetectable and HBV surface antibodies (HBsAb) and HBV e antibodies (HBeAb) will appear.

Fewer than 10% of immunocompetent adults will not produce antibody to HBsAg (Lee 1997) and fail to clear their HBV infection. Instead, they enter the chronic phase of disease. Those with chronic infection either will have progressive disease or will remain in a silent carrier state. Patients with ongoing disease stay positive for HBeAg and HBV DNA, and transaminase levels typically are elevated. These patients may complain of chronic fatigue or extrahepatic manifestations of hepatitis, such as glomerulonephritis or arthritis, but are usually asymptomatic until cirrhosis develops.

Precore and core mutations are relatively common and can be responsible for loss of HBeAg production. The most frequent of these, the precore stop codon mutation, halts HBeAg synthesis (Brunetto et al. 1991). It emerges during initiation of HBeAb production, when most patients begin to eliminate their HBV infection (Gandhe et al. 2003; Lee 1997). Although once believed to signify virulent disease (Brunetto et al. 1991), HBeAG-negative virus has recently been reported as common among asymptomatic carriers (Gandhe et al. 1993). The issue remains controversial.

Treatment

Before the era of combination retroviral therapy, the mortality of HIV was so high that treatment of HBV was not considered a priority. Given the impressive improvements in survival with combination antiretroviral therapy, the need for treatment of viral hepatitis has assumed far greater importance. Although treatment of HBV with interferon alfa has a reasonable success rate in immunocompetent patients, its value in HBV-infected patients with HIV is less clear. A large meta-analysis of studies showed that in immunocompetent patients, interferon alfa administered subcutaneously for 3 to 6 months, at dosages ranging from 7 to 30 million units weekly, has a response rate of 33% to 37% (loss of HBeAg), compared with 12% to 17% of untreated control patients, but the response is not as favorable among HIV patients (Wong et al. 1993). The current approved dose of interferon for chronic hepatitis B is 30 to 35 million international units per week (Intron-A 2004). Loss of HBsAg, HBeAg and detectable HBV DNA and normalization of ALT levels are more common in treated patients (Wong et al. 1993). As mentioned above, immunosuppressed HIV patients have higher levels of HBV DNA, lower pretreatment transaminase levels and less hepatic inflammation. These are all predictors of poor response to interferon alfa treatment against HBV (Brook et al. 1989). In one study, less than 10% of HIV-infected patients cleared HBeAg in response to interferon alfa (Zylberberg et al. 1996), a figure lower than that seen among HIV-seronegative patients.

The major side effect of interferon alfa therapy is a flu-like illness. Characteristic symptoms include fever, myalgias, arthralgias, chills, headache and fatigue. These usually begin within hours of each injection and last for a variable period of time. These symptoms may decrease over time, but they can severely decrease quality of life, necessitating treatment discontinuation. Discontinuation may also be necessary for severe granulocytopenia or thrombocytopenia, or depression that may accompany treatment. The advent of pegylated interferon as treatment for hepatitis C has led investigators to revisit interferon's usefulness in treating chronic hepatitis B. In one randomized trial, 307 singly infected (HIV-negative) hepatitis B patients were given either pegylated interferon alfa-2b alone (Peg-Intron in doses of 100 mcg weekly) or in combination with a daily dose of lamivudine (100 mg) for 52 weeks (Janssen et al. 2005). At the end of follow-up in week 78, 35% of the combination therapy group and 36% of the monotherapy group had a sustained response as measured by serum HBeAg loss. Another large multicenter, randomized trial of 537 singly infected hepatitis B patients compared results in those given 48 weeks of treatment with 1 of 3 regimens: 180 mcg of pegylated interferon alfa-2a (Pegasys) weekly plus placebo; 180 mcg of Pegasys once weekly plus 100 mg of lamivudine daily; and 100 mg of lamivudine daily (Marcellin et al. 2004). After 24 weeks of post-treatment follow-up (week 72), 59% of those on Pegasys monotherapy and 60% on Pegasys plus lamivudine experienced normalization of alanine aminotransferase levels, significantly more than the 44% of those on lamivudine alone. Loss of HBsAg occurred in 12 patients in the pegylated interferon groups compared with none in the group given only lamivudine. The lack of large, controlled trials in HIV/HBV-coinfected patients precludes definitive guidelines for use of pegylated interferon in this population.

Because HBV has a reverse transcription step in its life cycle, similar to HIV, nucleoside and nucleotide analogs have been used to treat HBV-infected patients. Lamivudine is a potent nucleoside analog inhibitor of both HIV and HBV. Lamivudine treatment of HIV-seronegative patients, at a dose of 100 mg daily for 1 year, suppresses HBV replication, reverses necroinflammatory activity, normalizes ALT levels in 72% of patients and improves liver histology, preventing further progression to cirrhosis (Lai et al. 1998). Success in treating HIV-infected patients for HBV with lamivudine compares favorably with the experience in HIV-uninfected patients (Hoff et al. 2001). Higher doses of lamivudine (150 mg twice daily) are typically used to treat HBV in HIV-infected patients (Pillay et al. 2000) compared with HIV-negative patients because of the risk that HIV will rapidly develop lamivudine resistance with lower doses.

Lamivudine is much better tolerated than is interferon alfa therapy, but development of YMDD mutations in the HBV viral polymerase gene leads to antiviral resistance in 14% to 47% of patients, with subsequent viral relapse within 1 year (Lau et al. 2000; Pillay et al. 2000). Additional data indicate that the frequency of resistance to lamivudine is even higher with further dosing beyond 1 year (Liaw 2001). Still, despite resistance and relapse of HBV DNA, improved liver function and histology as well as increased likelihood of HBeAg seroconversion may remain, perhaps due to decreased fitness of resistant virus (Pillay et al. 2000). Also, the immune response improves when HBV viral load declines after initiating lamivudine treatment. This leads to more HBeAb production, for example (Boni et al. 1998). The appearance of YMDD mutants in HBV may not mark the limit of benefit from this medication. However, one small study suggested that lamivudine-resistant HBV may be more difficult to treat with subsequent conventional interferon therapy (Danalioglu et al. 2004).

Adefovir (10 mg/day) is a nucleotide analog approved for HBV treatment (Gilson et al. 1999). In a recent study, 59 lamivudine-resistant monoinfected HBV patients were randomized to continue lamivudine alone, use adefovir alone or use adefovir along with continuing use of lamivudine (Peters et al. 2004). Median change from baseline in serum HBV DNA level at week 48 was 0.0 $\log_{10}$ copies/mL with lamivudine alone, -4.04 $\log_{10}$ copies/mL with adefovir alone, and -3.59 $\log_{10}$ copies/mL with the combination of adefovir and lamivudine. ALT level normalized in 10 of 19 (53%) and 9 of 19 (47%) recipients of adefovir/lamivudine and adefovir alone, respectively, compared with 1 of 19 (5%) recipients of lamivudine alone. These results show that adefovir, either alone or in combination with ongoing lamivudine therapy, achieves effective HBV suppression in many lamivudine-resistant, singly infected HBV-infected patients. An adefovir study in persons coinfected with HIV and lamivudine-resistant HBV observed a progressively decreasing HBV viral load in the course of nearly 3 years (Benhamou et al. 2003). Patients received adefovir on top of a lamivudine-containing antiretroviral regimen and experienced a mean -5.45 $\log_{10}$ decline in median HBV levels at the end of 144 weeks.

The main advantage of adefovir may be the low rate of resistance, reported in a recent review article to be less than 2% after 96 weeks' follow-up, compared with lamivudine resistance of 40% at 2 years and 67% at 4 years (Lim and Suh 2004). Because adefovir is no longer used in antiretroviral combinations to treat HIV, it may increase the total number of drugs taken. At least, its toxicity is greatly reduced at the 10-mg dose used for HBV (Lim and Suh 2004), compared with the higher doses (30-120 mg) formerly used against HIV.

Tenofovir (TDF), a drug similar to adefovir, is approved for HIV treatment and therefore is more likely to be used in combination with lamivudine for coinfected patients. Although not yet FDA-approved for this indication, it also may be an effective therapy for coinfected patients who have lamivudine-resistant HBV (Nelson et al. 2003; Ristig et al. 2002). One study looked at 88 coinfected individuals with detectable HBV (Piketty et al. 2004). Although 83 of these individuals were receiving lamivudine, adding tenofovir to their regimen yielded a 32% rate of undetectable HBV DNA after taking tenofovir for 1 to 24 months (median: 9). There was a mean reduction in HBV viral load of -3.8 $\log_{10}$ copies/mL. More recently, clinicians reported the experience of 30 coinfected patients who received anti-HIV regimens that included just lamivudine, tenofovir and lamivudine, or just lamivudine for at least a year with tenofovir added afterwards (Jain et al. 2004). Of the patients in each group, 30%, 25% and 100%, respectively, had received previous HIV treatment, possibly including lamivudine. After 1 to 2 years, HBV viral load was below detectable limits in 60% of the lamivudine-only recipients, 75% of the tenofovir-lamivudine recipients and 50% of those who received lamivudine plus deferred tenofovir. Treatment-naive patients had a significantly higher response rate than did treatment-experienced ones (83% versus 41%, respectively).

Few randomized studies have directly compared tenofovir and adefovir. One such trial is A5127, in which 52 participants HIV/HBV coinfected participants on stable HAART received either tenofovir or adefovir in blinded fashion (Peters et al. 2005). After a median of 75 weeks follow-up, the mean time-weighted average decline in HBV viral load was -4.44 $\log_{10}$ copies/mL in the tenofovir arm and -3.21 $\log_{10}$ copies/mL in the adefovir arm. Due to the study's small size, this difference was not statistically significant, but the results nonetheless suggest that tenofovir is at least as effective as adefovir.

Entecavir (Baraclude) is a newly approved HBV nucleoside analog (Baraclude 2005) that does not have activity against HIV. Although entecavir has shown activity against lamivudine-resistant virus, it has also triggered infrequent HBV resistance mutations leading to reduced susceptibility and treatment failure beyond 1 to 2 years of therapy (Tenney et al. 2004). In a 48-week phase III trial for nucleoside-naive, HBe-positive patients, HBV viral load was undetectable (below 400 copies/mL) in 69% of those on entecavir monotherapy compared with 38% of those on lamivudine (Chang et al. 2004). The response was poorer with either agent in the phase III trial for patients with lamivudine-refractory HBV: HBV was below 400 copies/mL in 21% and 1% of entecavir and lamivudine recipients, respectively (Sherman et al. 2004). Preliminary results from ETV-038, a phase II trial in 68 HIV/HBV-coinfected patients, also found that adding entecavir was superior to continuing on lamivudine alone (Pessoa et al. 2005). All trial partcipants were already receiving lamivudine, which they continued during the trial. The baseline prevalence of lamivudine resistance was 88%, and mean initial HBV viral load was 9.13 $\log_{10}$ copies/mL. At 24 weeks, HBV viral loads had declined by a mean -3.65 $\log_{10}$ copies/mL in the entecavir arm while they increased a mean 0.11 $\log_{10}$ copies/mL in the lamivudine-plus-placebo group. Only 6% of entecavir recipients reduced their viral loads to undetectable levels, compared with 0% of placebo recipients (Baraclude 2005).

Due to high rates of lamivudine-resistant HBV, combination therapy may be desirable. At the 2004 International AIDS Conference in Bangkok, the authors of the 903 trial reported data on its HBV-coinfected subset (Dore et al. 2004). In this 144-week, double-blind, active-controlled trial, antiretroviral-naive HIV-infected patients were randomized to receive lamivudine and efavirenz with either tenofovir or stavudine, of which only tenofovir and lamivudine have anti-HBV activity. Of 11 HIV/HBV-coinfected patients who completed the trial, 5 received tenofovir plus lamivudine, and 6 received lamivudine. All 11 patients had baseline serum HBV viral loads of at least 6 $\log_{10}$ copies/mL, and all completed 48 weeks. The mean decline from baseline HBV viral load was -4.5 $\log_{10}$ copies/mL in those receiving both tenofovir and lamivudine. Those who received only lamivudine experienced only a -2.2 $\log_{10}$ copies/mL decline. Two of 3 patients on both drugs maintained an HBV viral load below 1000 copies/mL at 144 weeks, but none did so in the lamivudine-alone arm. All patients receiving only lamivudine developed lamivudine-resistant HBV by week 96. This study, although small, suggests that combination therapy appears to have greater sustained anti-HBV activity than does lamivudine alone in treatment-naive patients. However, the data provide no information as to whether tenofovir alone is as active as tenofovir and lamivudine in combination. Also, there was a very high rate of discontinuation in this coinfected population, including discontinuation due to grade 3 ALT/AST elevations.

A number of additional nucleoside analogs are currently under development for HBV infection. One of these is emtricitabine (FTC, Emtriva), an approved HIV drug similar to lamivudine (Snow et al. 2004). In 14 of 17 coinfected patients receiving emtricitabine as part of anti-HIV clinical trials, HBV viral load had declined by greater than -5 $\log_{10}$ copies/mL or was undetectable after 48 weeks. Genotypic analysis in the 7 patients with detectable HBV found that 2 had developed the M204M/I resistance mutation in the YMDD region. In a 248-person randomized study of persons infected with HBV only, 56% had undetectable viral loads after

48 weeks compared with 7% on placebo (Shiffman et al. 2004). Drug resistance mutations were detectable in about one-eighth of trial participants.

Another experimental drug in advanced trials is telbivudine (LdT). In a year-long phase IIb trial for persons not infected with HIV, those receiving Ldt experienced a 1.5 log_{10} greater mean drop in HBV viral load than did those who received lamivudine (Lai et al. 2003). In the future, it may be possible to combine HBV agents for greater efficacy and durability, as occurs with HIV. This was not the case in the LdT trial, however. In that trial, LdT alone was as efficacious as LdT plus lamivudine (Lai et al. 2003).

Hepatitis C

Demographics

As HIV-related morbidity and mortality have declined in the era of combination antiretroviral therapy, the clinical impact of hepatitis C virus (HCV) coinfection among HIV-infected patients has increased. Several recent reports have underlined the significance of HIV/HCV coinfection. A study of HIV-infected patients enrolled in AIDS Clinical Trials Group studies found that 16.1% of subjects were coinfected with HCV, compared with an estimated overall prevalence of 1.8% in the United States (Sherman et al. 2002).

The prevalence of HIV/HCV coinfection varies considerably among different demographic groups. HIV-infected patients infected through the receipt of clotting factors or through injection-drug use are at highest risk for HCV. The prevalence of HCV among other HIV-infected patients (3.5%) is comparable to that of the general population (Sherman et al. 2002).

Testing

To screen HIV-infected patients for HCV, enzyme immunoassay (EIA) tests licensed to detect HCV antibody in blood should be used (USPHS/IDSA 2002), although many coinfected patients fail to produce detectable HCV antibodies. In one study, the standard second-generation EIA test did not find antibodies in 20 of 51 HIV patients who had HCV RNA detectable by an experimental whole blood HCV viral load assay (George et al. 2002). A sensitive HCV RNA assay should therefore be used to provide confirmatory evidence in patients with negative HCV EIA tests when there are strong grounds for suspicion of HCV infection, such as elevated ALT levels.

The decision to begin treatment is based on individual patient characteristics: the severity of disease, the risk of side effects, comorbid conditions and the likelihood of success (Strader et al. 2004). HCV-infected patients should have an HCV genotype performed before beginning therapy, because response to therapy is much better in patients infected with HCV genotypes 2 and 3 compared with genotype 1 (which unfortunately is the most common kind) (Strader et al. 2004; Zein 2000). In HCV-monoinfected patients with HCV genotype 2 or 3, 6 months of therapy will usually suffice, but a full year of therapy is required for genotype 1 (Strader 2004) There has been considerable debate on whether patients coinfected with HIV and HCV genotypes 2 or 3 should halt therapy at month 6. Most experts now recommend 48 weeks of treatment for coinfected patients who have genotype 2 or 3 (Strader et al. 2004).

Liver biopsies are useful for determining the need for treatment, especially in those with genotype 1 HCV and relatively low likelihood of achieving viral suppression (Strader et al. 2004). Liver function tests (showing plasma aminotransferase levels) do not necessarily indicate the severity of HCV disease or the degree of liver damage that has occurred. Prior to initiating therapy, HCV viral load assays help assess the likelihood of treatment response — high viral load indicates poor outcome — but this assay is a poor indicator of the condition of the liver. During therapy, HCV viral load reflects the degree of response (Strader 2004).

A potential alternative to liver biopsy for patients either unwilling or unable to undergo this procedure has emerged in the form of blood tests that use several different hepatic inflammatory markers in order to approximate hepatic inflammation and fibrosis on a graded scale. One study involved 130 HIV/HCV-coinfected patients and compared liver biopsies with a nonbiopsy evaluation system, an index incorporating age, sex, alpha(2)-macroglobulin, apolipoprotein A1, haptoglobin, bilirubin, and gamma-glutamyl-transpeptidase (GGT) (Myers et al. 2003). The serologic data appeared to correctly identify patients at extremes of the fibrosis scale (i.e., low grade or high grade), but had more difficulty with the moderate stages of liver damage. Although promising, the accuracy of these tests in HIV patients need to be further scrutinized, as many of the inflammatory markers used are abnormal at baseline in HIV patients due to certain HIV medications or HIV itself.

Coinfection complications

Although earlier studies indicated that HIV/HCV-coinfected patients progress more rapidly to liver cirrhosis and hepatic failure than do patients infected with HCV alone (Benhamou et al. 1999; Telfer et al. 1994), a more recent highly active antiretroviral therapy (HAART)-era study that prospectively followed HIV/HCV-coinfected and HCV-monoinfected patients for a mean of 4.2 years found similar rates of death or cirrhosis (Monto et al. 2004). Compared with singly infected HIV-positive patients, coinfected patients experience more AIDS-defining infections and death after initiating treatment for HIV (Greub et al. 2000). This is probably because their CD4 count rebound is lower even when combination antiretroviral therapy successfully suppresses their HIV (Greub et al. 2000).

HIV/HCV coinfection complicates the use of antiretroviral agents because rates of hepatotoxicity are higher in coinfected patients (Sulkowski et al. 2000). In addition, the use of didanosine (ddI) is not recommended in these patients due to an increased risk of hepatic decompensation (Mauss et al. 2004) and an interaction with ribavirin that increases ddI toxicity (Videx EC 2004). The initiation of combination antiretroviral therapy has also been associated with HCV "flares," in which HCV RNA levels and transaminase levels increase, and the clinician must therefore be aware that elevated liver function tests in this setting do not necessarily represent drug toxicity (Rutschmann et al. 1998).

Treatment

The previous standard of care for immunocompetent patients with HCV infection was interferon alfa plus the nucleoside analogue ribavirin (800-1200 mg/day). For those with HIV/HCV coinfection, this combination was less successful (Brau 2003). In general, coinfected patients' overall rates of sustained response (undetectable HCV viral load 6 months after treatment is over) to this combination have been only about 30%, compared with the 60% experienced by HIV-negative patients (Perez-Olmeda et al. 2003), with the sustained response rate still lower in HCV genotypes 1 and 4.

Recently, the combination of the newer pegylated interferon and ribavirin has become generally accepted as the treatment of choice in patients infected with HCV monoinfection due to the greater likelihood of a sustained virologic response (SVR) (Strader 2004). Pegylated interferon alfa-2a (Pegasys), alone or plus ribavirin, is now also officially indicated for use in HCV patients with stable HIV disease (Pegasys 2005).

In 3 controlled trials for HIV/HCV-coinfected patients, either pegylated interferon alfa-2a (180 mg once weekly) or pegylated interferon alfa-2b (1.5 mcg/kg Peg-Intron once weekly) plus ribavirin yielded higher SVR rates than standard interferon plus ribavirin given 3 times weekly (Chung et al. 2004; Perronne et al. 2004, Torriani et al. 2004). The overall sustained response rates ranged from 26% to 40%; for genotype 1, the sustained response rates ranged from 14% to 29%. The virologic response at week 12 of treatment was highly predictive of the sustained response and could be used to decide whether to keep patients on therapy (Perronne et al. 2004). A 412-patient coinfection study using Peg-Intron, the RIBAVIC trial, recently reported an overall SVR of 27% at 72 weeks, down from the 35% end-of-treatment response at 48 weeks (Carrat et al. 2004). The 134-patient coinfection trial using Pegasys, the AIDS Pegasys Ribavirin International Coinfection Trial (APRICOT), reported 72 week data showing a SVR rate of 40% for those given a combination of Pegasys with ribavirin compared with 20% for those given Pegasys monotherapy and 12% for those given conventional interferon with ribavirin (Torriani et al. 2004). In this trial, SVR was defined as undetectable HCV viral load (below 50 IU/mL) at the end of follow-up. The APRICOT study involved a higher initial dose of ribavirin (800 mg/day) than in the similar ACTG A5071 trial which used dose-escalating ribavirin starting at 600 mg/day for 4 weeks, then increasing to 800 mg/day for 4 weeks, and then going to 1000 mg/day for the remainder of the trial (Chung et al. 2004). Although both studies used 180 mcg/week of Pegasys as the pegylated interferon drug, it is difficult to say whether the higher initial ribavirin dose in the APRICOT study accounted for the difference in SVR (40% in APRICOT versus 27% in A5071). It is possible that the cumulative dose of ribavirin received by A5071 patients was insufficient to prevent relapse (Chung et al. 2004), and the researchers recommend studying dose optimization of ribavirin as one approach to improving response rates.

Two HIV/HCV coinfection studies reported in early 2005 that ribavirin plasma levels do indeed have a strong association with treatment response, at least when the drug is us ed in combination with Pegasys. In one study, a ribavirin plasma level of over 2.7 microgram/mL correlated with more frequent early virologic response as well as higher incidence of anemia (Rendón et al. 2005). In the second study, the observed ribavirin threshold for markedly improved sustained virologic response was 1 microgram/mL (Breilh et al. 2005).

Another area of research is determination of the optimal dose of pegylated interferon. In a recent study of 63 HIV/HCV-coinfected patients, low-dose pegylated interferon (1.0 mcg/kg/week) was comparable in efficacy to high-dose pegylated interferon (1.5 mcg/kg/week) (Hammoud et al. 2004).

Many patients receiving standard or pegylated interferon have improved liver histology without reaching undetectable HCV viral load (Chung et al. 2004). In the APRICOT study, a representative sample of biopsies showed histologic improvement in a substantial number of patients who did not achieve an SVR, leading the researchers to suggest that improvement in biopsies might be an alternative goal of therapy (Lissen et al. 2004). The histologic improvement in that study was greatest in those treated with the Pegasys/ribavirin combination. In a different study, HIV-coinfected patients taking protease inhibitors have decreased liver fibrosis and cirrhosis rates independent of CD4 count and HIV RNA changes (Benhamou et al. 2001). Protease inhibitors, along with improved CD4 counts and reduced alcohol consumption, could help prevent fibrosis. Combination antiretroviral therapy makes improvements in fibrosis rates even though it does not improve the virologic response to HCV treatment (Cooper et al. 2003).

The initial side effects of interferon treatment include "flu-like" symptoms. Cytopenias, irritability and depression may occur with sustained interferon treatment (Gervais et al. 2001). Retinal vein thrombosis has been reported with high-dose interferon use in patients with underlying risk factors for thrombosis (Nadir et al. 2000). In a recent study of 23 HIV/HCV-coinfected patients given pegylated interferon and ribavirin, 35% developed temporary eye problems, including cataracts, decreased color vision and cotton wool spots (Farel et al. 2004). In the 2 patients who developed cataracts, with continued therapy the cataracts did not worsen but did not resolve. In the 2 patients with color vision changes, 1 saw color vision return to normal during continued therapy, but the other discontinued therapy because of the severity of the change, with color vision returning to baseline 10 weeks after therapy cessation. In all 7 patients who developed cotton wool spots, the spots eventually disappeared despite continued therapy. It is thought desirable that a baseline ophthalmologic exam be obtained — particularly in HIV patients who have had retinal pathology with opportunistic infections such as CMV or toxoplasmosis — prior to the onset of therapy, if possible.

The major toxicity of ribavirin is dose-dependent hemolytic anemia (Gervais et al. 2001). Epoetin-alfa can improve ribavirin-induced anemia and help patients stay on therapy (Dietrich et al. 2004). In vitro studies have demonstrated that ribavirin reduces the activity and toxicity of zidovudine but boosts those of didanosine (Baba et al. 1987). Combining ribavirin with zidovudine is inadvisable, and coadministration of ribavirin and didanosine is not recommended (DHHS 2004). Didanosine's FDA-approved package inserts (Videx EC 2004) now carry a warning that coadministration with ribavirin is not recommended because of reports of fatal hepatic failure as well as peripheral neuropathy, pancreatitis and symptomatic hyperlactatemia/lactic acidosis.

Early response (after 12 weeks of treatment) can predict who will have a successful response at the end of treatment (Soriano et al. 2003). Those who do not have immediate HCV viral load reductions (over 2 $\log_{10}$ copies/mL) might justifiably terminate treatment early (Soriano et al. 2003). At the same time, extending therapy to 12 months for genotypes 2 and 3 and to 18 months for genotypes 1 and 4 has the potential to improve the poor sustained response rate experienced by coinfected patients after completing the standard course of therapy (Soriano et al. 2003).

Studies of induction dosing with current drugs and new drugs or drug combinations have shown preliminary results that may be promising in the general HCV-infected population (not specifically limited to the HIV-coinfected). Trials using either induction dosing (Diago et al. 2004), consensus interferon (CIFN) (Kaiser et al. 2004) or a combination of consensus interferon with gamma interferon (Leevy et al. 2004) have shown an SVR in a significant percentage of previous nonresponders. However, much additional research, especially in the coinfected, will be required to confirm the value of such approaches before any recommendation could be made for general use.

When to treat

Factors associated with poorer responses to anti-HCV therapy in coinfected patients include low CD4 counts, presence of HCV genotype 1, presence of multiple HCV quasispecies, higher HCV viral load, presence of cirrhosis and ongoing alcohol use (Sherman 2003). Poorer response rates have been seen in patients with CD4 counts below 200 to 350 cells/mm^3 (Sherman 2003). However, a newer pegylated interferon-ribavirin study in coinfected patients found that CD4 count, receipt of combination antiretroviral therapy or HIV viral load did not predict the response to 24 weeks of treatment, nor did HCV viral load (Hernández-Quero et al. 2003). Antiretroviral-naive patients should, in any case, begin combination antiretroviral therapy without delay when their CD4 counts decline to low levels. If they start interferon/ribavirin therapy, they risk reducing their CD4 count still further (Chung et al. 2004; Perronne et al. 2004).

There is still considerable debate as to when to start HCV therapy in relation to starting HIV antiretrovirals (ARVs). One common issue is the hepatotoxicity arising from ARV therapy. Arguments for treating HIV first include improving CD4 count to over 200 cells/mm^3 in order to minimize risk of subsequent opportunistic infections while on interferon since it can decrease the CD4 count by approximately 100-150 cells/mm^3 (Chung et al. 2004; Torriani et al. 2004). Initiating hepatitis C therapy first may be preferable for other reasons. One study reported a statistically significant decrease in the relative risk of ARV-associated hepatotoxicity among patients who initiated hepatitis C therapy first (Uberti-Foppa et al. 2003). In a prospective study, researchers assessed the incidence of severe hepatotoxicity (grade 3 or 4 change in alanine or aspartate transaminase levels) among 568 patients receiving nonnucleoside reverse transcriptase inhibitor (NNRTI)-containing antiretroviral therapy, with 312 prescribed efavirenz and 256 prescribed nevirapine (Sulkowski et al. 2002). Severe hepatotoxicity developed in 15.6% of those given nevirapine and 8.0% of those given efavirenz. Only 32% of nevirapine-associated hepatotoxicity cases and 50% of those associated with efavirenz developed in the first 12 weeks of therapy. The hepatotoxicity risk was 2-fold higher in the HBV- or HCV-coinfected and in those also using protease inhibitors. This study clearly showed that severe hepatotoxicity can occur at any point in the course of NNRTI therapy and is more common among those coinfected with HCV or HBV, those given nevirapine and those coadministered protease inhibitors.

The emergence of potentially "resistant" quasispecies of hepatitis C in longtime infected HIV patients has led to some concern that this might be a reason why heavily ARV-experienced patients responded poorly to interferon in initial studies. However a more recent study of 52 patients found that HCV pretherapeutic quasispecies complexity did not predict SVR in patients coinfected with HIV (Neau et al. 2003). No clear answer seems forthcoming, and therapy initiation should involve weighing the risks of an expected CD4 decline while on interferon, with the benefits of improving tolerance to HIV medications if hepatitis C is treated first.

References

Baba M, Pauwels R, Balzarini J, et al. Ribavirin antagonizes the inhibitory effects of pyrimidine 2',3'-dideoxynucleosides but enhances inhibitory effects of purine 2',3'-dideoxynucleosides on replication of human immunodeficiency virus in vitro. *Antimicrob Agents Chemother.* **1987**;31:1613-1617.

Baraclude (entecavir) [prescribing information]. Princeton, NJ: Bristol-Myers Squibb; March **2005**.

Bellini C, Keiser O, Chave JP, et al. Frequent liver dysfunction after lamivudine withdrawal in HIV- hepatitis B co-infection. *Antivir Ther.* **2003**;8(suppl 1):S464 [abstract 992].

Benhamou Y, Bochet M, Di Martino V, et al. Liver fibrosis progression in human immunodeficiency virus and hepatitis C virus coinfected patients. The Multivirc Group. *Hepatology.* **1999**;30:1054-1058.

Benhamou Y, Di Martino V, Bochet M, et al. Factors affecting liver fibrosis in human immunodeficiency virus-and hepatitis C virus-coinfected patients: impact of protease inhibitor therapy. *Hepatology.* **2001**;34:283-287.

Benhamou Y, Thibault V, Vig P, et al. Long term treatment with adefovir dipivoxil (ADV) for three years in patients with lamivudine-resistant (lam-r) HBV and HIV co-infection results in significant and sustained clinical improvement. In: Program and abstracts of the 54th Annual Meeting of the American Association for the Study of Liver Diseases (AASLD); October 24-28, **2003**; Boston, Massachusetts. Abstract 1158.

Boni C, Bertoletti A, Penna A, et al. Lamivudine treatment can restore T cell responsiveness in chronic hepatitis B. *J Clin Invest.* **1998**;102:968-975.

Brau N. Update on chronic hepatitis C in HIV/HCV-coinfected patients: viral interactions and therapy. *AIDS.* **2003**;17:2279-2290.

Brook MG, Karayiannis P, Thomas HC. Which patients with chronic hepatitis B virus infection will respond to alpha-interferon therapy? A statistical analysis of predictive factors. *Hepatology.* **1989**;10:761-763.

Breilh D, Neau D, Djabarouti S, et al. Plasma target concentration of ribavirin in HIV/HCV co-infected patients. In: Program and abstracts of the 12th Conference on Retroviruses and Opportunistic Infections; February 22-25, **2005**; Boston, Massachusetts. Abstract 928.

Brunetto MR, Giarin MM, Oliveri F, et al. Wild-type and e antigen-minus hepatitis B viruses and course of chronic hepatitis. *Proc Natl Acad Sci U S A.* **1991**;88:4186-4190.

Brunt EM. Nonalcoholic steatohepatitis. *Semin Liver Dis.* **2004**;24:3-20.

Carrat F, Bani-Sadr F, Pol S, et al. Pegylated interferon alfa-2b vs standard interferon alfa-2b, plus ribavirin, for chronic hepatitis C in HIV-infected patients. *JAMA.* **2004**;292:2839-2848.

Chang TT, Gish R, de Man R, et al. Entecavir is superior to lamivudine for the treatment of HBeAG(+) chronic hepatitis B: results of phase III study ETV-022 in nucleoside naive patients. In: Program and abstracts of the 55th Annual Meeting of the American Association for the Study of Liver Diseases (AASLD); October 29-November 2, **2004**; Boston, Massachusetts. Abstract 70.

Chung R, Andersen J, Volberding P, et al. A randomized, controlled trial of peg-interferon-alfa-2a plus ribavirin vs interferon-alfa-2a plus ribavirin for chronic hepatitis c virus infection in HIV-co-infected persons: follow-up results of ACTG A5071. In: Program and abstracts of the 11th Conference on Retroviruses and Opportunistic Infections; February 8-11, **2004**; San Francisco, California. Abstract 110.

Chung RT, Andersen J, Volberding P, et al. Peginterferon alfa-2a plus ribavirin versus interferon alfa-2a plus ribavirin for chronic hepatitis C in HIV-coinfected persons. *N Engl J Med*. **2004**;351:451-9.

Colin J-F, Cazals-Hatem D, Loriot MA, et al. Influence of human immunodeficiency virus infection on chronic hepatitis B in homosexual men. *Hepatology*. **1999**;29:1306-1310.

Cooper CL, LaRoche A, Kane M. Evaluation of the benefits of HAART in HIV-HCV co-infected subjects. In: Program and abstracts of the 43rd Interscience Conference on Antimicrobial Agents and Chemotherapy (ICAAC); September 14-17, **2003**; Chicago, Illinois. Abstract H-826.

Danalioglu A, Kaymakoglu S, Cakaloglu Y, et al. Efficacy of alpha interferon therapy for lamivudine resistance in chronic hepatitis B. *Int J Clin Pract*. **2004**;58:659-661.

Department of Health and Human Services (DHHS). Guidelines for the use of antiretroviral agents in HIV-1-infected adults and adolescents. October 29, **2004**. Available at: http://aidsinfo.nih.gov/guidelines/adult/AA_102904.pdf [accessed February 19, 2005].

Diago M, Romero-Gomez M, Crespo J, et al. Peginterferon alfa-2A (40KD) (Pegasys ®) and ribavirin (Copegus®) in patients infected with HCV genotype 1 who failed to respond to interferon and ribavirin: final results of the Spanish high-dose induction pilot trial. In: Program and abstracts of the 55th Annual Meeting of the American Association for the Study of Liver Diseases (AASLD); October 29-November 2, **2004**; Boston, Massachusetts. Abstract 522.

Dieterich D, Sulkowski M, Bini E, et al. Epoetin-alfa administered once weekly improves anemia in HIV/HCV co-infected patients treated with interferon/ribavirin therapy: a prospective, randomized study. In: Program and abstracts of the 11th Conference on Retroviruses and Opportunistic Infections; February 8-11, **2004**; San Francisco, California. Abstract 824.

Dore G, Cooper D, Pozniak AL, et al. Anti-hepatitis B Virus (HBV) activity in HBV/HIV co-infected patients treated with tenofovir DF (TDF) and lamivudine (LAM) versus LAM alone: 144-week follow-up. In: Program and abstracts of the XV International Conference on AIDS; July 11-14, **2004**; Bangkok, Thailand. Abstract MoPeB3308.

Farel C, Suzman DL, McLaughlin M, et al. Serious ophthalmic pathology compromising vision in HIV/HCV co-infected patients treated with peginterferon alpha-2b and ribavirin. *AIDS*. **2004**;18:1805-1809.

Gandhe SS, Chadha MS, Walimbe AM, Arankalle VA. Hepatitis B virus: prevalence of precore/core promoter mutants in different clinical categories of Indian patients. *J Viral Hepat*. **2003**;10:367-382.

George SL, Gebhardt J, Klinzman D, et al. Hepatitis C virus viremia in HIV-infected individuals with negative HCV antibody tests. *J Acquir Immune Defic Syndr.* **2002**;31:154-162.

Gervais A, Boyer N, Marcellin P. Tolerability of treatments for viral hepatitis. *Drug Safety.* **2001**;24:375-384.

Gilson RJ, Hawkins AE, Beecham MR, et al. Interactions between HIV and hepatitis B virus in homosexual men: effects on the natural history of infection. *AIDS*. **1997**;11:597-606.

Gilson RJC, Chopra KB, Newell AM, et al. A placebo-controlled phase I/II study of adefovir dipivoxil in patients with chronic hepatitis B virus infection. *J Viral Hepat*. **1999**;6:387-395.

Goldin RD, Fish DE, Hay A, et al. Histological and immunohistochemical study of hepatitis B virus in human immunodeficiency virus infection. *J Clin Pathol*. **1990**;43:203-205.

Greub G, Ledergerber B, Battegay M, et al. Clinical progression, survival, and immune recovery during antiretroviral therapy in patients with HIV-1 and hepatitis C virus coinfection: the Swiss HIV Cohort Study. *Lancet*. **2000**;356:1800-1805.

Hadler SC, Judson FN, O'Malley PM, et al. Outcome of hepatitis B virus infection in homosexual men and its relation to prior human immunodeficiency virus infection. *J Infect Dis*. **1991**;163:454-459.

Hammoud G, Li J, Vega K, et al. Low dose pegylated interferon alpha-2B is as effective as the high dose in HIV/HCV coinfected patients. In: Program and abstracts of the 55th Annual Meeting of the American Association for the Study of Liver Diseases (AASLD); October 29-November 2, **2004**; Boston, Massachusetts. Abstract 520.

Harrison SA, Ramrakhiani S, Brunt EM, Anbari MA, Cortese C, Bacon BR. Orlistat in the treatment of NASH: a case series. *Am J Gastroenterol*. **2003a**;98:926-930.

Harrison SA, Torgerson S, Hayashi P, Ward J, Schenker S. Vitamin E and vitamin C treatment improves fibrosis in patients with nonalcoholic steatohepatitis. *Am J Gastroenterol.* **2003b**;98:2485-2490.

Hernández-Quero J, Granados R, Pérez-Guzmán E, et al. Peginterferon alfa-2a (40kd) (Pegasys®) and ribavirin (Copegus®) in patients with HIV/HCV coinfection: interim results of a randomized, multicenter study from Spain. In: Program and abstracts of the 54th Annual Meeting of the American Association for the Study of Liver Diseases (AASLD). October 24-28, **2003**, Boston, Massachusetts. Abstract 987.

Hoff J, Bani-Sadr F, Gassin M, Raffi F. Evaluation of chronic hepatitis B virus (HBV) infection in co-infected patients receiving lamivudine as a component of anti-human immunodeficiency virus regimens. *Clin Infect Dis.* **2001**;32:963-969.

Intron-A [prescribing information]. Kenilworth, NJ: Schering Corporation; March **2004**.

Jain MK, Comanor L, White C et al. Hepatitis B virus (HBV) response to therapy with lamivudine (LAM) and tenofovir (TFV) in HBV/HIV co-infected patients: impact of genotype and treatment regimen. In: Program and abstracts of the 56th Annual Meeting of the American Association for the Study of Liver Diseases (AASLD); October 29-November 2, **2004**; Boston, Massachusetts. Abstract 1168.

Janssen HLA, Van Zonneveld M, Senturk H, et al. Pegylated interferon alfa-2b alone or in combination with lamivudine for HBeAg-positive chronic hepatitis B: a randomised trial. *Lancet.* **2005**;365:123-129.

Kaiser S, Hass H, Gregor M. Successful retreatment of chronic hepatitis C patients with a nonresponse to standard interferon/ribavirin using daily consensus interferon and ribavirin. In: Program and abstracts of the 55th Annual Meeting of the American Association for the Study of Liver Diseases (AASLD); October 29-November 2, **2004**; Boston, Massachusetts. Abstract 173.

Lai C-L, Chien R-N, Leung NWY, et al. A one-year trial of lamivudine for chronic hepatitis B. *N Engl J Med.* **1998**;339:61-68.

Lai C-L, Leung N, Teo EK, et al. A phase IIb comparative trial of LdT, lamivudine, and the combination in hepatitis B patients: greater antiviral effect with LdT. In: Program and abstracts of the 43rd Interscience Conference on Antimicrobial Agents and Chemotherapy (ICAAC); September 14-17, **2003**, Chicago, Illinois. Abstract V-1723.

Lau D T-Y, Khokhar MF, Doo E, et al. Long-term therapy of chronic hepatitis B with lamivudine. *Hepatology.* **2000**;32:828-834.

Lee WM. Hepatitis B virus Infection. *N Engl J Med.* **1997**;37:1733-1745.

Leevy II C, Blatt L, Chalmers C. Interim results of a pilot study of the combination of type 1 (IFN alfacon 1) and type 2 (IFN gamma 1b) interferons in chronic hepatitis C patients who have failed to respond to peg-interferon alfa 2a plus ribavirin. In: Program and abstracts of the 55th Annual Meeting of the American Association for the Study of Liver Diseases (AASLD); October 29-November 2, **2004**; Boston, Massachusetts. Abstract 530.

Liaw Y-F. Impact of YMDD mutations during lamivudine therapy in patients with chronic hepatitis B. *Antivir Chem Chemother.* **2001**;12(suppl 1):67-71.

Lim YS, Suh DJ. Current antiviral therapy for chronic hepatitis B. *J Korean Med Sci.* **2004**;19:489-494.

Lissen E, Clumeck N, Sola R, et al. Histological response to peginterferon alfa-2a (40kd) (Pegasys®) plus ribavirin (Copegus®) in patients with HIV-HCV co-infection: results of the AIDS Pegasys Ribavirin International Co-infection Trial (APRICOT). In: Program and abstracts of the 55th Annual Meeting of the American Association for the Study of Liver Diseases (AASLD); October 29-November 2, **2004**; Boston, Massachusetts. Abstract 174 .

Manegold C, Hannoun C, Wywiol A, et al. Reactivation of hepatitis B virus replication accompanied by acute hepatitis in patients receiving highly active antiretroviral therapy [brief report]. *Clin Infect Dis.* **2001**;32:144-148.

Marcellin P, Lau GKK, Bonino F, et al. Peginterferon alfa-2a alone, lamivudine alone, and the two in combination in patients with HBeAg-negative chronic hepatitis B. *N Engl J Med.* **2004**;351:1206-1217.

Marchesini G, Brizi M, Bianchi G, Tomassetti S, Zoli M, Melchionda N. Metformin in non-alcoholic steatohepatitis. *Lancet.* **2001**;358:893-894.

Martin-Carbonero L, Soriano V, Valencia E, Garcia-Samaniego J, Lopez M, Gonzalez-Lahoz J. Increasing impact of chronic viral hepatitis on hospital admissions and mortality among HIV-infected patients. *AIDS Res Human Retroviruses.* **2001**;17:1467-1471.

Mauss S, Valenti W, DePamphilis J, et al. Risk factors for hepatic decompensation in patients with HIV/HCV coinfection and liver cirrhosis during interferon-based therapy. *AIDS.* **2004**;18:F21-F25.

Medina J, Fernandez-Salazar LI, Garcia-Buey L, Moreno-Otero R. Approach to the pathogenesis and treatment of nonalcoholic steatohepatitis. *Diabetes Care.* **2004**;27:2057-2066.

Monto A, Dove LM, Seal KH, et al. HIV-HCV coinfected patients, followed prospectively for a mean of 4.2 years, have similar rates of death or cirrhosis compared to HCV monoinfected patients. In: Program and abstracts of the 55th Annual Meeting of the American Association for the Study of Liver Diseases (AASLD); October 29-November 2, **2004**; Boston, Massachusetts. Abstract 1212.

Myers RP, Benhamou Y, Imbert-Bismut F, et al. Serum biochemical markers accurately predict liver fibrosis in HIV and hepatitis C virus co-infected patients. *AIDS*. **2003**;17:721-725.

Nadir A, Amin A, Chalisa N, van Thiel DH. Retinal vein thrombosis associated with chronic hepatitis C: a case series and review of the literature. *J Viral Hepat*. **2000**;7:466-470.

Neau D, Jouvencel AC, Legrand E, et al. Hepatitis C virus genetic variability in 52 human immunodeficiency virus-coinfected patients. *J Med Virol*. **2003**;71:41-48.

Nelson MS, Portsmouth J, Stebbing, M, et al. An open-label study of tenofovir in HIV-1 and Hepatitis B virus co-infected individuals. *AIDS*. **2003**;17:F7-F10.

Neuschwander-Tetri BA, Brunt EM, Wehmeier KR, Oliver D, Bacon BR. Improved nonalcoholic steatohepatitis after 48 weeks of treatment with the PPAR-gamma ligand rosiglitazone. *Hepatology*. **2003**;38:1008-1017.

Neuschwander-Tetri BA, Caldwell SH. Nonalcoholic steatohepatitis: summary of an AASLD Single Topic Conference. *Hepatology*. **2003**;37:1202-1219.

National Institutes of Health (NIH). National Institutes of Health Consensus Development Conference Statement - Management of Hepatitis C: June 10-12, **2002**. Available at: http://consensus.nih.gov/cons/116/091202116cdc_statement.htm [accessed February 19, 2005].

Ockenga J, Tillmann HL, Trautwein C, Stoll M, Manns MP, Schmidt RE. Hepatitis B and C in HIV-infected patients: prevalence and prognostic value. *J Hepatol*. **1997**;27:18-24.

Pegasys (peginterferon alfa-2a) [prescribing information]. Nutley, NJ: Roche Pharmaceuticals; February **2005**.

Perez-Olmeda M, Nunez M, Romero M, et al. Pegylated IFN-alpha2b plus ribavirin as therapy for chronic hepatitis C in HIV-infected patients. *AIDS*. **2003**;17:1023-1028.

Perronne C, Carrat F, Bani-Sadr F, et al. Final results of ANRS HC02-RIBAVIC: a randomized controlled trial of pegylated-interferon-alfa-2b plus ribavirin vs interferon-alfa-2b plus ribavirin for the initial treatment of chronic hepatitis C in HIV co-infected patients. In: Program and abstracts of the 11th Conference on Retroviruses and Opportunistic Infections; February 8-11, **2004**; San Francisco, California. Abstract 117LB.

Pessoa W, Gazzard B, Huang A, et al. Entecavir in HIV/HBV-co-infected patients: safety and efficacy in a phase II study (ETV-038). In: Program and abstracts of the 12th Conference on Retroviruses and Opportunistic Infections; February 22-25, **2005**; Boston, Massachusetts. Abstract 123.

Peters M, Anderson J, Lynch P, et al. Tenofovir disoproxil fumarate is not inferior to adefovir dipivoxil for the treatment of hepatitis B virus in subjects who are co-infected with HIV: results of ACTG A5127. In: Program and abstracts of the 12th Conference on Retroviruses and Opportunistic Infections; February 22-25, **2005**; Boston, Massachusetts. Abstract 124.

Peters MG, Hann HW, Martin P, et al. Adefovir dipivoxil alone or in combination with lamivudine in patients with lamivudine-resistant chronic hepatitis B. *Gastroenterology*. **2004**;126:91-101.

Piketty C, Pellegrin I, Katlama C, et al. Efficacy of tenofovir disoproxil fumarate in hepatitis B virus in HIV-co-infected patients: the TECOVIR study. In: Program and abstracts of the 11th Conference on Retroviruses and Opportunistic Infections; February 8-11, **2004**; San Francisco, California. Abstract 834.

Pillay D, Cane PA, Ratcliffe D, Atkins M, Cooper D, for the CAESAR Co-ordinating Committee. Evolution of lamivudine-resistant hepatitis B virus and HIV-1 in co-infected individuals: an analysis of the CAESAR study. *AIDS*. **2000**;14:1111-1116.

Pol S, Lebray P, Vallet-Pichard A. HIV infection and hepatic enzyme abnormalities: intricacies of the pathogenic mechanisms. *Clin Infect Dis*. **2004**;38(suppl 2):S65-S72.

Promrat K, Lutchman G, Uwaifo GI, et al. A pilot study of pioglitazone treatment for nonalcoholic steatohepatitis. *Hepatology*. **2004**;39:188-196.

Rendón A, Nuñez M, Romero M, et al. Ribavirin plasma concentrations predict early virological response as well as anemia in anti-hepatitis C therapy. In: Program and abstracts of the 12th Conference on Retroviruses and Opportunistic Infections; February 22-25, **2005**; Boston, Massachusetts. Abstract 929.

Ristig MB, Crippin J, Aberg JA, et al. Tenofovir disoproxil fumarate therapy for chronic hepatitis B in human immunodeficiency virus/hepatitis B virus-coinfected individuals for whom interferon-alpha and lamivudine therapy have failed. *J Infect Dis*. **2002**;186:1844-1847.

Rodriguez-Mendez ML, Gonzalez-Quintela A, Aguilera A, Barrio E. Prevalence, patterns, and course of past hepatitis B virus infection in intravenous drug users with HIV-1 infection. *Am J Gastroenterol*. **2000**;95:1316-1322.

Rodriguez-Rosado R, Perez-Olmeda M, Garcia-Samaniego J, Soriano V. Management of hepatitis C in HIV-infected persons. *Antiviral Res.* **2001**;52:189-198.

Rutschmann OT, Negro F, Hirschel B, et al. Impact of treatment with human immunodeficiency virus (HIV) protease inhibitors on hepatitis C viremia in patients coinfected with HIV. *J Infect Dis.* **1998**;177:783-785.

Satapathy SK, Garg S, Chauhan R, et al. Beneficial effects of tumor necrosis factor-alpha inhibition by pentoxifylline on clinical, biochemical, and metabolic parameters of patients with nonalcoholic steatohepatitis. *Am J Gastroenterol.* **2004**;99:1946-1952.

Sherman KE, Rouster SD, Chung RT, Rajicic N. Hepatitis C Virus prevalence among patients infected with Human Immunodeficiency Virus: a cross-sectional analysis of the US adult AIDS Clinical Trials Group. *Clin Infect Dis.* **2002**;34:831-837.

Sherman KE. Implications of peginterferon use in special populations infected with HCV. *Semin Liver Dis.* **2003**;23(suppl 1):47-52.

Sherman M, Yurdaydin, C, Sollano J, et al. Entecavir is superior to continued lamivudine for the treatment of lamivudine-refractory, HBeAG(+) chronic hepatitis B: results of phase III study ETV-026. In: Program and abstracts of the 55th Annual Meeting of the American Association for the Study of Liver Diseases (AASLD); October 29-November 2, **2004**; Boston, Massachusetts. Abstract 1152.

Shiffman ML, Ng TM, Krastev Z et al. A double-blind, placebo-controlled trial of emtricitabine (FTC, Emtriva) administered once-daily for treatment of chronic hepatitis B virus (HBV) infection. In: Program and abstracts of the 55th Annual Meeting of the American Association for the Study of Liver Diseases (AASLD); October 29-November 2, **2004**; Boston, Massachusetts. Abstract 22.

Sinicco A, Raiteri R, Sciandra M, et al. Coinfection and superinfection of hepatitis B virus in patients infected with human immunodeficiency virus: no evidence of faster progression to AIDS. *Scand J Infect Dis.* **1997**;29:111-115.

Snow A, J Harris J, Borroto-Esoda K, et al. Emtricitabine therapy for hepatitis infection in HIV+ patients co-infected with hepatitis B virus: efficacy and genotypic findings in antiretroviral treatment-naïve patients. In: Program and abstracts of the 11th Conference on Retroviruses and Opportunistic Infections; February 8-11, **2004**; San Francisco, California. Abstract 836.

Soriano V, Garcia-Samaniego J, Perez-Olmeda M, et al. Pegylated interferon plus ribavirin for the treatment of chronic hepatitis C in HIV-infected patients. In: Program and abstracts of the 1st IAS Conference on HIV Pathogenesis and Treatment; July 8-11, **2001**; Buenos Aires, Argentina. Abstract 42.

Soriano V, Perez-Olmeda M, Camino N, et al. Clinical implications of the slower clearance of HCV-RNA under interferon (IFN) plus ribavirin (RBV) in patients coinfected with HIV and hepatitis C virus (HCV). In: Program and abstracts of the 43rd Interscience Conference on Antimicrobial Agents and Chemotherapy (ICAAC); September 14-17, **2003**; Chicago, Illinois. Abstract H-1718.

Strader DB, Wright T, Thomas L, Seeff LB. Diagnosis, management, and treatment of hepatitis C. *Hepatology.* **2004**;39:1147-1171.

Sulkowski MS, Thomas DL, Chaisson RE, Moore RD. Hepatotoxicity associated with antiretroviral therapy in adults infected with human immunodeficiency virus and the role of hepatitis C or B virus infection. *JAMA.* **2000**;283:74-80.

Sulkowski MS, Thomas DL, Mehta SH, Chaisson RE, Moore RD. Hepatotoxicity associated with nevirapine or efavirenz-containing antiretroviral therapy: role of hepatitis C and B infections. *Hepatology.* **2002**;35:182-189.

Telfer P, Sabin C, Devereux H, et al. The progression of HCV-associated liver disease in a cohort of haemophilic patients. *Br J Haematol.* **1994**;87:555-561.

Tenney DJ, Levine SM, Rose RE, et al. Clinical emergence of entecavir-resistant hepatitis B virus requires additional substitutions in virus already resistant to lamivudine. *Antimicrob Agents Chemother.* **2004**;48:3498-3507.

Thio CL, Seaberg EC, Skolasky R Jr, et al. HIV-1, hepatitis B virus, and risk of liver-related mortality in the Multicenter Cohort Study (MACS). *Lancet.* **2002**;360:1921-1926.

Thio CL. Hepatitis B virus infection in HIV-infected persons. *Current Hepatitis Reports.* **2004**;3:91-97.

Torriani FJ, Rodriguez-Torres M, Rockstroh JK, et al. Peginterferon alfa-2a plus ribavirin for chronic hepatitis C virus infection in HIV-infected patients. *N Engl J Med.* **2004**;351:438-450.

Uberti-Foppa C, De Bona A, Morsica G, et al. Pretreatment of chronic active hepatitis C in patients coinfected with HIV and hepatitis C virus reduces the hepatotoxicity associated with subsequent antiretroviral therapy. *J Acquir Immune Defic Syndr.* **2003**;33:146-152.

USPHS/IDSA Prevention of Opportunistic Infections Working Group. Guidelines for preventing opportunistic infections among HIV-infected persons—2002 recommendations of the U.S. Public Health Service and the Infectious Diseases Society of America. *MMWR Morbid Mortal Wkly Rep.* **2002**;51(RR-8).

Videx EC (didanosine) [prescribing information]. Princeton, NJ: Bristol-Myers Squibb; January **2004**.

Waite J, Gilson RJC, Weller IVD, et al. Hepatitis B virus reactivation or reinfection associated with HIV-1 infection. *AIDS*. **1988**;2:443-448.

Wong DK, Cheung AM, O'Rourke K, Naylor CD, Detsky AS, Heathcote J. Effect of alpha-interferon treatment in patients with hepatitis B e antigen-positive chronic hepatitis B: a meta-analysis. *Ann Intern Med.* **1993**;119:312-323.

Yu AS, Keeffe EB. Nonalcoholic fatty liver disease. *Rev Gastroenterol Disord.* **2002**;2:11-19.

Zein NN. Clinical significance of hepatitis C virus genotypes. *Clin Microbiol Rev.* **2000**;13:223-235.

Zylberberg H, Jiang J, Pialoux G, et al. Alpha-interferon for chronic active hepatitis B in human immunodeficiency virus-infected patients. *Gastroenterol Clin Biol.* **1996**;20:968-971.

(RLO-14)

III.58. SYPHILIS

LEARNING OBJECTIVE: Discuss current epidemiology (including behavioral and clinical factors associated with transmission), screening, clinical manifestations, indications for cerebrospinal fluid analysis, treatment and follow-up for syphilis in HIV infection.

Syphilis is a common concomitant disease in people with HIV. In this coinfected population, syphilis does not have a unique manifestation. Like any host–pathogen relationship, syphilis is influenced by the immune response of the host. Therefore, clinical manifestations may vary among HIV-infected patients compared with noninfected patients. Similarly, treatment response may also differ (Hook and Schwebke 2003).

The hallmark manifestation of primary syphilis is an ulcer or chancre at the site of infection, usually in the anogenital area, but chancres may also be seen orally or at any other site of organism inoculation. The lesion is classically single and painless, with clear exudates (described further below). As a genital ulcer disease, syphilis can have a marked impact on the rate of HIV transmission (Pao et al. 2002). Shortly after the initial infection causes an ulcer at the site of infection, the spirochetes disseminate throughout the body and over time may damage many organs.

Of special concern is the possibility that HIV-infected individuals treated for syphilis may have higher rates of syphilis treatment failure than their HIV-noninfected counterparts and may be more likely to develop neurologic complications, as suggested initially by a review of 4 case reports (Johns et al. 1987). Although those cases date from the period before the use of combination antiretroviral therapy, they continue to inform recommendations for syphilis treatment and follow-up in HIV-infected patients.

Epidemiology

Although rates of syphilis declined on a national level through the 1990s and rates continue to decline in women and non-Hispanic blacks, the incidence has recently risen in some urban areas among men, most commonly among men who have sex with men (MSM) (CDC 2004a). Preliminary data from CDC surveillance in 2003 indicate that this trend has continued nationally for a third consecutive year, primarily because of syphilis outbreaks among MSM, who in 2003 represented just over 60% of all new syphilis diagnoses (Heffelfinger 2004). Indeed, based on these data, the ratio of male:female new syphilis cases has reached 5:1 (Heffelfinger 2004), the highest ratio in more than 2 decades of STD surveillance (CDC 2004a).

This resurgence parallels growth in the amount of sexual risk-taking, with San Francisco offering the most dramatic example. The city saw early syphilis cases increase from 41 in 1998 to 496 in 2002 (CDC 2003), and among the 2002 cases, 434 were MSM, of whom 293 (67.5%) were also HIV-infected. In the spring of 2003, San Francisco clinicians found 15 new syphilis cases among 814 asymptomatic HIV-infected patients (Klausner et al. 2004).

What's New

The incidence of syphilis continues to rise in men, particularly men who have sex with men (MSM), resulting in a dramatic increase in the male:female case ratio. This global increase in syphilis cases sometimes occurs without a concomitant rise in HIV (as in San Francisco and Germany). European and American authorities are reporting an outbreak of lymphogranuloma venereum among MSM, most of them HIV-infected.

Key Points

- Syphilis is more common among persons with HIV, and HIV is relatively common among persons with syphilis.
- Syphilis does not have a unique manifestation or require special testing in HIV-infected patients, but clinical manifestations and response to treatment may vary with a patient's immune response.
- Neurosyphilis may be more common in people with HIV; cerebrospinal fluid should be examined for patients with neurologic manifestations, late latent syphilis or latent syphilis of unknown duration.
- HIV-infected patients with primary and secondary syphilis should receive clinical and serologic follow-up evaluations at 3, 6, 9, 12 and 24 months after therapy is completed; follow-up for those with latent syphilis is recommended every 6 months for 2 years after therapy.
- A European outbreak of proctitis induced by lymphogranuloma venereum (LGV) has also shown up in the United States. Patients are men who have sex with men and mainly HIV-infected. Physicians should include LGV when diagnosing proctitis and report possible cases to the CDC and local health authorities.

New York City has experienced a similar upward trend: 282 cases of primary and secondary syphilis were reported for 2001 (NYCDH 2002), more than double the 117 cases reported in 2000 (CDC 2002b). Sexual orientation was known for 188 male cases in 2002; 79% were MSM compared with 43% in a 1999 survey. Of the 86 MSM with known HIV status in 2002, 48% were HIV-infected compared with only 20% in 1999. In one New York City HIV clinic, the rates of syphilis diagnosis rose 54% from 2000 to 2003. Although men comprised 60% of the overall client population in this clinic, they represented 100% of the new syphilis diagnoses (Zweibel 2004).

Comparable trends have been observed in Seattle, Chicago, Los Angeles, Miami and other large cities in North America and Europe. A Dublin, Ireland, clinic reported that 125 (22%) of 561 syphilis patients seen between 2000 and 2003 were HIV-infected (Devitt et al. 2004). The syphilis coinfection rate among the clinic's MSM patients with HIV was 2% in 2000. It jumped to 23% to 29% during subsequent years. A newly implemented surveillance network in France reported a more than 10-fold increase in syphilis cases, from 37 cases in 2000 to 416 cases in 2002, with risk behaviors persisting among MSM (Troussier et al. 2004). In Germany, the number of syphilis cases among MSM rose from 200 in early 2001 to 550 by mid-2003; in contrast, HIV infections increased from 145 to 175 during that same time period (Marcus et al. 2004). A study of a cohort of HIV-negative MSM in Sydney, Australia, tracked HIV and STD seroconversion incidence from 2002 to 2003, and found a 1.5% incidence for new HIV and syphilis infections in this population (Jin et al. 2004).

Natural History of Syphilis

Early syphilis comprises primary, secondary, and latent stages; these stages typically occur within the first year after infection. Untreated patients may suffer relapses of secondary syphilis for more than 1 year after infection. An infected person who has not been treated may infect others during the first 2 stages and during the early latent phase. Thus, a person may be infectious for as long as 2 years after initial infection. This is true regardless of whether cutaneous lesions are present.

Late manifestations of syphilis (often defined as tertiary and quaternary) include gummatous syphilis (lesions of the skin and bone), cardiovascular syphilis, and neurosyphilis (Pao et al. 2002). Rapid progression to these late forms of syphilis, including neurosyphilis and ocular and gummatous syphilis, has been described in the HIV-infected population (Czelusta et al. 2000), although data to the contrary also exist (de Souza and Nitrini 1997). Symptomatic neurosyphilis does not appear to occur commonly during early syphilis (Flood et al. 1998) However, there is a relatively high prevalence of asymptomatic neurosyphilis in HIV-infected patients with latent syphilis, and the incidence of clinical neurosyphilis may be increased in HIV-infected patients versus HIV-uninfected patients (Hook and Schwebke 2003).

It is important to recognize that HIV-infected patients with early syphilis are at greater risk of neurologic complications than are HIV-negative patients (CDC 2002a). A patient who has clinical evidence of neurologic involvement, such as cognitive dysfunction, motor or sensory deficits, ophthalmic or auditory symptoms, cranial nerve palsies, and symptoms or signs of meningitis, should have a cerebrospinal fluid (CSF) evaluation (Lukehart et al. 1988). The range of neurologic manifestations during the course of syphilis is considerable. For example, early neurologic involvement can be asymptomatic or may include symptomatic meningitis (cranial nerve abnormalities, hydrocephalus) within the first year following primary infection. Meningovasculitis (presenting with strokes) generally occurs between 5 and 7 years after initial infection but may be seen sooner in HIV-infected persons. Late neurosyphilis is classically characterized by general paresis (forgetfulness, personality changes, psychiatric symptoms) or tabes dorsalis (e.g., sensory loss, ataxia, bladder dysfunction), and typically occurs 10 to 20 or more years after infection.

The diagnosis of neurosyphilis in HIV-infected persons can be difficult because HIV alone is often associated with neurologic abnormalities or with CSF pleocytosis and elevated CSF protein concentrations (Marra et al. 1996). In considering neurosyphilis in an HIV-infected patient, it is also important to be aware that case findings of neurosyphilis can be enhanced in this population because of such factors as a higher incidence of CSF evaluation for exclusion of opportunistic infections, and the fact that the U.S. Public Health Service guidelines and others recommend that a CSF evaluation for neurosyphilis be performed if the HIV patient has late latent syphilis (CDC 2002a; Flood et al. 1998). Two studies found syphilitic meningitis to be more common among HIV-infected individuals compared with those who were not HIV-infected (Katz et al. 1993; de Souza and Nitrini 1997); one of those studies reported finding parenchymal forms of neurosyphilis (general paresis and tabes dorsalis) more often in HIV-noninfected than HIV-infected persons (de Souza and Nitrini 1997), but it is possible that the shortened survival because of HIV/AIDS at the time of this study did not allow long-term effects of syphilis to develop in these patients.

Diagnosis

According to the U.S. Public Health Service, syphilis can be definitively diagnosed during the primary phase using dark-field examination and direct florescent antibody tests of lesion exudate or tissue (CDC 2002a). Failure to identify the spirochete in a specimen does not rule out the diagnosis of primary syphilis, however. The direct fluorescent antibody test for *Treponema pallidum* (DFA-TP) is an alternative technique used to identify the organism from lesion specimens, but few STD clinics have access to the DFA-TP.

In the absence of lesions, presumptive diagnoses can be made with 2 types of serologic tests: nontreponemal and treponemal tests. Common nontreponemal serologic tests are the Venereal Disease Research Laboratory (VDRL) test and the Rapid Plasma Reagin (RPR) test. There have been reports of unusual responses to these tests in people with HIV, such as false-negative reactions and high titers relative to HIV-seronegative people; however, most experts now consider these tests to be reliable for both screening diagnosis and follow-up (Hook and Schwebke 2003; CDC 2002a). Most often, specimens found to have a reactive nontreponemal test will undergo confirmatory testing using a treponemal test. The confirmatory treponemal tests are the FTA-ABS (fluorescent treponemal antibody absorption) test and the TP-PA (*Treponema pallidum* particle agglutination) test; both are immunoassays (CDC 2002a). It is important to note that patients usually become nonreactive to nontreponemal tests at some point in time after treatment. However, in some people who appear to have been treated successfully, low titers of nontreponemal antibodies may persist; these people are said to be "serofast." With the treponemal test, conversely, once a patient has had a reactive test, they typically remain reactive regardless of reinfection, although some patients can revert to seronegativity.

False-positive and false-negative tests occur with both nontreponemal and treponemal tests (Larsen 1989). Various febrile illnesses and immunizations can result in false-positive treponemal tests; test abnormalities attributed to these conditions typically last no longer than 6 months. False-positive tests are associated with a variety of conditions, including autoimmune or connective tissue disease, genital herpes and narcotic addiction (Hart 1986) and HIV infection (Rompalo et al. 1992).

The most common cause of false-negative syphilis serology is testing before diagnostic antibodies develop (Hart 1986). However, some patients with very-late-stage HIV infection have delayed or absent serologic responses to syphilis (i.e., false-negative tests) (Tikjob et al. 1991; Hicks et al. 1987) or are more likely to lose their reactivity after appropriate syphilis therapy (Johnson et al. 1991; Haas et al. 1990). The possibility of either false-positive or false-negative syphilis serologies in HIV-infected individuals may be related to abnormally active B-cell function during early HIV infection and B-cell failure during late-stage HIV infection.

When serologic findings are negative or the interpretation is unclear, but syphilis is suspected, the U.S. Public Health Service recommends that alternative diagnostic tests be considered, such as lesion biopsy, dark-field examination or direct fluorescent antibody staining of lesion matter (CDC 2002a).

Treatment of Primary and Secondary Syphilis in HIV-Infected Persons

The U.S. Public Health Service recommends, and recent research confirms, that treatment for primary or secondary syphilis in HIV-infected patients be 2.4 million units of benzathine penicillin G administered by intramuscular injection in a single dose, as for HIV-noninfected patients (Hook and Schwebke 2003; CDC 2002a). Most HIV-infected patients respond appropriately to standard treatment (Hopkins et al. 2004), particularly if receiving combination antiretroviral therapy. However, the U.S. Public Health Service guidelines note that some specialists advocate more aggressive treatment approaches (e.g., additional weekly doses of benzathine penicillin G up to a total of 3 doses, as suggested for late syphilis) (CDC 2002a).

CSF abnormalities are common among both asymptomatic HIV-infected patients in the absence of syphilis and HIV-noninfected patients who have primary or secondary syphilis. Such abnormalities in patients with primary or secondary syphilis are of unknown prognostic significance. Some experts recommend intensified penicillin treatment when neurologic symptoms of syphilis are suspected, but this should be considered only after CSF examination.

Testing for suspected central nervous system invasion of syphilis is somewhat controversial. Some clinicians believe that an examination of CSF before treatment is prudent for all HIV-infected patients (CDC 2002a), although recent studies of early syphilis in HIV-infected patients do not support this (Hook and Schwebke 2003). However, most clinicians agree that CSF examination is important for HIV-infected patients with neurologic manifestations, late latent syphilis, and latent syphilis of unknown duration (positive serologic test without syphilis treatment history) (Hook and Schwebke 2003; CDC 2002a). Furthermore, current CDC guidelines recommend CSF examination in persons with syphilis and any of the following (CDC 2002a):

- Neurologic or ophthalmic signs or symptoms
- Evidence of active tertiary syphilis
- Treatment failure
- HIV infection with late latent syphilis or syphilis of unknown duration

In a study to identify clinical and laboratory factors related to neurosyphilis in individuals with a syphilis diagnosis, 326 individuals with reactive serum treponemal and nontreponemal serologic tests underwent lumbar puncture. Of these 326 individuals, 65 were diagnosed with neurosyphilis as determined by CSF white blood cell count greater than 20 cells/mm^3 or a reactive CSF VDRL test. Factors associated with a diagnosis of neurosyphilis were a high serum RPR titer and HIV infection with a CD4 count below 350 cells/mm^3 (Marra et al. 2004). Another recent study found that the risk for neurosyphilis rose in tandem with the RPR level for all those with titers of 1/32 or higher (Libois et al. 2004).

After therapy, HIV-infected patients should be evaluated, both clinically and serologically, for treatment failure at 3, 6, 9, 12 and 24 months. Although definitive criteria have not been established in HIV or non-HIV populations, a few indications can help in assessing treatment failure: signs and symptoms that continue or recur, or a sustained fourfold increase in nontreponemal test titers (compared with baseline or maximum titer at time of treatment) can be considered to indicate treatment failure or even, in some cases, reinfection (CDC 2002a). HIV-infected patients who meet the criteria for treatment failure should be managed the same as HIV-uninfected patients (i.e., a CSF examination and re-treatment). For patients whose nontreponemal test titer does not decrease fourfold within 6 to 12 months, CSF examination and re-treatment also should be strongly considered. If CSF examinations are normal, retreating patients with 7.2 million units of benzathine penicillin G (administered as 3 weekly doses of 2.4 million units each) is recommended by most experts (CDC 2002a).

HIV-infected patients who have primary or secondary syphilis and are allergic to penicillin should be managed according to the recommendations for penicillin-allergic HIV-uninfected patients. However, the efficacy of nonpenicillin regimens in HIV-infected patients has not been well studied. Although data supporting alternatives to penicillin in treating early syphilis are limited, two therapies have been used for many years and might be considered effective for nonpregnant, penicillin-allergic patients with primary or secondary syphilis: doxycycline (100 mg orally twice daily for 14 days) and tetracycline (500 mg four times daily for 14 days) (CDC 2002a).

Treatment of Late Latent Syphilis in HIV-Infected Persons

A patient with late latent syphilis or syphilis of unknown duration and a normal CSF examination can be treated with 7.2 million units of benzathine penicillin G (as 3 once-weekly doses of 2.4 million units each). Patients who have CSF consistent with neurosyphilis symptoms (cognitive dysfunction, motor or sensory deficits, ophthalmic or auditory symptoms, cranial nerve palsies, and signs or symptoms of meningitis) should be treated with 18 to 24 million units of aqueous crystalline penicillin G per day, administered as 3 to 4 million units intravenously every 4 hours or by continuous infusion, for 10 to 14 days (CDC 2002a). An alternative regimen is procaine penicillin 2.4 million units intramuscularly once daily plus probenecid 500 mg orally four times daily, both for 10 to 14 days (Hook and Schwebke 2003; CDC 2002a).

For patients allergic to penicillin with late latent syphilis or latent syphilis of unknown duration, the U.S. Public Health Service considers the only acceptable alternatives for the treatment to be doxycycline (100 mg orally twice daily) or tetracycline (500 mg orally four times daily), both for 28 days, and only in conjunction with close serologic and clinical follow-up. For HIV-infected patients, the efficacy of these alternative regimens has not been studied and so should be considered only with extreme caution (CDC 2002a).

HIV-infected patients with late latent syphilis should receive clinical and serologic follow-up evaluations every 6 months for 2 years after therapy is completed; if clinical symptoms fail to subside or if they recur, or if nontreponemal titers rise fourfold during treatment or fail to decline fourfold after treatment has been completed, a repeat CSF examination should be performed and treatment administered accordingly (CDC 2002a).

Lymphogranuloma Venereum (LGV)

As of September 2004, a total of 92 reported cases of Lymphogranuloma venereum (LGV) had occurred in Dutch MSM over the previous 17 months; usually, there are only about 5 LGV cases per year in the Netherlands (CDC 2004b). Of the 30 patients with known HIV status, 23 (77%) were HIV-infected. The majority of these patients had participated in unprotected anal intercourse or other unprotected anal penetration in the 12 months before onset of symptoms. Their clinical symptoms were unusual. Patients presented with painful proctitis, constipation, and a bloody purulent or mucous anal discharge. The inguinal lymphadenopathy characteristic of LGV was missing in all but one of the cases. Further investigation found that all cases resulted from infection by *Chlamydia trachomatis* serovar 2, one of the three that causes LGV.

There have been reports of similar cases of *Chlamydia trachomatis* serovar 2 from the United Kingdom (29 as of the end of January 2005 [Ison et al. 2005]), and from cities in Western Europe. Seventeen (89%) of the 29 U.K. cases also had HIV. There have been descriptions of LGV-associated proctitis in the United States since the late seventies (Bolan et al. 1982), and the recent CDC warning triggered a handful of reports from San Francisco, Atlanta and New York (Stagg 2005). HIV clinicians across the U.S. should be aware of this spreading outbreak and add LGV to their differential diagnosis for any patients with proctitis.

The CDC treatment recommendations (CDC 2004b) describe effective treatment for LGV with a 21-day course of doxycycline 100 mg twice daily. An alternative treatment is erythromycin 500 mg four times daily for 21 days. Azithromycin 1 gram weekly for 3 weeks may also be effective, but clinical data are lacking. Patients' sexual partners over the past 30 days should undergo evaluation and receive treatment if symptomatic. If asymptomatic, they should be treated prophylactically for 7 days with either doxycycline 100 mg twice daily or 1 gram of azithromycin as a single dose.

In the Dutch cases, serology tests supported the evaluation of symptoms when making the diagnosis. A polymerase chain reaction (PCR) confirmed the presence of *C. trachomatis* in rectal samples, but urethral swabs yielded negative results. Subsequent genotyping determined the serovar (CDC 2004b).

The CDC is requesting that physicians report possible LGV cases to both their local health departments as well as to the CDC (404-639-2059).

References

Bolan RK, Sands M, Schachter J, Miner RC, Drew WL. Lymphogranuloma venereum and acute ulcerative proctitis. *Am J Med.* **1982**;72:703-706.

Centers for Disease Control and Prevention (CDC). Sexually transmitted diseases treatment guidelines 2002. *MMWR Morb Mortal Wkly Rep.* **2002a**;51(RR-6).

Centers for Disease Control and Prevention (CDC). Primary and secondary syphilis among men who have sex with men—New York City, 2001. *MMWR Morb Mortal Wkly Rep.* **2002b**;51:853-856.

Centers for Disease Control and Prevention (CDC). Internet use and early syphilis infection among men who have sex with men – San Francisco, California, 1999-2003. *MMWR Morb Mortal Wkly Rep.* **2003**;52:1229-1232.

Centers for Disease Control and Prevention (CDC). National STD Surveillance Report 2003. **2004a**. Available at: http://www.cdc.gov/std/stats/ [accessed April 22, 2003].

Centers for Disease Control and Prevention (CDC). Lymphogranuloma venereum among men who have sex with men — Netherlands, 2003-2004. *MMWR Morb Mortal Wkly Rpt.* **2004b**;53;985-988.

Czelusta A, Yen-Moore A, van der Straten M, et al. An overview of sexually transmitted diseases. Part 3. Sexually transmitted diseases in HIV-infected patients. *J Am Acad Dermatol.* **2000**;43:409-432.

de Souza MC and Nitrini R. Effects of human immunodeficiency virus infection on the manifestations of neurosyphilis [letter]. *Neurology.* **1997**;49:893-894.

Devitt E, Hopkins S, Mulcahy F, Bergin C. Rising numbers of HIV infection after a syphilis epidemic. In: Program and abstracts of the 11th Conference on Retroviruses and Opportunistic Infections; February 8-11, **2004**; San Francisco, California. Abstract 848.

Flood JM, Weinstock HS, Guroy ME, et al. Neurosyphilis during the AIDS epidemic, San Francisco, 1985-1992. *J Infect Dis.* **1998**;177:931-940.

Haas JS, Bolan G, Larsen SA, Clement MJ, Bacchetti P, Moss AR. Sensitivity of treponemal tests for detecting prior treated syphilis during human immunodeficiency virus infection. *J Infect Dis.* **1990**;162:862-866.

Hart G. Syphilis tests in diagnostic and therapeutic decision making. *Ann Intern Med.* **1986**;104:368-376.

Heffelfinger JD. Syphilis trends in the United States. Emerging patterns and trends in nationally notifiable sexually transmitted diseases. In: Program and abstracts of the 2004 National STD Prevention Conference; March 8-11, 2004; Philadelphia, Pennsylvania. Symposium A7. Available at: http://www.cdc.gov/std/2004STDConf/#A [accessed February 21, **2005**].

Hicks CB, Benson PM, Lupton GP, Tramont EC. Seronegative secondary syphilis in a patient with the human immunodeficiency virus (HIV) with Kaposi sarcoma: A diagnostic dilemma. *Ann Intern Med.* **1987**;107:492-495.

Hook EW III, Schwebke JR. Sexually transmitted diseases. In: Dolin R, Masur H, Saag MS. eds. *AIDS Therapy.* 2nd ed. Philadelphia: Churchill-Livingstone; **2003**:674-681

Hopkins S, Khalid A, Courtney G, Mulcahy F, Bergin C. Syphilis treatment outcomes in HIV-infected and -non-infected individuals. In: Program and abstracts of the 11th Conference on Retroviruses and Opportunistic Infections; February 8-11, **2004**; San Francisco, California. Abstract 771.

Ison CA, Macdonald N, Martin IMC, et al. Enhanced surveillance for lymphogranuloma venereum (LGV) in England. In: Program and abstracts of the 11th annual conference of the British HIV Association [BHIVA] with the British Association for Sexual Health and HIV [BASHH]; April, 20-23, **2005**; Dublin, Ireland. Abstract O37.

Jin FY, Prestage G, Van de Ven P, et al. Prevalence, incidence and risk factors for HIV, syphilis, gonorrhoea and chlamydia in an HIV negative cohort of homosexual men. In: Program and abstracts of the XV International AIDS Conference; July 11-16, **2004**; Bangkok, Thailand. Abstract ThPeC7358.

Johns DR, Tierney M, Felsenstein D. Alteration in the natural history of neurosyphilis by concurrent infection with the human immunodeficiency virus. *N Engl J Med.* **1987**;316:1569-1572.

Johnson PD, Graves SR, Stewart L, Warren R, Dwyer B, Lucas CR. Specific syphilis serological tests may become negative in HIV infection. *AIDS.* **1991**;5:419-423.

Katz DA, Berger JR, Duncan RC. Neurosyphilis. A comparative study of the effects of infection with human immunodeficiency virus. *Arch Neurol.* **1993**;50:243-249.

Klausner J, Stanley H, Kohn R, Stansell J. Syphilis, gonorrhea, and chlamydia screening in HIV-infected patients in care, San Francisco, 2003. In: Program and abstracts of the 11th Conference on Retroviruses and Opportunistic Infections; February 8-11, **2004**; San Francisco, California. Abstract 869.

Larsen SA. Syphilis. *Clin Lab Med.* **1989**;9:545-557.

Libois A, De Wit S, Poll B, et al. HIV and syphilis: when to perform a lumbar puncture? In: Program and abstracts of the7th International Congress on Drug Therapy in HIV Infection; November 14-18, **2004**; Glasgow, United Kingdom. Abstract PL9.5.

Lukehart SA, Hook EW, Baker-Zander SA, Collier AC, Critchlow CW, Handsfield HH. Invasion of central nervous system by Treponema pallidum: implications for diagnosis and treatment. *Ann Intern Med.* **1988**;109:855-862.

Marcus U, Hamouda O, Voss L, Bremer V, Kollan C. Large increase of syphilis incidence among MSM in Germany since 2000 accompanied by only small increase of newly diagnosed HIV infections. In: Program and abstracts of the XV International AIDS Conference; July 11-16, **2004**; Bangkok, Thailand. Abstract ThPeC7332.

Marra CM, Gary DW, Kupers J, et al. Diagnosis of neurosyphilis in patients infected with human immunodeficiency virus type 1. *Infect Dis.* **1996**;174:219-221.

Marra CM, Maxwell CL, Smith SL, et al. Cerebrospinal fluid abnormalities in patients with syphilis: association with clinical and laboratory features. *J Infect Dis.* **2004**;189:369-376.

New York City Department of Health (NYCDOH). NYC Department of Health presents 2001 data on syphilis [press release]. New York: Office of Public Affairs; March 6, **2002**. Available at: http://www.nyc.gov/html/doh/html/public/press02/pr11-306.html [accessed February 21, 2005].

Pao D, Goh BT, Bingham JS. Management issues in syphilis. *Drugs.* **2002**;62:1447-1461.

Rompalo AM, Cannon RO, Quinn TC, Hook EW III. Association of biologic false-positive reactions for syphilis with human immunodeficiency virus infection. *J Infect Dis.* **1992**;165:1124-1126.

Stagg Elliott V. CDC sounds doctor alert about rare STD: Lymphogranuloma venereum is tough to diagnose, easy to treat and making inroads here. *AMNews.* Feb. 28, **2005**. Available at: http://www.ama-assn.org/amednews/2005/02/28/hlsc0228.htm [accessed April 28, 2005].

Tikjob G, Russel M, Peterson CS, et al. Seronegative secondary syphilis in a patient with AIDS: Identification of Treponema pallidum in a biopsy specimen. *J Am Acad Dermatol.* **1991**; 24:506-508.

Troussier T, Delatour F, Couturier E, et al. Syphilis control in France 2000 to 2004. In: Program and abstracts of the XV International AIDS Conference; July 11-16, **2004**; Bangkok, Thailand. Abstract ThPeC7377.

Zweibel M. Increasing rates of syphilis in an urban HIV clinic. In: Program and abstracts of the XV International AIDS Conference; July 11-16, **2004**; Bangkok, Thailand. Abstract ThPeC7389.

PRINCIPLES OF ANTIRETROVIRAL THERAPY

This section covers the most recent information developments in antiretroviral therapy.

Upon completion of this section, clinicians should be able to describe FDA-approved antiretroviral agents, including dosing, common side effects and contraindications; discuss when and how to use, monitor and modify combination antiretroviral therapy with approved agents; identify experimental antiretrovirals in advanced stages of development; discuss the manifestations and management of complications resulting from antiretroviral treatment; and describe new genetic approaches to HIV therapy.

At-a-glance

What's New - Overview

Tipranavir is undergoing FDA licensing review, and five other compounds are in phase III study. Testing companies have established new clinical cutoffs to define resistance in their phenotype and virtual phenotype assays. New studies suggest that replication capacity may predict outcome independent of HIV RNA level and CD4 cell count. There is a high rate of virologic failure with tenofovir/didanosine/efavirenz when used as initial HAART. Severe hypersensitivity reactions to nevirapine are up to 12-fold more common in women with low CD4 counts. Patients receiving antiretroviral therapy are at a higher risk for cardiovascular events.

(RLO-15)

IV.1. TREATMENT OF ACUTE HIV

LEARNING OBJECTIVE: Debate the advantages and disadvantages of very early treatment of acute HIV infection.

Interest in early treatment has been strengthened by anecdotes of individuals who were treated during primary infection and then sustained viral control off treatment (Lisziewicz et al. 1999), although other anecdotal reports failed to demonstrate consistent virologic control (Daar et al. 1998). Despite initial hopes, it does not appear that early antiretroviral therapy will prevent viral dissemination and seeding of reservoirs (Finzi et al. 1997).

There has been evidence that early treatment may offer a unique opportunity to preserve HIV-specific immune responses (Jansen et al. 2004 Rosenberg et al. 2000). During the first four weeks of infection, patients produce a high number of activated CD4 effector cells, though these decline in subsequent weeks to preinfection levels (Zaunders et al. 2005). In the intestinal mucosa, restoration of the CD4 cell population is more complete among patients starting on HAART in primary infection compared with those who initiate treatment during chronic infection (Guadalupe et al. 2005). Restoration still takes years, and anti-HIV responses remain much weaker in the blood than in the GI tract.

It had been hoped that treatment during primary or acute infection may allow certain patients to later discontinue antiretroviral therapy while sustaining virologic control. Recent data have raised questions about this conclusion, as the HIV-specific immune responses engendered by early treatment do not appear to support viral control. In a pilot study of treatment interruptions subsequent to acute HIV treatment, 14 patients were able to temporarily hold their viral loads below 5000 copies/mL, but CD4+ T cells slowly declined and HIV eventually rebounded at latest observation in all but two of the 14 (Kaufmann et al. 2004). Only three of the 14 study participants were able to remain off therapy for more than 1000 days without viral rebound. Patients did develop robust anti-HIV immune responses, but these did not correlate with their ability to control HIV without therapy. Moreover, with successive treatment interruptions, there was no trend toward longer time off therapy.

Two other recent studies failed to observe strong benefit from initiating HAART during acute infection. The French PRIMSTOP trial enrolled 26 patients undergoing acute HIV infection (Hoen et al. 2004). They received 34 weeks of therapy. Twenty-two of these, with viral loads below 50 copies/mL, underwent three 2-week treatment interruptions each separated by 12 weeks on HAART and then a permanent discontinuation at week 84. Only one maintained virologic suppression through week 108. The median viral load at that point was 10,000 copies/mL, and protease resistance mutations had appeared in 3 patients. Another French study, SEROCO, compared 58 patients who began therapy within six months of acquiring HIV with another 58 patients who were untreated (Desquilbet et al. 2004). The treated group received HAART for 24 months. At month 36, viral loads were similar in both study arms.

New efforts are attempting to combine immune suppressants with antiretrovirals during acute HIV. The immune suppressant may help protect CD4 cells and retard HIV replication

What's New

The most recent reports on treatment during acute infection are less optimistic than previous reports.

Key Points

Advantages

- Reduction in the severity of acute disease.
- Reduced risk of HIV transmission.
- Preservation of HIV-specific immune responses, which might allow patients to discontinue therapy with sustained viral control.
- Possible establishment of more favorable viral setpoint, which could slow the rate of disease progression.

Disadvantages

- Limited data supporting antiretroviral treatment during this stage.
- Little indication of what type of strategy, if any, might support and preserve effective anti-HIV immune responses.
- No apparent inhibition of viral dissemination or seeding of reservoirs.
- Early exposure to antiretroviral therapy's cost and toxicities.
- High patient adherence needed to avoid development of drug-resistant virus and the closing off of treatment options later in disease.

by reducing cellular activation. After a time, HAART is interrupted (but not necessarily the immune suppressant) to test the extent of patients' control of their HIV. New trials have taken place using HAART plus hydroxyurea and mycophenolate. The hydroxyurea trial observed no difference in virologic control between the hydroxyurea and control arms after 12 months of treatment and then multiple treatment interruptions (Bloch et al. 2005). In the mycophenolate study, patients had been on successful HAART for many years after acute infection (Ciufredda et al. 2005). The trial added the mycophenolate two weeks before stopping the antiretrovirals. Viral load rebound was reduced in all 15 patients on mycophenolate compared with 6 controls off all drugs. After a mean two years after stopping antiretrovirals, 12 of the 15 still had viral loads less than 10,000 copies/mL.

The mycophenolate researchers also tried adding 8 weeks of cyclosporin A to the regimen of 34 patients initiating HAART during primary infection (Khonkarly et al. 2005). There was no treatment interruption in this trial, and median follow-up was 28 months. Compared to a 43-person control group, the 34-person cyclosporin group contained a significantly greater percentage of persons with viral loads below 50 copies/mL through 36 weeks of follow-up. Otherwise, viral suppression was similar in the two arms. Mean increase in CD4 counts was higher in the cyclosporin arm, though this may merely reflect a difference in cell activation and lymph node sequestration.

The U.S. government HIV treatment guidelines consider therapy during early HIV to be "optional" (DHHS 2004). Persons diagnosed with primary infection should be counseled regarding the current rationale for early treatment, but they should also understand that the data supporting antiretroviral treatment during this stage of disease remain limited (DHHS 2004). Counseling should address the reality that, if the issue of treatment of primary HIV infection were set aside, many of these individuals may be able to defer therapy for chronic HIV infection for many years, depending upon their plasma HIV RNA "setpoints" (Mellors et al. 1995).

Patients should be informed that the basis for treating during acute HIV remains speculative. Treatment is expensive and associated with potential short-term and long-term toxicities. While on treatment, patients must strictly adhere to the regimen or risk developing drug-resistant virus that may limit future therapeutic options. Given the possibility of acquiring drug-resistant HIV from the source contact (Little et al. 2002), baseline resistance testing should also be strongly considered (see Objective IV.20 on Resistance Testing in this Update). If the decision has been made to treat early, initiation of therapy should not be delayed until resistance testing results are available. Because of the possibility of infection with NNRTI-resistant virus, consideration should be given to treating with a boosted-PI-based regimen or a regimen containing NRTIs, PIs, and NNRTIs, pending resistance test results.

Data are stronger for treatment during acute viremia, often before Western blot seroconversion (Hecht et al. 2005; Smith et al. 2003; Berrey et al. 2001), but the guidelines also recommend consideration of treatment for recent seroconverters (DHHS 2004). The rationale is that patients in this state may have immune systems that have not yet developed their best control over HIV.

An important remaining argument for treatment during acute or early HIV is that the high viral loads present during this period greatly increase an individual's infectiousness. Also, the virus of a patient with acute HIV infection is homogenous and genetically close to the acquired strain, which is presumably easily transmissible. Infectious fluids during this period do not contain antibodies that might interfere with transmission. In a mathematical model of heterosexual transmission, the per exposure risk of heterosexual transmission decreased 8-9 times between the peak risk at day 20 after infection and when the model predicted that the virologic setpoint would be reached (day 54) (Pilcher et al. 2004).

References

Berrey MM, Schacker T, Collier AC, et al. Treatment of primary human immunodeficiency virus type 1 infection with potent antiretroviral therapy reduces frequency of rapid progression to AIDS. *J Infect Dis.* **2001**;183:1466-1475.

Bloch M, Smith D, Grey P, et al. The role of hydroxyurea in enhancing the virological control achieved through structured treatment interruption in primary HIV infection: final results from a randomized clinical trial. In: Program and abstracts of the 12th Conference on Retroviruses and Opportunistic Infections; February 22-25, **2005**; Boston, Massachusetts. Abstract 569.

Ciuffreda D, Rizzardi GP, Tassan-Din C, et al. Single supervised treatment interruption coupled with mycophenolate mofetil therapy induces control of HIV-1 RNA replication in patients treated with ART since primary HIV-1 infection: 102-week follow-up. In: Program and abstracts of the 12th Conference on Retroviruses and Opportunistic Infections; February 22-25, **2005**; Boston, Massachusetts. Abstract 514.

Daar ES, Bai J, Hausner MA, Majchrowicz M, Tamaddon M, Giorgi JV. Acute HIV syndrome after discontinuation of antiretroviral therapy in a patient treated before seroconversion. *Ann Intern Med.* **1998**;128:827-829.

Department of Health and Human Services (DHHS). Guidelines for the use of antiretroviral agents in HIV-1-infected adults and adolescents. October 29, **2004**. Available at: http://AIDSinfo.nih.gov [accessed January 12, 2005].

Desquilbet L, Goujard C, Deveau C, et al. HIV-1 RNA viral load dynamics after discontinuation of early and effective HAART initiated during primary HIV-1 infection. In: Program and abstracts of the 11th Conference on Retroviruses and Opportunistic Infections; February 8-11, **2004**; San Francisco, California. Abstract 397.

Finzi D, Hermankova M, Pierson T, et al. Identification of a reservoir for HIV-1 in patients on highly active antiretroviral therapy. *Science.* **1997**;278:1295-1300.

Guadalupe M, Reay E, Sankaran S, et al. Mucosal CD4+ T-cell restoration and antigen-specific T-cell responses in HIV-1-infected individuals initiating therapy during primary vs chronic infection. In: Program and abstracts of the 12th Conference on Retroviruses and Opportunistic Infections; February 22-25, **2005**; Boston, Massachusetts. Abstract 314.

Hecht F, Wang L, Collier A, et al. Outcomes of HAART for acute/early HIV-1 infection after treatment discontinuation. In: Program and abstracts of the 12th Conference on Retroviruses and Opportunistic Infections; February 22-25, **2005**; Boston, Massachusetts. Abstract 568.

Hoen B, I Fournier I, Charreau I, et al. Structured treatment interruptions in primary HIV infection: final results of the multicenter prospective PRIMSTOP pilot trial. In: Program and abstracts of the 11th Conference on Retroviruses and Opportunistic Infections; February 8-11, **2004**; San Francisco, California. Abstract 395.

Jansen C, De Cuyper I, Steingrover R, et al. Differential effect of HAART during acute HIV infection on HIV-specific CD4+ T-cell proliferative capacity and function. In: Program and abstracts of the 11th Conference on Retroviruses and Opportunistic Infections; February 8-11, **2004**; San Francisco, California. Abstract 241.

Kaufmann DE, Lichterfeld M, Altfeld M, et al. Limited durability of viral control following treated acute HIV infection. *PLoS Med.* **2004**;1:e36

Khonkarly M, Tambussi G, Ciuffreda D, et al. Long-term benefit of cyclosporin A coupled with highly active antiretroviral therapy in primary HIV-1 infection. In: Program and abstracts of the 12th Conference on Retroviruses and Opportunistic Infections; February 22-25, **2005**; Boston, Massachusetts. Abstract 567.

Lisziewicz J, Rosenberg E, Lieberman J, et al. Control of HIV despite the discontinuation of antiretroviral therapy [letter]. *N Engl J Med.* **1999**;340:1683-1684.

Little SJ, Holte S, Routy J-P, et al. Antiretroviral-drug resistance among patients recently infected with HIV. *N Engl J Med.* **2002**;347:385-394.

Mellors JW, Kingsley LA, Rinaldo CR Jr, et al. Quantitation of HIV-1 RNA in plasma predicts outcome after seroconversion. *Ann Intern Med.* **1995**;122:573-579.

Pilcher CD, Tien HC, Eron JJ Jr, et al. Brief but efficient: acute HIV infection and the sexual transmission of HIV. *J Infect Dis*. **2004**; 189:1785-1792.

Rosenberg ES, Altfeld M, Poon SH, et al. Immune control of HIV-1 after early treatment of acute infection. *Nature*. **2000**;407:523-526.

Smith DE, Kaufmann GR, Kahn JO, et al. Greater reversal of CD4+ cell abnormalities and viral load reduction after initiation of antiretroviral therapy with zidovudine, lamivudine, and nelfinavir before complete HIV type 1 seroconversion. *AIDS Res Hum Retrovirus*. **2003**;19:189-199.

Zaunders J, Kaufmann D, Munier M, et al. Early proliferation and apparent loss of CCR5+ CD38+++ antigen-specific CD4+ Th1 effector cells during primary HIV-1 infection. In: Program and abstracts of the 12th Conference on Retroviruses and Opportunistic Infections; February 22-25, **2005**; Boston, Massachusetts. Abstract 286.

(RLO-16)

IV.2. INDICATIONS FOR INITIATING THERAPY

LEARNING OBJECTIVE: Summarize the latest guidelines for initiating HIV therapy by the Department of Health and Human Services (DHHS) and the International AIDS Society-USA Panel (IAS-USA).

U.S. Public Health Service Guidelines

The most recent DHHS guidelines continue to recommend therapy for all symptomatic patients and asymptomatic patients with CD4 counts below 200 cells/mm^3 (DHHS 2004). A greater emphasis is placed on CD4 count as a better prognostic predictor than viral load for those commencing therapy. Viral load is a comparatively minor factor in deciding to initiate therapy. The optimal CD4 threshold for beginning therapy in asymptomatic patients is unknown, but the available data indicate that it is in the range of 200-350 cells/mm^3. The DHHS guidelines therefore recommend that asymptomatic patients initiate therapy when their CD4 counts fall into this zone. They further recommend deferral of therapy in asymptomatic patients with CD4 counts above 350 cells/mm^3 and a viral load below 100,000 copies/mL. This advice is based on current data on the risk of disease progression after therapy commences. For asymptomatic patients with CD4 counts above 350 cells/mm^3 who have higher viral loads, the guidelines note that some physicians advocate initiating therapy, but most defer therapy and monitor the CD4 count and viral load every three months.

CD4 percentage may provide additional information regarding when to start HAART in patients with borderline absolute CD4 counts. In one study, an initial CD4 fraction less than 15% was found to be an independent predictor of mortality in 1623 patients starting HAART with CD4 cell counts between 200 and 340 cells/mm^3 (Moore et al. 2005).

Delayed initiation of HIV therapy is supported by the robust immune reconstitution that occurs in patients who wait until their CD4 count falls to 200-350 cells/mm^3 before initiating therapy. Deferring therapy preserves treatment options for the time when they are most needed, helps avoid drug toxicities and treatment fatigue, and gives a chance for research to develop better treatments and management techniques (DHHS 2004). However, no CD4 threshold is written in stone, and there are a number of reasons why some experts are beginning to think about earlier therapy (Holmberg et al. 2004). These include: (1) some cohort studies suggest benefit from earlier therapy (see Objective IV.4 on Delaying Initiation in this Update) and that longer-term follow-up may yield still better results; (2) current regimens are easier and better tolerated than earlier ones; (3) preservation of options for intermittent therapy, should that approach become standard; (4) the reduced cost of treating patients earlier in the disease process; and (5) reduced risk of HIV transmission.

Given the renewed emphasis on CD4 count, the recommendations for starting antiretroviral therapy are now the same for women as for men (DHHS 2004). Rates of disease progression are similar for men and women. Although some studies have indicated that women tend to have lower viral loads than men at the same CD4 count, this is only the case for the first five or six years of infection. CD4 counts in both men and women are generally too high to support initiating therapy during this early period. Pregnancy, however,

What's New

The DHHS and IAS-USA have revised their treatment guidelines.

Key Points

- For symptomatic patients and those with CD4 counts below 200 cells/mm^3, initiation of antiretroviral therapy is recommended.
- For asymptomatic patients with CD4 counts between 200 and 350 cells/mm^3, therapy should be considered especially if viral load is high or CD4 count decline is rapid.
- Therapy is not usually initiated in asymptomatic patients with CD4 counts above 350 cells/mm^3. Some clinicians consider therapy if such patients' viral load is above 100,000 copies/mL.
- Treatment guidelines do not delineate different sex-based thresholds for initiating therapy.
- Pregnancy is an indication for antiretroviral therapy regardless of CD4 count or HIV RNA. The purpose is to prevent perinatal HIV transmission.

is reason to at least temporarily initiate therapy regardless of CD4 count. The goal is to prevent mother-to-child-transmission. The typical regimen is combination antiretroviral therapy, although the U.S. Public Health Service Task Force (PHS) guidelines mention that women with viral loads below 1000 copies/mL may use the traditional three-part zidovudine regimen from ACTG trial 076 (PHS 2004).

For further discussion on delaying antiretroviral therapy, see Objective IV.4 on Delaying Initiation in this Update.

International AIDS Society-USA Panel Guidelines

Similar to the DHHS guidelines, the International AIDS Society-USA Panel (IAS-USA) guidelines (Yeni et al. 2004) recommend initiation of treatment for all symptomatic patients and those with CD4 counts below 200 cells/mm^3. For patients with CD4 counts from 200-350 cells/mm^3, the panel recommends that physicians "consider" treatment. Factors that enter into the individual decision to initiate therapy include CD4 count close to 200 cells/mm^3, high rate of CD4+ T cell loss (over 100 cells/mm^3/year), high viral load (over 100,000 copies/mL) and patient readiness. Therapy is generally not recommended when CD4 count is below 350 cells/mm^3. It may nonetheless merit consideration when viral load is high or CD4 count is declining rapidly.

Table IV.2-1 summarizes and compares the treatment guidelines from DHHS and IAS-USA.

Table IV.2-1. Summary of DHHS and IAS-USA guidelines for initiating antiretroviral therapy.

Disease type	DHHS recommendations	IAS-USA recommendations
Symptomatic HIV disease	Treatment recommended	Treatment recommended
Asymptomatic HIV disease, CD4 count <200 cells/mm^3	Treatment recommended	Treatment recommended
Asymptomatic HIV disease, CD4 count 201-350 cells/mm^3	Treatment should be offered following discussion with patient of risks and benefits	Treatment should be considered within the context of the individual patent's risk of progression
Asymptomatic HIV disease, CD4 count >350 cells/mm^3	Defer therapy if HIV RNA is <100,000 copies/mL; if HIV RNA >100,000 copies/mL, most experts would defer therapy while monitoring more closely	Continue monitoring; counsel on preventing HIV transmission; in patients with CD4 counts between 350 and 500 cells/mm^3, consider treatment if viral load is high or CD4+ T cell loss is rapid

Adapted from DHHS (2004, Table 4) and Yeni et al. (2004, Table 1).

References

Department of Health and Human Services (DHHS). Guidelines for the use of antiretroviral agents in HIV-1-infected adults and adolescents. October 29, **2004**. Available at: http://AIDSinfo.nih.gov [accessed November 9, 2004].

Holmberg SD, Palella FJ Jr, Lichtenstein KA, Havlir DV. The case for earlier treatment of HIV infection. *Clin Infect Dis*. **2004**;39:1699-1704.

Moore D, Hogg R, Yip B, et al. Baseline CD4 percentage is predictive of survival in patients starting antiretroviral therapy, including those with CD4 cell counts between 200 and 350 cells/microL. In Program and Abstracts of the 12th Conference on Retroviruses and Opportunistic Infections; February 22-25, **2005**; Boston, Massachusetts. Abstract 589.

Public Health Service (PHS). Recommendations for use of antiretroviral drugs in pregnant HIV-1-infected women for maternal health and interventions to reduce perinatal HIV-1 transmission in the United States. June 23, **2004**. Available at: http://AIDSinfo.nih.gov [accessed November 9, 2004].

Yeni PG, Hammer SM, Carpenter CCJ, et al. Treatment for adult HIV infection. 2004: recommendations of the International AIDS Society-USA Panel. *JAMA*. **2004**;292:222-235.

(RLO-17)

IV.4. DELAYING INITIATION

LEARNING OBJECTIVE: Identify advantages and disadvantages of delaying initiation of therapy in a patient with chronic HIV infection.

Changes Since the Introduction of HAART

In the past, there was concern that delayed initiation of therapy for chronic HIV could result in irreversible loss of specific components of the immunologic repertoire, such that later therapy-induced immune reconstitution might not result in protective immunity against, for example, specific opportunistic infections (Connors et al. 1997). However, subsequent experience has demonstrated effective immune reconstitution even in patients with advanced immunosuppression at the time they initiate therapy (as long as they are highly adherent to therapy). This is reflected in current guidelines on opportunistic infections from the U.S. Public Health Service, which endorse the discontinuation of primary and, in many cases, secondary prophylaxis against opportunistic infections after patients surpass specific CD4 count thresholds (CDC 2002).

A meta-analysis of four studies conducted early in the HAART era and using the same antiretroviral regimen (zidovudine, lamivudine and indinavir) at different stages of HIV infection (acute, early [CD4 count above 500 cells/mm^3], mid [CD4 count between 50 and 400 cells/mm^3] and late [CD4 count below 50 cells/mm^3]) found that a much larger proportion of patients with higher CD4 counts attained plasma viremia below 50 copies/mL, compared with those who had lower CD4 counts (Meibohm et al. 2000).

Later studies with various regimens have not borne out this finding. For example, the efavirenz- and lopinavir/ritonavir-based regimens currently preferred by the DHHS Guidelines (DHHS 2004) have both shown similar or comparable efficacy in patients with viral loads above and below 100,000 copies/mL (King et al. 2002; Staszewski et al. 1999). Nevertheless, investigators found that the risk of disease progression increased when treatment was initiated at CD4 counts below 200 cells/mm^3 (Ferrer et al. 2003; Sterling et al. 2003, 2001; Hogg et al. 2001). Two large observational studies – one including nearly 12,500 patients and the other 2700 – have reported no significant difference in 3-year risk of progression to AIDS or death between those starting therapy at CD4 counts between 200 and 350 cells/mm^3 and those starting with CD4 counts above this range (Egger et al. 2002; Kaplan et al. 2003). In both of these studies, the prognosis tended to be poorer for patients who started treatment with viral loads over 100,000 copies/mL.

Several smaller observational studies did find that earlier initiation of antiretroviral therapy led to improved long-term survival. These include the HOPS cohort, which found that 605 patients starting any antiretroviral therapy with a CD4 count between 200 and 350 cells/mm^3, experienced over 70% reduction in risk of death compared with patients who further deferred therapy (Palella et al. 2003). The Swiss HIV Cohort observed a similar 3-year reduction in AIDS or death among 283 patients who commenced HAART at a CD4 count greater than 350 cells/mm^3 (Opravil et al. 2002). Finally, a Johns Hopkins study of intravenous-drug users detected a doubling in mortality risk for patients who deferred

What's New

Several new cohort studies have again found that CD4 count at initiation of therapy ceases to be an important predictor of outcome above 200 cells/mm^3, although high viral load (over 100,000 copies/mL) may be an independent predictor of response to therapy. Some studies indicate better clinical outcome with treatment initiation at greater than 350 cells/mm^3. A crucial factor in persons starting therapy with low CD4 counts is adherence: Those who are adherent to therapy are likely to have an excellent response despite low baseline CD4 count.

Key Points

Advantages of deferring therapy:

- Deferred side effects and toxicities.
- Deferred development of resistance.
- Deferred costs.
- Drug efficacy retained in later disease.

Disadvantages of deferring therapy:

- If therapy is delayed until CD4 count is below 200 cells/mm^3, immunologic reconstitution and clinical outcomes on therapy may be compromised compared with earlier initiation.
- Therapy is tolerated less well in patients with more advanced HIV disease.
- Greater possibility of HIV transmission if therapy is delayed.
- Greater likelihood of transformation to X4-tropic or dual-tropic virus, thereby decreasing the benefit from CCR5 antagonists.

Key Points (cont.)

- Limited options for intermittent ("CD4-guided") therapy with prolonged treatment interruptions

therapy until their CD4 counts were less than 350 cells/mm^3 (Wang et al. 2004). Such findings suggest that there may be a benefit to even earlier initiation of therapy (i.e., with CD4 counts greater than 350 cells/mm^3) (see Objective IV. 2 on Indications for Initiating Therapy in this Update).

Adherence and Durable Response

For patients commencing therapy at a low CD4 count, the definitive factor might be adherence: In a study of some 1400 patients commencing antiretroviral therapy, British Columbian investigators observed that the 4-year survival rate was the same for nearly everyone with good adherence (whether defined as taking 75% or 95% of pills during the first year of therapy) (Wood et al. 2003). The sole exception was patients who began treatment after their CD4 counts had fallen to less than 200 cells/mm^3. Those with CD4 counts below 200 cells/mm^3 and adherence over 75% had an 80% survival rate compared with 91% and above for adherent patients in higher CD4 strata. But the patients with CD4 counts below 200 cells/mm^3 still had a lower risk of death than those with poor (less than 75%) adherence and higher pretreatment CD4 counts.

A follow-up analysis found that all patients initiating therapy with good adherence, even those with pretreatment CD4 counts below 50 cells/mm^3, had about the same rate of achieving a CD4 count increase of over 50 cells/mm^3 (Wood et al. 2004). Adherence of greater than 75% was the major determining factor (the only other observed significant factor was male sex). In contrast, CD4 counts changed little overall in the nonadherent subgroups. Substantial, durable increases in CD4 counts were observed in all of the adherent subgroups, including those starting treatment with less than 50 cells/mm^3, but the actual value of the week-75 CD4 count did vary according to pretreatment CD4.

In a EuroSIDA report involving almost 2400 patients, the risk of immunologic failure (at least 1 CD4 count less than or equal to the pre-HAART CD4 count) was greater in persons with higher pretreatment CD4 counts (Dragsted et al. 2004). The factors are complex. They may include lower adherence among patients commencing treatment at higher CD4 counts. Such patients may be less motivated to rigorously continue treatment because of their lower risk of disease progression. An inverse relationship between adherence and pretreatment CD4 count was an effect noted by the British Columbia researchers (Wood et al. 2004).

In those who do achieve sustained CD4+ T cell increases, the question remains as to whether immune status is the same at a given CD4 count regardless of the pretreatment CD4 nadir. A small study looked at 29 patients with posttreatment CD4 counts over 450 cells/mm^3 and viral loads under 400 copies/mL for at least a year. It found that response to vaccination varied according to pretreatment CD4 count. The results suggest that delaying therapy results in an attenuation of functional immune restoration (Lange et al. 2003).

Looking at virologic response, Johns Hopkins researchers found that those with a durable viral load reduction (majority of viral loads under 400 copies/mL) had no difference in disease progression, again, unless they started treatment with a CD4 count below 200, and particularly below 50 cells/mm^3 (Sterling et al. 2003). These late initiators also had a lower virologic suppression rate – 48% compared with about 60% for those starting treatment at

CD4 counts above 200 cells/mm^3. It should be borne in mind, though, that the later initiators contained a disproportionate number of injection-drug users. Egger and colleagues (2002) also found that injection drug use was an independent factor associated with disease progression after starting therapy.

Deferred Therapy and Treatment Interruptions

A hypothetical disadvantage of delayed therapy is that it may reduce the ability to interrupt therapy in the future. Most treatment interruption strategies are viewed with increasing skepticism (see Objective IV.29 on Treatment Interruptions in this Update). One approach to interrupted therapy, CD4-guided intermittent therapy, still attracts great interest. In the BASTA trial, 46 participants with CD4 counts greater than 800 cells/mm^3 and viral loads less than 50 copies/mL discontinued therapy until their CD4 counts fell below 400 cells/mm^3 irrespective of viral load (Maggiolo et al. 2004a). (There were 76 treatment interrupters in a later presentation from this trial [Maggiolo et al. 2004b].) These trial participants were supposed to again discontinue therapy once their CD4 count rebounded to greater than 800 cells/mm^3, but this phase of the trial has yet to be reported. The goal was to minimize time on treatment while maintaining CD4 counts within a more or less normal range. Time off therapy during the first interruption was highly dependent on nadir CD4 count before HAART (Maggiolo et al. 2004a). By month 17, none of the patients with nadir viral loads over 500 copies/mL had restarted treatment and only 10% of those with a nadir between 350 and 500 copies/mL had restarted. In contrast 40% of those with CD4 nadirs of 200-300 cells/mm^3 had restarted treatment by week 14, and all those with nadirs below 200 cells/mm^3 were back on treatment by month 10. Viral load rebounds were somewhat lower in patients with CD4 nadirs above 350 cells/mm^3.

Despite being allowed to remain off therapy, those with higher nadir CD4 consistently lost CD4+ T cells. Trial participants with CD4 nadirs above 500 cells/mm^3 dropped from a mean of 1200 cells/mm^3 to 850 cells/mm^3 over the first 48 weeks. The BASTA participants with higher CD4 nadirs have been able to endure longer treatment interruptions, but their CD4 trend is downward. The question remains: Did these early initiators gain any benefit from starting treatment in the first place? Without a deferred therapy control arm, treatment interruption trials cannot answer this central question.

The federal guidelines do not address whether patients who defer therapy are more likely to acquire X4-tropic or dual R5/X4-tropic HIV (Moyle et al. 2004). Such patients may lose the option of using the CCR5 antagonists now under development as entry blockers (see Objective IV.32 on Investigational Antiretroviral Agents in this Update).

Federal Treatment Guidelines

Current antiretroviral guidelines for adults and adolescents from the U.S. Public Health Service (DHHS 2004) recommend initiating therapy if patients' CD4 counts fall below 200 cells/mm^3 and that therapy should be "offered" to patients with 200-350 cells/mm^3 after considering all of the available data. The guidelines note that although therapy can be considered for patients with viral loads above 100,000 copies/mL, most clinicians would not initiate therapy at CD4 counts above 350 cells/mm^3 regardless of viral load. Instead, they would monitor patients more frequently if viral loads rise above 100,000 copies/mL.

The following risks and benefits should be considered before deferring therapy for asymptomatic HIV-infected persons who have higher CD4 counts (DHHS 2004).

Potential risks of deferred therapy include:

- The possibility that damage to the immune system, which might otherwise be salvaged by earlier therapy, is irreversible
- The increased possibility of progression to AIDS
- The increased risk for HIV transmission to others during a longer untreated period

Potential benefits of deferred therapy include:

- Avoidance of treatment-related negative effects on quality of life and drug-related toxicities
- Preservation of treatment options
- Delay in development of drug resistance if there is incomplete viral suppression
- More time for the patient to have a greater understanding of treatment demands
- Decreased total time on medication with reduced chance of treatment fatigue
- More time for the development of more potent, less toxic and better studied combinations of antiretrovirals

See also Objective IV. 2 on Indications for Initiating Therapy, and Objective IV. 1 on Treatment of Acute HIV, in this Update.

References

Centers for Disease Control (CDC). Guidelines for preventing opportunistic infections among HIV-infected persons — 2002 recommendations of the U.S. Public Health Service and the Infectious Diseases Society of America. *MMWR Morb Mortal Wkly Rep.* **2002**;51(RR-8).

Connors M, Kovacs JA, Krevat S, et al. HIV infection induces changes in CD4+ T-cell repertoire that are not immediately restored by antiviral or immune-based therapies. *Nature Med.* **1997**;3:533-540.

Department of Health and Human Services (DHHS). Guidelines for the use of antiretroviral agents in HIV-1-infected adults and adolescents. October 29, **2004**. Available at: http://AIDSinfo.nih.gov [accessed January 10, 2005].

Dragsted UB, Mocroft A, Vella S, et al. Predictors of immunological failure after initial response to highly active antiretroviral therapy in HIV-1-infected adults: a EuroSIDA study. *J Infect Dis.* **2004**;190:148-155.

Egger M, May M, Chene G, et al. Prognosis of HIV-1-infected patients starting highly active antiretroviral therapy: a collaborative analysis of prospective studies. *Lancet.* **2002**;360:119-129.

Ferrer E, Santamarina E, Santin M, et al. Progression to AIDS/death is higher in patients initiating antiretroviral therapy with CD4 counts below 350 cells/microL. In: Program and abstracts of the 10th Conference on Retroviruses and Opportunistic Infections; February 10-14, **2003**; Boston, Massachusetts. Poster 910.

Hogg RS, Yip B, Chan KJ, et al. Rates of disease progression by baseline CD4 cell count and viral load after initiating triple-drug therapy. *JAMA.* **2001**;286:2568-2577.

Kaplan JE, Hanson DL, Cohn DL, et al. When to begin highly active antiretroviral therapy? Evidence supporting initiation of therapy at CD4+ lymphocyte counts <350 cells/microL. *Clin Infect Dis.* **2003**;37:951-958.

King M, Bernstein B, Cernohous P, Moseley J, Bauer E, Sun E. Impact of baseline CD4 cell count and viral load on durability of virologic response through 96 weeks for lopinavir/ritonavir (LPV/r) and nelfinavir (NFV) in a phase III clinical trial. In: Program and abstracts of the 9th Conference on Retroviruses and Opportunistic Infections; February 24-28, **2002**; Seattle, Washington. Poster 470-M.

Lange CG, Lederman MM, Medvik K, et al. Nadir CD4+ T-cell count and numbers of CD28+ CD4+ T-cells predict functional responses to immunizations in chronic HIV-1 infection. *AIDS.* **2003**;17:2015-2023.

Maggiolo F, Ripamonti D, Gregis G, Quinzan G, Callegaro A, Suter F. Effect of prolonged discontinuation of successful antiretroviral therapy on CD4 T cells: a controlled, prospective trial. *AIDS.* **2004a**;18:439-446.

Maggiolo F, Ripamonti D, Trabattoni D, et al. Immunologic determinants of failure in individualized structured treatment interruptions. Should the timing of HAART be reconsidered? In: Program and Abstracts of the 11th Conference on Retroviruses and Opportunistic Infections; February 8-11, **2004b**; San Francisco, California. Abstract 238.

Meibohm A, Alexander J Jr, Robertson M, et al. Early versus late initiation of indinavir (IDV) in combination with zidovudine (ZDV) and lamivudine (3TC) in HIV-1-infected adults. In: Program and abstracts of the 7th Conference on Retroviruses and Opportunistic Infections; January 30-February 2, **2000**; San Francisco, California. Abstract 521.

Moyle G, Wildfire A, Mandalia S, et al. Prevalence and predictive factors for CCR5 and CXCR4 co-receptor usage in a large cohort of HIV positive individuals. In: Program and abstracts of the 44th Interscience Conference on Antimicrobial Agents and Chemotherapy; October 30-November 2, **2004**; Washington, DC. Abstract H-566/359.

Opravil M, Ledergerber B, Furrer H, et al. Clinical efficacy of early initiation of HAART in patients with asymptomatic HIV infection and CD4 cell count > 350 x 10(6) /l. *AIDS.* **2002**;16:1371-1381.

Palella FJ Jr, Deloria-Knoll M, Chmiel JS, et al. Survival benefit of initiating antiretroviral therapy in HIV-infected persons in different CD4+ cell strata. *Ann Int Med.* **2003**;138:620-626.

Staszewski S, Morales-Ramirez J, Tashima KT, et al. Efavirenz plus zidovudine and lamivudine, efavirenz plus indinavir, and indinavir plus zidovudine and lamivudine in the treatment of HIV-1 infection in adults. *N Engl J Med.* **1999**;341:1865-1873.

Sterling TR, Chaisson RE, Moore RD. HIV-1 RNA, CD4 T-lymphocytes, and clinical response to highly active antiretroviral therapy. *AIDS.* **2001**;15:2251-2257.

Sterling TR, Chaisson RE, Keruly J, Moore RD. Improved outcomes with earlier initiation of highly active antiretroviral therapy among human immunodeficiency virus-infected patients who achieve durable virologic suppression: longer follow-up of an observational cohort study. *J Infect Dis.* **2003**;188:1659-1665.

Wang C, Vlahov D, Galai N, et al. Mortality in HIV-seropositive versus -seronegative persons in the era of highly active antiretroviral therapy: implications for when to initiate therapy. *J Infect Dis.* **2004**;190:1046-1054.

Wood E, Hogg RS, Yip B, Harrigan PR, O'Shaughnessy MV, Montaner JS. Effect of medication adherence on survival of HIV-infected adults who start highly active antiretroviral therapy when the CD4+ cell count is 0.200 to 0.350 x 10(9) cells/L. *Ann Int Med.* **2003**;139:810-816.

Wood E, Hogg RS, Yip B, Harrigan PR, O'Shaughnessy MV, Montaner JS. The impact of adherence on CD4 cell count responses among HIV-infected patients. *J Acquir Immune Defic Syndr.* **2004**;35:261-268.

(RLO-18)

IV.6. ANTIRETROVIRAL DOSING FOR FDA-APPROVED AGENTS

LEARNING OBJECTIVE: Describe the usual dosing, dose modifications for weight or impaired renal or liver clearance, and contraindications for current FDA-approved antiretroviral therapies.

Table IV.6-1. Currently FDA-approved antiretrovirals*.

NRTIs and NtRTIs
abacavir, Ziagen (ABC) abacavir/lamivudine, Epzicom, Kivexa abacavir/lamivudine/zidovudine, Trizivir didanosine, Videx and Videx EC (ddI) emtricitabine, Emtriva (FTC) emtricitabine/tenofovir DF, Truvada lamivudine, Epivir (3TC) lamivudine/zidovudine, Combivir stavudine, Zerit (d4T) tenofovir DF, Viread (TDF) zalcitabine, Hivid (ddC) zidovudine, Retrovir (AZT)
NNRTIs
delavirdine, Rescriptor (DLV) efavirenz, Sustiva, Stocrin (EFV) nevirapine, Viramune (NVP)
Protease inhibitors
amprenavir, Agenerase (APV) fosamprenavir, Lexiva, Telzir (fAPV or FPV) atazanavir, Reyataz (ATV) indinavir, Crixivan (IDV) lopinavir/ritonavir, Kaletra (LPV/RTV) nelfinavir, Viracept (NFV) ritonavir, Norvir (RTV) saquinavir, Invirase, Fortovase (SQV)
Fusion inhibitors
enfuvirtide, Fuzeon (ENF, T-20)

*as of February 2005

Hypersensitivity

There are few absolute contraindications listed in the package inserts for antiretrovirals currently approved by the U.S. Food and Drug Administration. Allergy or a hypersensitivity to the drug in question is always listed as an absolute contraindication. The FDA-approved package inserts for abacavir, abacavir/lamivudine (Epzicom) (Epzicom 2004); abacavir/lamivudine/zidovudine (Trizivir) (Trizivir 2003); and nevirapine (Viramune 2005) have black box warnings informing clinicians that hypersensitivity reactions are more frequent with these agents and can sometimes be fatal. As with any drug, the recently approved fixed-dose combinations of antiretrovirals are contraindicated for patients with previously demonstrated hypersensitivity to any components of these agents (Truvada 2005; Epzicom 2004).

What's New

Recognition of potential drug-drug interactions with other medications, both antiretroviral and non-antiretroviral, is important for optimal therapeutic potency and side-effect mitigation. Updated guidelines for tenofovir dosing in patients with renal insufficiency are included here. Dosing of the recently approved fixed-dose combinations abacavir/lamivudine (Epzicom) and emtricitabine/tenofovir DF (Truvada) require special attention in patients with renal impairment. Also, abacavir/lamivudine (Epzicom) is contraindicated for patients with hepatic impairment because the dose cannot be adjusted.

Key Points

- Abacavir, abacavir/lamivudine (Epzicom), lamivudine/zidovudine/abacavir (Trizivir) and nevirapine carry warnings about possibly severe hypersensitivity reactions. Stavudine combined with didanosine has been associated with potentially fatal lactic acidosis, particularly during pregnancy.
- Tenofovir DF, emtricitabine and emtricitabine/tenofovir DF (Truvada) require dose interval adjustments in patients with renal insufficiency.
- Administration of tenofovir DF or emtricitabine/tenofovir DF (Truvada) with didanosine requires reduced doses of didanosine and should be avoided altogether in therapy-naive persons.
- When atazanavir is coadministered with emtricitabine/tenofovir DF (Truvada), concomitant ritonavir is recommended (300 mg ATV and 100 mg RTV).

Key Points (cont.)

- The combination of fosamprenavir and lopinavir/ritonavir (Kaletra) should be used with caution, and preferably only with therapeutic drug monitoring (TDM). There are negative bidirectional drug interactions with this combination and the optimal dose has not been determined.
- Table IV.6-3 gives current guidance for usual dosing and dosing adjustments in the presence of renal or hepatic failure for most antiretroviral agents.

Hepatic Metabolism Alterations

Certain antiretrovirals induce or inhibit hepatic metabolism of coadministered agents, resulting in the following contraindications listed in the package inserts:

- Efavirenz is contraindicated in the presence of ergotamine derivatives (e.g., Cafergot), the gastrointestinal motility agent cisapride (Propulsid), the benzodiazepine sedative/hypnotics midazolam (Versed) and triazolam (Halcion), the neuroleptic pimozide (Orap), and the now-discontinued antihistamines astemizole (Hismanal) and terfenadine (Seldane).
- The protease inhibitors currently approved by the U.S. Food and Drug Administration (FDA) are all contraindicated in the presence of ergotamine derivatives, cisapride (Propulsid), midazolam (Versed) and triazolam (Halcion).
- All protease inhibitors except nelfinavir are also contraindicated with pimozide (Orap) and the discontinued antihistamines astemizole (Hismanal) and terfenadine (Seldane).
- Ritonavir and lopinavir/ritonavir are also contraindicated with the antiarrhythmics flecainide (Tambocor) and propafenone (Rythmol). Ritonavir at treatment doses is contraindicated in the presence of the antiarrhythmic bepridil (Vascor).
- Both nelfinavir and ritonavir are contraindicated in the presence of quinidine preparations and amiodarone (Cordarone).
- Atazanavir and fosamprenavir are contraindicated with many common medications. See Table IV.6-2 below for a complete list.
- As of January 2005, use of nevirapine is contraindicated in adult females with CD4 cell counts greater than 250 cells/mm^3 and in adult males with CD4 cell counts greater than 400 cells/mm^3. The product labeling recommends starting nevirapine in these populations only if the benefit outweighs the risk of severe hepatotoxicity (Viramune 2005). For more on nevirapine toxicity, see Objective IV.8 on Common Antiretroviral Toxicities in this Update.

Table IV.6-2. Drugs that should not be co-administered with atazanavir and fosamprenavir.

Drug class of contraindicated agents	Atazanavir sulfate (Reyataz 2004)	Fosamprenavir calcium (Lexiva 2004)
Ergot derivatives	Dihydroergotamine Ergonovine Ergotamine Methylergonovine	
GI motility agents	Cisapride	
Benzodiazepines (sedatives/hypnotics)	Midazolam Triazolam	
HMG Co-A reductase inhibitors	Lovastatin Simvastatin	
Antimycobacterials	Rifampin*	
Herbal products	St. John's wort *(Hypericum perforatum)*	
Neuroleptics	Pimozide	
Proton-pump inhibitors	Proton-pump inhibitors	
Antineoplastics	Irinotecan	
Antiarrhythmics		If coadministered with ritonavir: flecainide and propafenone
NNRTIs		Delavirdine
Protease inhibitors	Indinavir	

* Concurrent rifampin substantially reduces atazanavir levels even when administering elevated doses of ritonavir-boosted atazanavir (Burger 2005).

Antiretroviral Drugs and Renal Impairment

Most NRTIs and NtRTIs require dose adjustment in persons with baseline renal dysfunction; see Table IV.6-3.

Recent reports on the renal impairment associated with tenofovir DF are contradictory. Some report no renal impairment, while others report modest declines in renal function (see Objective IV. 8 on Common Antiretroviral Toxicities in this Update). Kearney et al. (2002) concluded from Study 919 that tenofovir DF was generally well tolerated and that tenofovir pharmacokinetics are such that dose modification is not required in patients with creatinine clearance of at least 50 mL/min. Those with a creatinine clearance below 50 mL/min have higher systemic exposures (C_{max} and area under the curve), necessitating a longer dosing interval (see Table IV.6-3).

Table IV.6-3. Dosing adjustments in the presence of renal or hepatic failure.

Drug name	Usual adult dose	Renal insufficiency			Dosing in hemodialysis	Hepatic failure*
AZT (Retrovir)	300 mg b.i.d.	"Severe renal disease" – 100 mg t.i.d. or 300 mg q.d.			100 mg t.i.d. or 300 mg q.d.[a]	Usual dose
ddI (Videx)	Weight >60 kg: 400 mg q.d. Weight <60 kg: 250 mg q.d.	**CrCl†**	**>60 kg**	**<60 kg**	Same as for CrCl <10[a]	Usual dose
		30-59	200 mg/d	125 mg/d		
		10-29	125 mg/d	100 mg/d		
		<10	125 mg/d	75 mg/d		
d4T (Zerit)	Weight >60 kg: 40 mg b.i.d. Weight <60 kg 30 mg b.i.d.	**CrCl†**	**>60 kg**	**<60 kg**	Same as for CrCl 10-25[a]	Usual dose
		26-50	20 mg b.i.d.	15 mg b.i.d.		
		10-25	20 mg q.d.	15 mg q.d.		
ddC (Hivid)	0.75 mg t.i.d.	**CrCl†**			No data	Usual dose
		10-40	0.75 mg b.i.d.			
		<10	0.75 mg q.d.			
3TC (Epivir)	300 mg q.d. or 150 mg b.i.d.	**CrCl†**			No data	Usual dose
		30-49	150 mg q.d.			
		15-29	150 mg first dose, then 100 mg q.d.			
		5-14	150 mg first dose, then 50 mg q.d.			
		<5	50 mg first dose, then 25 mg q.d.			
FTC (Emtriva)	200 mg q.d.	**CrCl†**			200 mg q96h[a]	Usual dose
		30-49	200 mg every 48 hr			
		15-29	200 mg every 72 hr			
		<15	200 mg every 96 hr			
TDF (Viread)	300 mg q.d.	**CrCl†**			300 mg/wk[a]	Usual dose
		30-49	300 mg every 48 hr			
		10-29	300 mg b.i.w.			
		<10	300 mg/wk			
		Dosing for GFR >50 mL/min	**Dosing for GFR 10-50 mL/min**	**Dosing for GFR <10 mL/min**		
ABC (Ziagen)	300 mg b.i.d.	Usual dose	Usual dose	Usual dose	Usual dose	Usual dose
EFV (Sustiva, Stocrin)	600 mg q.d.	Usual dose likely[b]	Usual dose	Usual dose likely[b]	Usual dose	Use with caution
NVP (Viramune)	200 mg q.d. for 14 days, then 200 mg b.i.d.	Usual dose[b]	Usual dose	Usual dose	Usual dose	Avoid use with severe liver disease
DLV (Rescriptor)	400 mg t.i.d.	Usual dose	Usual dose likely[b]	Usual dose likely[b]	Usual dose	Use with caution
NFV (Viracept)	750 mg t.i.d. or 1250 mg b.i.d.	Usual dose	Usual dose	Usual dose	Usual dose[a]	Use with caution
IDV (Crixivan)	800 mg t.i.d	Usual dose	Usual dose	Usual dose	Usual dose	600 mg q8h

Table IV.6-3. Dosing adjustments in the presence of renal or hepatic failure *(continued)*.

Drug name	Usual adult dose	Renal insufficiency			Dosing in hemodialysis	Hepatic failure*
		Dosing for GFR >50 mL/min	Dosing for GFR 10-50 mL/min	Dosing for GFR <10 mL/min		
RTV (Norvir)	600 mg b.i.d.	Usual dose	Usual dose	Usual dose	Usual dose	Use with caution
SQV (Invirase, Fortovase)	*Invirase used only with RTV:* 1000/100 mg b.i.d. or 2000/100 mg q.d. *Fortovase:* 1200 mg t.i.d.	Usual dose	Usual dose	Usual dose	Usual dose	Use with caution
APV (Agenerase)[c]	1200 mg b.i.d.	Usual dose	Usual dose likely[b]	Usual dose likely[b]	Usual dose likely[b] (no data)	**CP score**[‡] 5-8: 450 mg b.i.d. 9-12: 300 mg b.i.d.[b]
fAPV (Lexiva, Telzir)	1400 mg b.i.d.	Usual dose	Usual dose	Usual dose	Usual dose	**CP score**[‡] 6-8: 700 mg b.i.d. 9-12: Avoid
ATV (Reyataz)	400 mg q.d.	Usual dose	Usual dose	Usual dose	Usual dose	**CP score**[‡] 7-9: 300 mg q.d. >9: Avoid
LPV/RTV (Kaletra)	400/100 mg b.i.d.	Usual dose	Usual dose likely	Usual dose likely	Usual dose	Use with caution
T-20, ENF (Fuzeon)	90 mg SQ b.i.d.	Usual dose	Usual dose	Usual dose	Usual dose	Usual dose

* Lactic acidosis syndrome should be ruled out before treating for hepatic failure.

† CrCl = creatinine clearance in mL/min.

For men CrCl equals (140 – age in years) x wt (kg)/72 x serum creatinine
For women, multiply this value x 0.85

‡ CP score=Child-Pugh score

[a] Administer post dialysis on dialysis days. Hemodialysis removes significant amounts of ddI, d4T, ddC, 3TC, TDF and NFV. Hemodialysis removes little or no AZT, ABC, EFV, NVP, IDV, RTV, SQV and LPV/r. There is little information on removal by peritoneal dialysis. Removal is anticipated or established with d4T as well as ddC, which should be dosed post dialysis. TDF is not recommended with peritoneal dialysis. Others are not removed or are not expected to be removed.

[b] Avoid APV liquid due to its propylene glycol content.

[c] Agenerase 150mg capsules are no longer available (GlaxoSmithKline 2004).

Reprinted with permission from Bartlett and Gallant 2004.

Antiretroviral Interactions

Several of the newest antiretrovirals require boosting with ritonavir to counter drug-drug interactions. When atazanavir is administered with tenofovir DF, whether alone or in combination with emtricitabine in the form of Truvada, ritonavir boosting is recommended (ATV/RTV 300/100 mg once daily) due to the induced decrease in atazanavir levels (Truvada 2005; Reyataz 2004). For the same reason, atazanavir should be boosted with ritonavir when combined with efavirenz (300/100 mg once daily for treatment-naive patients, but no dosing recommendations as yet for treatment-experienced patients) (Reyataz 2004). The same issue has come up with nevirapine: Data indicate that trough plasma levels of atazanavir are significantly decreased in patients concurrently taking nevirapine (Winston 2005). No dosing recommendations have been established for this combination (Reyataz 2004).

When fosamprenavir and ritonavir are given once daily with efavirenz, an additional 100 mg/day (300 mg total) of ritonavir is recommended (Lexiva 2004), but this is not required when lopinavir/ritonavir (Kaletra) is given twice daily.

Didanosine levels increase when coadministered with tenofovir, causing or worsening didanosine-related toxicities (pancreatitis [Martinez et al. 2004], lactic acidosis [Murphy 2003] and peripheral neuropathy [Videx 2004]). When administering both didanosine and tenofovir, it is recommended that the didanosine EC dose be decreased to 250 mg once daily (in adults weighing over 60 kg with creatinine clearance over 60 mL/min) or to 200 mg (in adults weighing under 60 kg with creatinine clearance over 60 mL/min) (Videx 2004). However, recent studies caution against the coadministering of tenofovir with didanosine as the nucleoside backbone in antiretroviral-naive patients due to higher rates of virologic failure and lower CD4 gains — see Objective IV.15 on Antiretroviral Interactions, and Objective IV.18 on Not-Recommended Antiretroviral Combinations, in this Update.

A number of additional clinically significant drug-drug interactions are detailed elsewhere in this Update: Objective IV.9 on Antiretroviral Interactions with Non-Antiretroviral Drugs; Objective IV.15 on Antiretroviral Interactions; and, Objective IV.17 on Boosted Protease Inhibitors.

References

Bartlett JG, Gallant JE. *Medical Management of HIV Infection*. Baltimore, Md: Johns Hopkins University School of Medicine; **2004**: table 4-23.

Bristol-Myers Squibb. Healthcare provider important drug warning letter. January 5, **2001**. Available at: http://www.fda.gov/medwatch/Safety/2001/Zerit&Videx_letter.htm [accessed February 12, 2005].

Burger D, Agarwala S, Child M, Wang Y, Grasela D. Effect of rifampin on steady-state pharmacokinetics of atazanavir and ritonavir in healthy subjects. In: Program and abstracts of the 12th Conference on Retroviruses and Opportunistic Infections; February 22-25, **2005**; Boston, Massachusetts. Abstract 657.

Epzicom (abacavir and lamivudine) [prescribing information]. Research Triangle Park, NC: GlaxoSmithKline. August **2004**.

GlaxoSmithKline. Dear Health Care Professional letter, September **2004**. Available at: http://www.fda.gov/cder/drug/shortages/AgeneraseLetter_E2.pdf [accessed April 20, 2005].

Kearney BP, Liaw S, Yale K, et al. Pharmacokinetics following single dose administration of tenofovir DF in subjects with renal impairment. In: Program and abstracts of the 6th International Congress on Drug Therapy in HIV; November 17-20, **2002**; Glasgow, Scotland. Poster P4.

Lexiva (fosamprenavir) [prescribing information]. Research Triangle Park, NC: GlaxoSmithKline. December **2004**.

Martinez E, Milinkovic A, de Lazzari E, et al. Pancreatic toxic effects associated with co-administration of didanosine and tenofovir in HIV-infected adults. *Lancet*. **2004**;364:65-67.

Murphy MD, O'Hearn M, Chou S. Fatal lactic acidosis and acute renal failure after addition of tenofovir to an antiretroviral regimen containing didanosine. *Clin Infect Dis*. **2003**;36:1082-1085.

Reyataz (atazanavir) [prescribing information]. Princeton, NJ: Bristol-Myers Squibb Company. October **2004**.

Trizivir (abacavir sulfate, lamivudine, and zidovudine) [prescribing information]. Research Triangle Park, NC: GlaxoSmithKline. November **2003**.

Truvada (emtricitabine and tenofovir DF) [prescribing information]. Foster City, Calif: Gilead Sciences, Inc. January **2005**.

Videx EC (didanosine) [prescribing information]. Princeton, NJ: Bristol-Myers Squibb; January **2004**.

Viramune (nevirapine) [prescribing information]. Ridgefield, Conn: Boehringer Ingelheim. January **2005**.

Winston A, Bloch M, Carr A, et al. The clinical correlations of trough plasma atazanavir levels in a cohort of HIV-1-positive individuals receiving HAART. In: Program and abstracts of the 12th Conference on Retroviruses and Opportunistic Infections; February 22-25, **2005**; Boston, Massachusetts. Abstract 656.

(RLO-19)

IV.7. PHARMACOGENOMICS

LEARNING OBJECTIVE: Discuss recent data on how pharmacogenomics may affect antiretroviral management in clinical practice, e.g., abacavir hypersensitivity reaction, atazanavir-induced hyperbilirubinemia and efavirenz pharmacokinetics.

Pharmacogenomics is the study of the molecular basis of drug therapy outcomes. The pharmacogenomic study of HIV treatments is relatively recent but has already proven critical to understanding and preventing genomically determined drug toxicity. In other therapeutic areas, such as oncology and organ transplantation, pharmacogenomics has substantially improved clinical outcomes. The survival rate in childhood acute lymphocytic leukemia was substantially increased following the identification of polymorphisms responsible for the metabolism of chemotherapeutics (reviewed in McLeod et al. 2000). In solid organ transplantation, pharmacogenomic study has shown that rejection rates are a function of the donor organ P-glycoprotein genotype that is encoded by the *MDR1* gene that influences the drug concentrations in the transplanted organ. Genetic testing for *MDR1* allows for individualized dosing of antirejection agents intended to increase survival rates (reviewed in Staatz et al. 2004).

Therapies for HIV are complex, involving multiple agents that often interact, directed at different drug targets. Enzymes responsible for metabolism (e.g., cytochrome P450) and drug transporters involved in cellular entry (i.e., influx pump and efflux pump [e.g., P-glycoprotein]) have variable expression and function among individuals. Sex-related (Fletcher et al. 2004) and race-related (Hernandez et al. 2003) differences in antiretroviral drug disposition may underlie differences in treatment response. Additionally, variability in drug receptor targets (Turriziani et al. 2003) and host immune characteristics (Boehringer Ingelheim 2004) suggest that genetic factors may have a clinical affect on agents commonly used to treat HIV.

Overview

Pharmacogenomics can be divided into two broad categories: immunogenetics and pharmacogenetics. Immunogenetics uses both genetics and immunology to determine the genetics responsible for antibody formation and the immune response. Host immune factors appear to determine the hypersensitivity reaction (HSR) associated with some antiretroviral agents, such as abacavir (Martin et al. 2004) and nevirapine (Martin et al. 2005). The interaction between host genetic and environmental factors is illustrated in the complexity of the nevirapine reactions where haplotype (HLA; i.e., one set of alleles of linked genes) (Martin et al. 2005) and immune competence, (i.e., CD4 count) determine the likelihood of drug toxicity (Baylor and Johann-Liang 2004; Boehringer Ingelheim 2004).

Pharmacogenetics is an amalgamation of pharmacology and genetics dealing with genetically determined responses to drug therapy. An example of pharmacogenetic factors leading to drug toxicity is the presence of one or more variant alleles that significantly predict a higher probability of unconjugated hyperbilirubinemia associated with atazanavir treatment (O'Mara 2003, 2000).

What's New

This learning objective is new to the AAHIVM Core Curriculum. See Key Points below for highlights.

Key Points

- Genetic variability of drug-metabolizing enzymes, targets and transporters, and immune characteristics have a clinical effect on agents commonly used to treat HIV.
- Immunogenetic factors are the basis for drug-induced hypersensitivity reactions associated with abacavir and nevirapine treatment.
- Pharmacogenetic factors are the basis for hyperbilirubinemia associated with atazanavir treatment.

Immunogenetic Factors

Several immunogenic mechanisms can underlie HSRs. The most likely is the introduction of a drug or a reactive metabolite to endogenous peptides prior to T-cell presentation. The resulting release of inflammatory and proinflammatory cytokines and chemokines initiates a cascade of molecular events ultimately manifesting in the clinical features of HSR. In addition to abacavir and nevirapine, HSRs have been associated with several other agents commonly used in HIV treatment, such as sulfamethoxazole (Septra 2004), dapsone (Dapsone 1997), enfuvirtide (Fuzeon 2003), efavirenz (Sustiva 2004) and amprenavir (Agenerase 2004).

Abacavir hypersensitivity

Abacavir hypersensitivity occurs in approximately 8% of patients (Ziagen 2004). The immunogenetic basis for abacavir-induced HSR was suspected when a familial pattern of occurrence (Hetherington et al. 2002) and a reduced frequency in men and black populations was observed (Hernandez et al. 2003). The ancestral haplotype (i.e., major histocompatibility alleles inherited in blocks) HLA-B*5701 has been implicated with differing frequencies depending on the racial mix of the study population (Martin et al. 2004; Hetherington et al. 2002). In the racially homogeneous population of Western Australia, HLA-B*5701 occurred in 78% of patients presenting with HSR (Mallal et al. 2002), while in the racially diverse population in the United States, the HLA-B57 rate was 46% (Hetherington et al. 2002). Isolation of additional genetic loci has improved the identification of genetic characteristics of those at risk. The combination of HLA-B*5701, HLA-DR7 and HLA-DQ3 resulted in a positive predictive value of 100% and a negative predictive value of 97% to predict abacavir HSR (Mallal et al. 2002).

Although the precise mechanism of HSR remains unknown, it appears that HLA genetic predisposition is associated with a second loci, a variant allele within the heat shock proteins also carried on the ancestral HLA-B*5701 haplotype (Martin et al. 2004).

Genetic testing for abacavir HSR before treatment initiation can identify patients at risk of developing HSR. Such genetic testing is routinely used in Western Australia, where predictive value is high, and may reduce the rate of HSR to 2% to 5% (Mallal et al. 2002). However, in a racially mixed society, such as the United States, the likely lower predictive value of the test has precluded routine use.

For information on the clinical management of abacavir hypersensitivity, see Objective IV.8 on Common Antiretroviral Toxicities in this Update.

Nevirapine hypersensitivity

Nevirapine HSR includes rash, constitutional symptoms and hepatitis, either alone or in combination. Recent research suggests an HLA-mediated mechanism for these toxicities (Martin et al. 2005), as the presence of both HLA-DRB1*0101 and greater than 25% CD4+ T cells had a 40% positive and 96% negative predictive value of hepatic/systemic nevirapine reactions. Other research has shown that nevirapine hepatotoxicity is related to sex and CD4 count, e.g. risk of severe hepatotoxicity is increased 12-fold in women with CD4 counts greater than 250 cells/mm^3 (Boehringer Ingelheim 2004) and the risk increased in men with CD4 counts above 400 cells/mm^3 (Dieterich et al. 2004).

Pharmacogenetic Factors

In the 1970s, genetic determinants of pharmacokinetics were discovered when variation in the conjugative enzyme *n*-acetyltransferase (then termed slow and fast acetylators) was found to be associated with drug toxicity (Drayer et al. 1977; Ellard et al. 1975). Variability in drug-metabolizing enzyme expression is considerable and affects both the phase I or cytochrome P450 enzyme system, and a number of phase II or conjugative enzymes. This variability in enzyme expression, i.e., the genotype, underlies the response to therapy, i.e., the phenotype, for many drug classes. The genetic factors most responsible for differences in therapeutic response are variants in the drug-metabolizing enzyme systems and drug transporters. Genetic variation may take the form of amino acid substitutions in proteins, known as single nucleotide polymorphism (SNP; pronounced "snip"), or at a level involving an association of genes, i.e., haplotype.

Pharmacogenomic studies use both haplotype and SNP approaches. SNPs associated with drug-metabolizing enzymes or drug transporters are a common phenomenon but do not always result in a significant pharmacodynamic outcome. The following examples demonstrate the importance of haplotype and SNP variations.

Atazanavir and hyperbilirubinemia

Atazanavir, a recently approved protease inhibitor, inhibits the conjugative enzyme uridine diphosphate-glucuronosyltransferase (UGT1A1) (Reyataz 2004; O'Mara 2003). This enzyme is responsible for the metabolism of bilirubin (O'Mara et al. 2003). In individuals with UGT1A1 deficiency, unconjugated bilirubin accumulates and can induce jaundice. Any underlying deficiency of the UGT1A1 enzyme determines the occurrence of the hyperbilirubinemia (Bosma et al. 1995) and/or jaundice. The rates of wild type (6/6) and allelic variants (6/7 or 7/7, hetero- and homozygous variants, respectively) vary widely in the population, and the risk of hyperbilirubinemia appears to correlate not only with higher atazanavir exposure but also with the presence of specific alleles of the gene responsible for UGT1A1 expression (O'Mara et al. 2003, 2000; Raijmakers et al. 2000; Monaghan et al. 1996; Bosma et al. 1995).

Note that this toxicity does not represent hepatotoxicity because no elevation of aminotransferase (AST/ALT) levels is present. Should jaundice result, discontinuation of atazanavir will result in normalization of serum bilirubin levels and resolution of icterus (Reyataz 2004).

Efavirenz pharmacokinetics

Pharmacogenomic evaluation of efavirenz found that a SNP at position 516 of the CYP2B6 enzyme is associated with decreased clearance and possibly central nervous system (CNS) adverse events (Haas et al. 2004). The allelic variant, genotype T/T, more common among African Americans, is associated with increased plasma levels of efavirenz and a near threefold increase in the area under the time-concentration curve (Haas et al. 2004). All is not so straightforward, however. Further study by Haas and colleagues found that the T/T genotype, while decreasing efavirenz clearance, is not associated with treatment outcome (Haas et al. 2005). Moreover, a study of patients in the Johns Hopkins AIDS clinic observed twofold greater efavirenz discontinuation among African Americans compared with whites due to more frequent virologic failure, not toxicity (Moore et al. 2005). This would not seem to be the result of the higher efavirenz plasma levels that Haas and colleagues detected.

Conclusions

Pharmacogenomics is a powerful tool to investigate variable responses to pharmacotherapies and adverse effects, such as the HSRs associated with abacavir and nevirapine, the hyperbilirubinemia associated with atazanavir, and the CNS effects possibly associated with efavirenz. The study of pharmacogenomics has evolved from the phenotype-to-genotype approach to a genotype-to-clinical phenotype method. Advances in molecular biology have made it possible to identify variant alleles in a wide variety of drug-metabolizing enzymes, transporters and targets. These polymorphic genotypes are matched, where possible, with examples of clinically variant responses to therapy. The potential of pharmacogenomics to *individualize* therapy based on genetic constitution has been touted as the "promise of the human genome project."

References

Agenerase (amprenavir) [prescribing information]. Research Triangle Park, NC: GlaxoSmithKline; February **2004**.

Baylor MS, Johann-Liang R. Hepatotoxicity associated with nevirapine use. *J Acquir Immune Defic Syndr.* **2004**;35:538-539.

Beutler E, Gelbart T, Demina A. Racial variability in the UDP-glucuronosyltransferase 1 (UGT1A1) promoter: a balanced polymorphism for regulation of bilirubin metabolism? Proc Natl Acad Sci U S A. **1998**;95:8170-8174.

Boehringer Ingelheim. Important new safety information re: Clarification of risk factors for severe, life-threatening and fatal hepatotoxicity with VIRAMUNE (nevirapine)[letter]. February **2004**. Available at: http://www.fda.gov/medwatch/SAFETY/2004/viramune_deardoc_Feb04.pdf [accessed February 14, 2005].

Bosma PJ, Chowdhury JR, Bakker C, et al. The genetic basis of the reduced expression of bilirubin UDP-glucuronosyltransferase 1 in Gilbert's syndrome. *N Engl J Med.* **1995**;333:1171-1175.

Dapsone [prescribing information]. Princeton, NJ: Jacobus Pharmaceutical Co, Inc; June **1997**.

Dieterich DT, Robinson PA, Love J, Stern JO. Drug-induced liver injury associated with the use of nonnucleoside reverse-transcriptase inhibitors. *Clin Infect Dis.* **2004**;38(suppl 2):S80-S89.

Drayer DE, Reidenberg MM. Clinical consequences of polymorphic acetylation of basic drugs [commentary]. *Clin Pharmacol Ther.* **1977**;22:251-258.

Ellard GA, Gammon PT, Titinen H. Determination of the acetylator phenotype using matrix isoniazid. *Tubercle.* **1975**;56:203-209.

Fletcher CV, Jiang H, Brundage RC, et al. Sex-based differences in saquinavir pharmacology and virologic response in AIDS Clinical Trials Group Study 359. *J Infect Dis.* **2004**;189:1176-1184.

Fuzeon (enfuvirtide) [prescribing information]. Nutley, NJ: Roche Pharmaceuticals and Durham, NC: Trimeris; March **2003**.

Haas D, Ribaudo H, Kim R, et al. A common CYP2B6 variant is associated with efavirenz pharmacokinetics and central nervous system side effects: AACTG Study NWCS214. In: Program and abstracts of the 11th Conference on Retroviruses and Opportunistic Infections; February 8-11, **2004**; Boston, Massachusetts. Abstract 133.

Haas DW, Smeaton L, R Shafer R, et al. Pharmacogenetics of long-term response to efavirenz- and nelfinavir-containing regimens: NWCS213, an analysis of ACTG 384. In: Program and Abstracts of the 12th Conference on Retroviruses and Opportunistic Infections. Boston, MA; February 22-25, **2005**. Abstract 81.

Hernandez JE, Cutrell A, Edwards M, et al. Clinical risk factors for hypersensitivity reactions to abacavir: retrospective analysis of over 8,000 subjects receiving abacavir in 34 clinical trials. In: Program and abstracts of the 43rd Annual Interscience Conference on Antimicrobial Agents and Chemotherapy; September 14-17, **2003**; Chicago, Illinois. Abstract H-2013.

Hetherington S, Hughes AR, Mosteller M, et al. Genetic variations in HLA-B region and hypersensitivity reactions to abacavir. *Lancet.* **2002**;359:1121-1122.

McLeod HL, Krynetski EY, Relling MV, Evans WE. Genetic polymorphism of thiopurine methyltransferase and its clinical relevance for childhood acute lymphoblastic leukemia. *Leukemia.* **2000**;14:567-572.

Mallal S, Nolan D, Witt C, et al. Association between presence of HLA-B*5701, HLA-DR7 and HLA-DQ3 and hypersensitivity to HIV-1 reverse-transcriptase inhibitor abacavir. *Lancet.* **2002**;359:727-732.

Martin AM, Nolan D, Gaudieri S, et al. Predisposition to abacavir hypersensitivity conferred by HLA-B*5701 and a haplotypic Hsp70-Hom variant. Proc Natl Acad Sci U S A. **2004**;101:4180-4185.

Martin AM, Nolan D, James I, et al. Predisposition to nevirapine hypersensitivity associated with HLA-DRB1*0101 and abrogated by low CD4 T-cell counts [letter]. *AIDS.* **2005**;19:97-99.

Monaghan G, Ryan M, Seddon R, Hume R, Burchell B. Genetic variation in bilirubin UPD-glucuronosyltransferase gene promoter and Gilbert's syndrome. *Lancet.* **1996**;347:578-581.

Moore R, Keruly J, Gebo K, Lucas G. Racial differences in efavirenz discontinuation in clinical practice. In: Program and abstracts of the 12th Conference on Retroviruses and Opportunistic Infections. Boston, MA; February 22-25, **2005**. Abstract 619.

O'Mara E, Mummaneni V, Randall D, Geraldes M. Relationship between uridine diphosphate-glucuronosyl transferase (UDP-GT) 1A1 genotype and total bilirubin elevations in healthy subjects receiving BMS-232632 and saquinavir. In: Program and abstracts of the 40th Interscience Conference on Antimicrobial Agents and Chemotherapy; September 17-20, **2000**; Toronto, Ontario, Canada. Abstract 1645.

O'Mara E Jr. Genetic factors in protease inhibitor hyperbilirubinemia. In: Program and abstracts of the 43rd International Conference on Antimicrobial Agents and Chemotherapy; September 14-17, **2003**; Chicago, Illinois. Abstract 1133.

Raijmakers MT, Jansen PL, Steegers EA, Peters WH. Association of human liver bilirubin UDP-glucuronyl transferase activity with a polymorphism in the promoter region of the UGT1A1 gene. *J Hepatol.* **2000**;33:348-351.

Reyataz (atazanavir sulfate) [prescribing information]. Princeton, NJ: Bristol-Myers Squibb; October **2004**.

Septra (sulfamethoxazole and trimethoprim) [prescribing information]. Bristol, Tenn: King Pharmaceuticals; February **2004**.

Staatz CE, Tett SE. Clinical pharmacokinetics and pharmacodynamics of tacrolimus in solid organ transplantation. *Clin Pharmacokinet.* **2004**;43:623-653.

Sustiva (efavirenz) [prescribing information]. Princeton, NJ: Bristol-Myers Squibb; December **2004**.

Turriziani O, Scagnolari C, Bellomi F, Solimeo I, Focher F, Antonelli G. Cellular issues relating to the resistance of HIV to antiretroviral agents. *Scand J Infect Dis Suppl.* **2003**;35(suppl 106):45-48.

Ziagen (abacavir sulfate) [prescribing information]. Research Triangle Park, NC: GlaxoSmithKline; August **2004**.

(RLO-20)

IV.8. COMMON ANTIRETROVIRAL TOXICITIES

LEARNING OBJECTIVE: Describe the important toxicities and their management for all current FDA-approved antiretroviral therapies.

Antiretroviral toxicities are one of the most important barriers to successful therapy of HIV infection. It is vitally important for prescribers to know about these toxicities, not only to make the appropriate treatment decisions but also to educate patients on self-monitoring for these side effects. Recent data suggest that the rate of adverse effects may be decreasing when compared with previous experience, and it is speculated that this decrease results from increased provider awareness, increased options for therapy or optimization of therapy (Keiser et al. 2004).

Nucleoside Reverse Transcriptase Inhibitors (NRTIs)

Class effects

All antiretrovirals now carry a warning that they may be associated with lipodystrophy, as mandated by the U.S. Food and Drug Administration (FDA), even though the cause of lipodystrophy is unclear (see Objective IV.47 on Morphologic Changes in this Update).

All the NRTIs contain warnings about the possible development of lactic acidosis and severe hepatomegaly with steatosis. Lactic acidosis is a serious complication that is managed by discontinuation of all NRTIs and supportive care (see Objective IV.49 on Metabolic Complications in this Update). Rare occurrences of rapidly progressive neuromuscular weakness with features that overlap with those of Guillain-Barré syndrome have been reported in individuals receiving stavudine in combination with other nucleoside analogues (Simpson et al. 2004; Marcus et al. 2002).

Nonalcoholic steatohepatitis (NASH) has been reported in 16% of patients with evidence of antiretroviral therapy-associated metabolic abnormalities, such as hyperlipidemia, diabetes and hyperinsulinemia (Bruno et al. 2002). NASH closely resembles alcoholic liver disease in being characterized by the accumulation of fat in the liver (steatosis) accompanied by inflammation, cell injury and fibrosis (hepatitis), but NASH occurs in patients who drink little or no alcohol (Neuschwander-Tetri 2002). The natural history and prognosis of NASH are poorly understood. Stavudine use with protease inhibitor therapy was associated with a higher risk of fatty liver in one study (Sulkowski et al. 2004). (See Objective III.42 on Hepatitis in this Update.)

"d" drugs

The "d" drugs—didanosine, stavudine, zalcitabine (ddI, d4T, ddC)—carry warnings on their labels regarding peripheral neuropathy, the most common serious side effect for all of these drugs. The development of neuropathy is usually managed by discontinuing the offending NRTI and administering gabapentin (Neurontin), amitriptyline (Elavil) and pain relief as necessary for patient comfort. Some providers will rechallenge patients with lower doses of the NRTI if symptoms resolve. The addition of hydroxyurea to stavudine- and/or didanosine-containing regimens is associated with higher rates of peripheral neuropathy (Moore et al. 2000) and should be avoided.

Didanosine, stavudine and zalcitabine also carry warnings regarding pancreatitis. It is important that these drugs be stopped immediately and not restarted if a patient presents with pancreatitis. The prescribing information for stavudine

What's New

Emtricitabine has been associated with skin discoloration, especially in nonwhite patients. This usually manifests as hyperpigmentation of the palms and soles and is reported to occur in up to 8% of African American patients. Tenofovir appears to have mild potential for renal toxicity that can become clinically relevant in some patients with underlying renal disease and/or risk factors for renal dysfunction. Severe hypersensitivity reactions to nevirapine are up to 12-fold more common in women with CD4 counts above 250 cells/mm^3 compared with women with lower counts. The risk for men with CD4 counts above 400 is also elevated. These populations should avoid nevirapine. Enfuvirtide causes injection-site reactions in virtually all patients, although only rarely do these cause discontinuation of the drug.

Key Points

- Hepatotoxicity may occur with any antiretroviral agent. Among the protease inhibitors, the risk is highest with ritonavir. That risk increases in a dose-dependent fashion for those on ritonavir. Nevirapine carries the highest risk among NNRTIs. Among NRTIs, stavudine has been associated with hepatic steatosis.
- Signs of hepatotoxicity should be closely monitored for up to 18 weeks after starting nevirapine. Women with CD4 counts above 250 cells/mm^3 appear more commonly affected by serious, potentially fatal nevirapine hepatotoxicity. Elevated risk is also seen in men with CD4 cell counts above 400 cells/mm^3.
- Coinfection with HBV and/or HCV clearly raises the risk of hepatotoxicity with all antiretrovirals, but should not be considered an absolute contraindication for any specific antiretroviral.

Key Points (cont.)

- All antiretrovirals now carry a warning that they may be associated with lipodystrophy.
- All nucleoside reverse transcriptase inhibitors (NRTIs) contain warnings about the possible development of lactic acidosis and subsequent toxicity to cellular mitochondria.
- Didanosine, stavudine and zalcitabine carry warnings about pancreatitis. Stavudine, didanosine and zalcitabine carry warnings regarding peripheral neuropathy — the most common serious side effect for all of these drugs. Coadministration of didanosine and tenofovir can lead to elevated didanosine levels with a resulting increased risk of pancreatitis and neuropathy.
- Zidovudine carries a warning regarding bone marrow suppression (most usually resulting in anemia) and myopathy.
- Abacavir is associated with a serious hypersensitivity reaction in 5% to 8% of patients.
- All three FDA-approved nonnucleoside reverse transcriptase inhibitors (NNRTIs) may cause a rash early in treatment; efavirenz carries warnings regarding psychiatric and nervous system symptoms and reproductive risk; nevirapine is also rarely associated with a severe hypersensitivity reaction.
- Toxicities commonly associated with protease inhibitors are gastrointestinal symptoms, malaise, hyperlipidemia, and insulin resistance. The last of these may induce diabetes mellitus.
- Atazanavir and, to a lesser extent, indinavir are associated with an asymptomatic indirect hyperbilirubinemia, which may cause jaundice.

also notes that after a confirmed diagnosis of pancreatitis, reinstitution of stavudine should be undertaken with particular caution and close patient monitoring (Zerit 2004). Patients should be managed supportively with gastrointestinal rest, as for other causes of pancreatitis. Didanosine also carries a warning regarding possible retinal changes and optic neuritis in adults and children, which would require discontinuation. Didanosine can cause nausea, dyspepsia, and diarrhea, but the incidence of these gastrointestinal side effects is greatly reduced using the enteric-coated (EC) formulation.

Didanosine levels increase when coadministered with tenofovir, causing or worsening didanosine-related toxicities (pancreatitis (Martinez et al. 2004), lactic acidosis (Murphy 2003) and peripheral neuropathy) (Videx 2004). When administering both didanosine and tenofovir, it is recommended that the didanosine EC dose be decreased to 250 mg once daily (in adults weighing over 60 kg with creatinine clearance over 60 mL/min) or to 200 mg (in adults weighing under 60 kg with creatinine clearance over 60 mL/min) (Videx 2004). However, recent studies caution against the coadministering of tenofovir with didanosine as the nucleoside backbone in antiretroviral-naive patients due to higher rates of virologic failure and lower CD4 gains — see Objective IV.15 on Antiretroviral Interactions in this Update. (See below for more on tenofovir-related toxicity.)

Zalcitabine has further warnings on its label regarding oral and esophageal ulceration, cardiomyopathy and anaphylactic reaction. All require discontinuation of the drug and conventional medical care of the respective problem. Given the availability of other, less toxic agents in this class, there is virtually no indication for zalcitabine therapy (DHHS 2004).

Zidovudine

Zidovudine is commonly associated with nausea, headache and fatigue, which are rarely treatment limiting and frequently resolve with continued treatment. The drug's label warns of bone marrow suppression (most usually resulting in anemia) and myopathy. Discontinuation is the usual management, given the variety of other treatment options available. The risk of anemia is greatest in patients with advanced HIV disease (Retrovir 2003). The occasional patient who requires continued zidovudine could be supported with coadministered erythropoietin.

Zidovudine should not be used in conjunction with cytotoxic chemotherapy. Such cancer treatment also causes bone marrow suppression, and its concomitant use with zidovudine often leads to profound anemia and neutropenia (Gill et al. 1987). It is therefore contraindicated.

Both Combivir (zidovudine/lamivudine) and Trizivir (zidovudine/lamivudine/abacavir) contain zidovudine and should therefore also be avoided during chemotherapy. Other antiretroviral agents can safely be administered with cytotoxic chemotherapy; for example, CHOP chemotherapy has been successfully coadministered with stavudine/lamivudine/indinavir (Ratner et al. 2001).

Macrocytosis (mean corpuscular volume [MCV] greater than100 fL) is a more benign red blood cell-related toxicity associated with zidovudine and stavudine. A study found that macrocytosis was incident in 39 of 50 (78%) patients who had commenced zidovudine therapy at least 8 weeks prior to evaluation (Romanelli et al. 2002). It was present in only 30 of 92 controls (33%) with at least 8 weeks free of zidovudine. Twenty-seven of these 30 were on stavudine. The overall macrocytosis rate for the 41 control group members on stavudine was 66%. Far from recommending that patients stop either drug, the study authors suggested using MCV as a marker for patient adherence to dosing schedules.

Abacavir

Abacavir is now associated in about 5% to 8% of patients with a serious hypersensitivity reaction, which consists of fever, marked malaise, fatigue, gastrointestinal symptoms and sometimes rash or dyspnea, and a higher incidence of severe reactions has been noted when abacavir is given once-daily compared with twice-daily dosing (James and Johann-Liang 2005). If this syndrome occurs, the drug should be permanently discontinued and never reinstituted, because cases of severe hypotension and death have occurred in patients who have been rechallenged. Physicians should note (and counsel patients) that this reaction may occur, rarely, for the first time after resumption of the drug in a patient who previously tolerated abacavir but discontinued it for a reason other than a drug reaction. Because of the serious nature of this uncommon adverse effect, good communication between patient and physician, especially during the first 6 weeks of treatment, is important to determine whether this reaction is occurring. Abacavir may also be associated with a mild-to-moderate maculopapular rash, which is not a part of the more serious systemic hypersensitivity described above and which usually resolves with continued treatment.

A retrospective study of over 8000 abacavir-treated patients found that African ethnicity, male sex, and an AIDS diagnosis were associated with a reduced risk for a hypersensitivity reaction when initiating abacavir therapy (Hernandez 2003). Abacavir hypersensitivity has been found to occur more frequently among patients with HLA-B*5701, HLA-DR7 and HLA-DQ3 tissue types (Hetherington et al. 2002; Mallal et al. 2002); however, the use of HLA screening to determine individual patients' risk for abacavir hypersensitivity is not recommended by current guidelines. (See also Objective IV.7 on Pharmacogenmics in this Update.)

Tenofovir

Rare cases of renal failure, resulting from proximal tubular necrosis, have been associated with tenofovir (Schaaf et al. 2003), including cases with Fanconi syndrome (Creput et al. 2003), metabolic acidosis (Eg Hansen et al. 2004) and diabetes insipidus (Karras et al. 2003; Verhelst et al. 2002). Another study observed creatinine elevations over 1.5 times baseline within 6 months in 7.1% of patients receiving tenofovir compared with 3.1% of those receiving abacavir (Harris et al. 2003). In this study, tenofovir was discontinued by over 1% of patients because of elevated creatinine levels within 12 months of initiation. Kidney biopsies from patients with suspected tenofovir-induced renal dysfunction have shown acute tubular necrosis (Creput et al. 2003; Karras et al. 2003).

A 144-week, prospective randomized trial (Gilead 903) compared tenofovir plus efavirenz and lamivudine with stavudine plus efavirenz and lamivudine in patients with normal baseline renal function (Gallant et al. 2004). No significant renal toxicity was noted in either treatment group during up to 3 years follow-up. A modest difference in kidney function was evident in a cohort of 658 clinic patients, approximately half on tenofovir-containing regimens (Gallant et al. 2005). Cohort members were unrestricted as to renal risk factors. After a mean 319 days since starting treatment, the patients receiving tenofovir on average experienced a 10% decrease in creatinine clearance. Those on other NRTIs had a 6% loss.

In clinical trials of tenofovir, renal toxicities usually resolved after stopping the drug (Creput et al. 2003; Karras et al. 2003; Schaaf et al. 2003; Verhelst et al. 2002). One study's authors recommend periodic screening of patients on long-term tenofovir therapy. They advised measuring serum phosphate, checking renal function and looking for evidence of glycosuria and proteinuria (Reynes et al. 2003). Other than discontinuing the drug, there are no specific therapies for renal toxicities related to tenofovir. Patients prescribed tenofovir should be regularly monitored with serum creatinine measurements and urinalyses. The drug should be used with caution in patients having underlying renal disease or other risk factors for nephrotoxicity, and it also requires dose adjustment in those

Key Points (cont.)

- Indinavir can cause flank/back pain from crystal accumulation (kidney stones) because of its relative insolubility in urine; it is also associated with skin, hair and toenail effects secondary to its effects on retinoid metabolism.
- Enfuvirtide causes injection-site reactions in greater than 98% of recipients. The reactions are usually tender, erythematous nodules that rarely cause discontinuation of therapy.

who already have low renal capacity (Viread 2004). (See also Objective IV.6 on Antiretroviral Dosing in this Update.)

Emtricitabine

Emtricitabine has been associated with a slightly higher incidence of skin discoloration when compared with control regimens in phase III trials (Emtriva 2004; Mondou et al. 2004). The skin discoloration is usually described as hyperpigmentation of the palms and/or soles and has only rarely resulted in discontinuation of the drug. The risk for skin discoloration is highest in nonwhite patients: up to 8% of African American patients, 4% of Asian patients and 3% of Hispanic patients (Mondou et al. 2004).

Nonnucleoside Reverse Transcriptase Inhibitors (NNRTIs)

All antiretrovirals now carry an FDA-mandated warning that they may be associated with lipodystrophy, even though the cause of lipodystrophy is unclear (see Objective IV.47 on Morphologic Changes in this Update).

Class effects

All three FDA-approved NNRTIs—efavirenz, nevirapine, delavirdine—may cause a rash, which generally occurs in the first month or 2 of treatment and is self-limited. Prophylactic prednisone or antihistamine does not decrease the incidence of rash with nevirapine (Launay et al. 2004; Montaner et al. 2003). Most rashes from the NNRTIs will resolve without stopping these medications. Treatment is supportive and does not often involve discontinuing the drug. All NNRTIs could cause Stevens-Johnson syndrome (although this happens rarely)—nevirapine more commonly than the others (Fagot et al. 2001). If there is any fever and mucous membrane involvement with a rash associated with NNRTI therapy, the NNRTI should be immediately and permanently discontinued.

Efavirenz

There have been reports linking efavirenz with serious psychiatric symptoms (severe depression, suicidal ideation, aggressive behavior, paranoia and manic reactions), central nervous system (CNS) symptoms (dizziness, insomnia, impaired concentration, somnolence, abnormal dreams) and teratogenic risks (Sustiva 2004). The prescribing information also indicates that CNS symptoms have occurred in 53% of patients who have received efavirenz in clinical trials. CNS-related adverse events resulted in treatment interruption in 6% of patients in a large, open-label prospective and observational study in Spain conducted between October 1999 and April 2000 (Perez-Molina 2002). A substudy of a large, randomized trial (ACTG 5095) evaluated neuropsychological performance, mood and sleep in patients after weeks 1, 4, 12 and 24 on efavirenz (Clifford et al. 2003). In this study, the drug was associated with increased neurologic symptoms and "bad dreams" (but not depression or anxiety) at week 1; however, these had resolved by week 4. A small Spanish study found a significant incidence of dizziness, abnormal dreams, lightheadedness and difficulty sleeping at 4 weeks in patients initiating an efavirenz-containing regimen; these effects resolved by week 24 in most but not all patients (Fumaz et al. 2002).

However, other studies have reported that moderate-to-severe neuropsychiatric side effects of efavirenz can persist beyond the initial month of treatment (Lochet et al. 2003); may not emerge until after the first 3 months of treatment (Reynes et al. 2002); and may be so severe as to require discontinuation of the drug (Puzantian 2002).

Pregnant women should avoid efavirenz, especially during the first trimester, because animal studies have shown teratogenic effects (Sustiva 2004, Perinatal

HIV Guidelines Working Group 2004). (See Objective IV.35 on Antiretroviral Agent Toxicity and Contraindication in Pregnancy in this Update.)

Nevirapine

Nevirapine can trigger a severe hypersensitivity reaction, presenting as a rash and fever associated with severe hepatic necrosis. When this occurs, it is often during the first 6 weeks of therapy (Viramune 2005; Stern et al. 2002). Patients should be warned to present immediately if they feel ill soon after starting nevirapine. Symptoms may include rash (in about half of all cases), fever, flu-like symptoms, fatigue, malaise, anorexia, nausea, jaundice, liver tenderness or hepatomegaly, with or without initially abnormal serum transaminase. Liver function should be monitored closely, and the drug should be permanently discontinued at once if there is an increase in transaminase levels combined with rash or systemic symptoms (Viramune 2005). Based on postmarketing surveillance data and the manufacturer's clinical trial database for nevirapine, the product labeling has been amended to include updated information about hepatotoxicity (Viramune 2005). The risk of severe and fatal hepatic events, often associated with rash (as mentioned above), has been found to continue beyond 6 weeks, and patients should be monitored closely for the first 18 weeks of treatment. In addition, women with CD4 counts above 250 cells/mm^3 are at 12-fold higher risk of serious hepatotoxicity. Men with a CD4 count above 400 cells/mm^3 have a fivefold greater risk. As of January 2005, the product labeling now states, "Viramune should not be initiated in adult females with CD4 counts greater than 250 cells/mm^3 or in adult males with CD4 counts greater than 400 cells/mm^3 unless the benefit outweighs the risk" (Viramune 2005).

Nevirapine has recently been associated with serious liver toxicity in studies of HIV-infected pregnant women (Hitti et al. 2004; Lyons et al. 2003). A cohort of 139 women received nevirapine as part of combination therapy for a median duration of 68 days during pregnancy (Lyons et al. 2003). Nearly all women studied were black Africans and 6 (4.3%) had abnormal liver enzymes at baseline. During the study, ACTG-graded abnormal liver enzymes were detected in 35 women (28%): 19 (15%) had grade 1; 9 (7%) had grade 2; and 7 (6%) had grade 3 or 4. All women with grade 3 or 4 events had higher CD4 counts than those with normal liver enzymes, with these events detected within 8 weeks of receiving nevirapine. Two women (1.4%) died of fulminant hepatitis despite careful monitoring during the early treatment period. Both women had high CD4 counts and had no detectable hepatitis B surface antigen (HBsAg) or HCV RNA. Nevirapine therapy should therefore be used with caution in HIV-infected pregnant women.

Some studies have found that nevirapine-associated liver toxicity occurs at rates similar to those seen with many other antiretrovirals (reviewed in Dieterich et al. 2004). However, other studies have found that nevirapine can be associated with a higher incidence of severe hepatotoxicity (Law et al. 2003; Wit et al. 2002). One small pharmacokinetic study demonstrated that coadministration of fluconazole and nevirapine resulted in both increased nevirapine levels and rates of hepatotoxicity (Geel et al. 2004). A small study from Spain found that treatment with nevirapine was associated with a faster progression of liver fibrosis in patients with chronic hepatitis C than other HAART regimens, especially compared with those containing protease inhibitors (Macias et al. 2004).

The 2NN trial was the first large-scale randomized study comparing nevirapine and efavirenz. A total of 1216 treatment-naive patients were randomized into 1 of 4 treatment arms: nevirapine once daily, nevirapine twice daily, efavirenz, or nevirapine once daily plus efavirenz. The NRTI backbone consisted of stavudine and lamivudine but could be changed for toxicity reasons (van Leth et al. 2004). The results showed that nevirapine and efavirenz had comparable efficacy over 48 weeks in terms of HIV viral load suppression and immunologic effect. The incidence of clinical adverse events was also similar, although there was a statistically significant higher incidence in liver-associated laboratory adverse events in the nevirapine once-daily treatment arm.

There was also a trend toward higher rates of clinical CNS adverse events in the efavirenz-containing arms. The combination of nevirapine and efavirenz did not improve therapy outcome; in fact, patients randomized to the dual-NNRTI arm did not do as well as those in other study arms because of more treatment discontinuations from a higher incidence of adverse events in this group.

Protease Inhibitors (PIs)

All antiretrovirals now carry a warning that they may be associated with lipodystrophy, as mandated by the FDA, even though the cause of lipodystrophy is unclear (see Objective IV.47 on Morphologic Changes in this Update).

The most common toxicities associated with PIs are gastrointestinal symptoms (e.g., nausea, abdominal bloating and diarrhea), malaise and dyslipidemia. Diarrhea may be managed with the use of medications such as loperamide or pancreatic enzyme supplements. Bulking agents such as Metamucil and calcium tablets have also been helpful for some patients.

Metabolic effects

Hyperlipidemia may become so severe as to require discontinuation of PI therapy and switching to an alternative antiretroviral regimen; if less severe, it may be managed by diet, exercise and lipid-lowering fibrates and statins (see also Objective IV.9 on Antiretroviral Interactions with Non-Antiretroviral Drugs in this Update). Atazanavir, when administered without ritonavir boosting, has been associated with more favorable alterations in lipid parameters in comparison to efavirenz and nelfinavir (Reyataz 2004).

PIs have a tendency to cause insulin resistance (Murata et al. 2000; Wang et al. 2003), which can lead to diabetes mellitus. This may be managed by discontinuing the PI (Murata et al. 2000) or by using oral hypoglycemic medications (reviewed in Grinspoon and Carr 2005). Investigators have found that even a single, 1200-mg dose of indinavir reduces glucose disposal (Noor et al. 2002) in a study of HIV-negative men. At the same time, indinavir also increases fasting glucose production (Schwartz 2004). Atazanavir appears to have the least effect on glucose metabolism (Wang et al. 2003). In HIV-negative healthy volunteers, lopinavir/ritonavir significantly reduced insulin-mediated glucose disposal rates and induced insulin resistance to a greater extent than atazanavir (Noor et al. 2004).

See also Objective IV.49 on Metabolic Complications in this Update.

Hepatotoxicity

Hepatotoxicity is a potential toxicity common to all currently available members of the PI class of drugs. Full-dose ritonavir appears to be the PI associated with the highest rates of hepatotoxicity, but it is still unclear whether the other members of this class differ in hepatotoxicity, especially in the setting of HBV and/or HCV coinfection (Sulkowski 2004).

Other effects

Indinavir is unique among the PIs in causing nephrolithiasis, or a syndrome of flank/back pain from crystal accumulation, because of its relative insolubility in urine. This complication may also be associated with reduction in renal function (Crixivan

2004). Patients should be advised to drink plenty of fluids to keep themselves adequately hydrated when taking indinavir.

Atazanavir and, to a lesser extent, indinavir are associated with elevations of total unconjugated bilirubin, which may cause mild jaundice (Crixivan 2004; Reyataz 2004). Total bilirubin levels greater than 2.5 times the upper limit of normal have been observed in almost 50% of patients after 48 and 120 weeks of therapy with boosted or unboosted atazanavir, respectively (Reyataz 2004). It occurs in approximately 14% of indinavir-treated patients (Crixivan 2004). The increased bilirubin can be of cosmetic concern (Reyataz 2004) but is rarely so severe as to cause discontinuation of the drug (Squires et al. 2004). It rapidly reverses after drug discontinuation.

Indinavir may cause retinoid-like side effects (dry skin, dry lips, hair loss, and ingrown toenails) secondary to its effects on retinoid metabolism (Garcia-Silva et al. 2002); these adverse effects are augmented when the drug is boosted with ritonavir.

Fusion Inhibitors

Enfuvirtide is a synthetic peptide that inhibits the fusion of HIV with CD4+ T cells. It is administered via subcutaneous injection. The most common adverse reaction to this drug is an injection site reaction (ISR), which occurs in almost every patient during the first week of treatment (Fuzeon 2004; Lalezari et al. 2003a; Lazarrin et al. 2003) and can continue to occur throughout treatment (Fuzeon 2004). The ISRs are usually painful, indurated, erythematous nodules (Fuzeon 2004) and are more common in the abdomen than in the upper extremities (Lalezari et al. 2003b). Biopsies of the ISRs show an inflammatory infiltrate consistent with a localized hypersensitivity reaction (Ball et al. 2003). The ISRs are rarely severe enough to cause discontinuation of the drug (Lalezari et al. 2003a,b; Lazarrin et al. 2003), with most individual ISRs reported to last less than 1 week (Fuzeon 2004).

References

Ball RA, Kinchelow T for the ISR Substudy Group. Injection site reactions with the HIV-1 fusion inhibitor enfuvirtide. *J Am Acad Dermatol.* **2003**;49:826-831.

Boehringer Ingelheim. Important new safety information [letter]. February **2004**. Available at: http://www.fda.gov/medwatch/SAFETY/2004/viramune_deardoc_Feb04.pdf [accessed February 21, 2005].

Bruno R, Sacchi P, Gazzaruso C, et al. Non-alcoholic steatohepatitis (NASH) in a cohort of HIV patients with metabolic syndrome. In: Program and abstracts of the XIV International AIDS Conference; July 7-12, **2002**; Barcelona, Spain. Abstract TuPeB4521.

Clifford DB, Evans S, Yang Y, Acosta E, Goodkin K, Gulick RM. ACTG 5097s: impact of efavirenz (EFV) on neuropsychological performance, mood, and sleep behaviour in HIV-positive individuals [abstract 54]. *Antiviral Ther.* **2003**;8(suppl 1):S196-S197.

Creput C, Gonzalez-Canali G, Hill G, Piketty C, Kazatchkine M, Nochy D. Renal lesions in HIV-1-positive patient treated with tenofovir. *AIDS.* **2003**;17:935-937.

Crixivan (indinavir) [prescribing information]. Whitehouse Station, NJ: Merck; May 2004.

Department of Health and Human Services (DHHS). Guidelines for the use of antiretroviral agents in HIV-1-infected adults and adolescents. October 29, **2004**. Available at: http://aidsinfo.nih.gov/guidelines [accessed February 21, 2005].

Dieterich DT, Robinson PA, Love J, Stern JO. Drug-induced liver injury associated with the use of nonnucleoside reverse-transcriptase inhibitors. *Clin Infect Dis.* **2004**;38(suppl 2):S80-S89.

Eg Hansen AB, Mathiesen S, Gerstoft J. Severe metabolic acidosis and renal failure in an HIV-1 patient receiving tenofovir [case report]. *Scand J Infect Dis.* **2004**;36:389-392.

Emtriva (emtricitabine) [prescribing information]. Foster City, CA: Gilead Sciences; September **2004**.

Fagot JP, Mockenhaupt M, Bouwes-Bavinck JN, et al. Nevirapine and the risk of Stevens-Johnson syndrome or toxic epidermal necrolysis. *AIDS.* **2001**;15:1843-1848.

Fumaz CR, Tuldra A, Ferrer MJ, et al. Quality of life, emotional status, and adherence of HIV-1-infected patients treated with efavirenz versus protease inhibitor-containing regimens. *J Acquir Immune Defic Syndr.* **2002**;29:244-253.

Fuzeon (enfuvirtide) [prescribing information]. Nutley, NJ: Roche Laboratories, and Durham, NC: Trimeris; October **2004**.

Gallant JE, Staszewski S, Pozniak AL, et al. Efficacy and safety of tenofovir DF vs stavudine in combination therapy in antiretroviral-naive patients: a 3-year randomized trial. *JAMA.* **2004**;292:191-201.

Gallant JE, Parish MA, Keruly JC, Moore RD. Changes in renal function associated with tenofovir disoproxil fumarate treatment, compared with nucleoside reverse-transcriptase inhibitor treatment. *Clin Infect Dis.* **2005**;40:1194-1198.

Garcia-Silva J, Almagro M, Pena-Penabad C, Fonseca E. Indinavir-induced retinoid-like effects: incidence, clinical features and management. *Drug Saf.* **2002**;25:993-1003.

Geel J, Pitt JA, Orrell CJ, Van Dyk M, Wood R. Effect of fluconazole on nevirapine pharmacokinetics. In: Program and abstracts of the XV International AIDS Conference; July 11-16, **2004**. Bangkok, Thailand. Abstract TuPeB4606.

Gill PS, Rarick MU, Brunes RK, Causey D, Levine AM. Azidothymidine (AZT) and bone marrow failure in AIDS. *Ann Intern Med.* **1987**;107:502-505.

Grinspoon S and Carr A. Cardiovascular risk and body-fat abnormalities in HIV-infected adults. *N Engl J Med.* **2005**;352:48-62.

Harris M, Yip B, Montaner J, et al. Increases in creatinine during therapy with tenofovir DF. *Antiviral Ther.* **2003**;8(suppl 1):S196-S197.

Hernandez JE, Cutrell A, Edwards M, Fleming J, Powell W, Scott T. Clinical risk factors for hypersensitivity reactions to abacavir: retrospective analysis of over 8,000 subjects receiving abacavir in 34 clinical trials. In: Program and abstracts of the 43rd Annual Interscience Conference on Antimicrobial Agents and Chemotherapy. September 14-17, **2003**. Chicago, Illinois. Abstract H-2013.

Hetherington S, Hughes A, Mosteller M, et al. Genetic variations in HLA-B region and hypersensitivity reactions to abacavir. *Lancet.* **2002**;359:1121-1122.

Hitti J, Frenkel L, Stek AM, et al. Maternal toxicity with continuous nevirapine in pregnancy: results from PACTG 1022. *J Acquir Immune Defic Syndr.* **2004**;36:772-776.

James A, Johann-Liang R. Increased rate and severity of abacavir-associated hypersensitivity reaction in randomized controlled clinical trials. In: Program and abstracts of the 12th Conference on Retroviruses and Opportunistic Infections; February 22-25, **2005**; Boston, Massachusetts. Abstract 835.

Karras A, Lafaurie M, Molina JM, et al. Tenofovir-related nephrotoxicity in human immunodeficiency virus-infected patients: three cases of renal failure, Fanconi syndrome, and nephrogenic diabetes insipidus. *Clin Infect Dis.* **2003**;36:1070-1073.

Keiser O, Rickenbach M, Telenti A, et al. Did the burden of adverse events due to antiretroviral treatment change over the last four years?: The Swiss HIV Cohort study. In: Program and abstracts of the XV International AIDS Conference; July 11-16, **2004**. Bangkok, Thailand. Abstract WePeB5949.

Lalezari JP, Henry K, O'Hearn M, et al. Enfuvirtide, an HIV-1 fusion inhibitor, for drug-resistant HIV infection in North and South America. *N Engl J Med.* **2003a**;348:2175-2185.

Lalezari JP, Patel IH, Zhang X, et al. Influence of subcutaneous injection site on the steady-state pharmacokinetics of enfuvirtide (T-20) in HIV-1-infected patients. *J Clin Virol.* **2003b**;28:217-222.

Launay O, Roudiere L, Boukli N, et al. Assessment of cetirizine, an antihistamine, to prevent cutaneous reactions to nevirapine therapy: results of the Viramune-Zyrtec double-blind, placebo-controlled trial. *Clin Infect Dis.* **2004**;38:e66-e72.

Law WP, Dore GJ, Duncombe CJ, et al. Risk of severe hepatotoxicity associated with antiretroviral therapy in the HIV-NAT Cohort, Thailand, 1996-2001. *AIDS.* **2003**;17:2191-2199.

Lazzarin A, Clotet B, Cooper D, et al. Efficacy of enfuvirtide in patients infected with drug-resistant HIV-1 in Europe and Australia. *N Engl J Med.* **2003**;348:2186-2195.

Lochet P, Peyriere H, Lotthe A, Mauboussin JM, Delmas B, Reynes J. Long-term assessment of neuropsychiatric adverse reactions associated with efavirenz. *HIV Medicine.* **2003**;4:62-66.

Lyons F, Hopkins S, McGeary A, Sheehan G, Bergin C, Mulcahy F. Nevirapine tolerability in HIV infected women in pregnancy – a word of caution. In: Program and abstracts of the 2nd IAS Conference on HIV Pathogenesis and Treatment; July 13-16, **2003**; Paris, France. Abstract LB27.

Macias J, Castellano V, Merchante N, et al. Effect of antiretroviral drugs on liver fibrosis in HIV-infected patients with chronic hepatitis C: harmful impact of nevirapine. *AIDS*. **2004**;18:767-774.

Mallal S, Nolan D, Witt C, et al. Association between presence of HLA-B*5701, HLA-DR7, and HLA-DQ3 and hypersensitivity to HIV-1 reverse-transcriptase inhibitor abacavir. *Lancet*. **2002**;359:727-732.

Marcus K, Truffa M, Boxwell D, Toerner J. Recently identified adverse events secondary to NRTI therapy in HIV-infected individuals: cases from the FDA's adverse event reporting system (AERS). In: Program and abstracts of the 9th Conference on Retroviruses and Opportunistic Infections; February 24-28, **2002**; Seattle, Washington. Abstract LB14.

Martinez E, Milinkovic A, de Lazzari E, et al. Pancreatic toxic effects associated with co-administration of didanosine and tenofovir in HIV-infected adults. *Lancet*. **2004**;364:65-67.

Mondou E, Hinkle J, Shaw A, Quinn J, Adda N, Rousseau F. Incidence of skin discoloration across phase 3 clinical trials of emtricitabine (FTC). In: Program and abstracts of the XV International AIDS Conference; July 11-16, **2004**. Bangkok, Thailand. Abstract WePeB5916.

Montaner JS, Cahn P, Zala C, et al. Randomized, controlled study of the effects of a short course of prednisone on the incidence of rash associated with nevirapine in patients infected with HIV-1. *J Acquir Immune Defic Syndr.* **2003**;33:41-46.

Moore RD, Wong WM, Keruly JC, McArthur JC. Incidence of neuropathy in HIV-infected patients on monotherapy versus those on combination therapy with didanosine, stavudine and hydroxyurea. *AIDS*. **2000**;14:273-278.

Murata H, Hruz PW, Mueckler M. The mechanism of insulin resistance caused by HIV protease inhibitor therapy. *J Biol Chem*. **2000**;275:20251-20254.

Murphy MD, O'Hearn M, Chou S. Fatal lactic acidosis and acute renal failure after addition of tenofovir to an antiretroviral regimen containing didanosine. *Clin Infect Dis*. **2003**;36:1082-1085.

Noor MA; Seneviratne T, Aweeka FT, et al. Indinavir acutely inhibits insulin-stimulated glucose disposal in humans: A randomized, placebo-controlled study. *AIDS*. **2002**;16:F1-F8.

Noor MA, Parker RA, O'Mara E, et al. The effects of HIV protease inhibitors atazanavir and lopinavir/ritonavir on insulin sensitivity in HIV-seronegative healthy adults. *AIDS*. **2004**;18:2137-2144.

Neuschwander-Tetri BA. Evolving pathophysiologic concepts in nonalcoholic steatohepatitis. *Curr Gastroenterol Rep*. **2002**;4:31-36.

Perez-Molina JA. Safety and tolerance of efavirenz in different antiretroviral regimens: results from a national multicenter prospective study in 1,033 HIV-infected patients. *HIV Clin Trials*. **2002**;3:279-286.

Perinatal HIV Guidelines Working Group. Recommendations for Use of Antiretroviral Drugs in Pregnancy HIV-1-infected women for maternal health and interventions to reduce perinatal HIV-1 transmission in the United States. December 17, **2004**. Available at: http://www.aidsinfo.nih.gov/guidelines [accessed February 19, 2005].

Puzantian T. Central nervous system adverse effects with efavirenz: case report and review. *Pharmacother.* **2002**;22:930-933.

Retrovir (zidovudine) [prescribing information]. Research Triangle Park, NC: GlaxoSmithKline; April **2003**.

Reyataz (atazanavir) [prescribing information]. Princeton, NJ: Bristol-Myers Squibb; October **2004**.

Reynes J, Peyriere H, deBoever CM, LeMoing V. Renal tubular injury and severe hypophosphoremia (Fanconi syndrome) associated with tenofovir therapy. In: Program and abstracts from the 10th Conference on Retroviruses and Opportunistic Infections; February 10-14, **2003**; Boston, Massachusetts. Abstract 717.

Romanelli F, Empey K, Pomeroy C. Macrocytosis as an indicator of medication (zidovudine) adherence in patients with HIV infection. *AIDS Patient Care STDs*. **2002**;16:405-411.

Schaaf B, Aries SP, Kramme E, Steinhoff J, Dalhoff K. Acute renal failure associated with tenofovir treatment in a patient with acquired immunodeficiency syndrome. *Clin Infect Dis*. **2003**;37:e41-e43.

Schwarz J-M, Lee GA, Park, S, et al. Indinavir increases glucose production in healthy HIV-negative men. *AIDS*. **2004**;18:1852-1854.

Simpson D, Estanislao L, Evans S, et al. HIV-associated neuromuscular weakness syndrome. *AIDS*. **2004**;18:1403-1412.

Squires K, Lazzarin A, Gatell JM, et al. Comparison of once-daily atazanavir with efavirenz, each in combination with fixed-dose zidovudine and lamivudine, as initial therapy for patients infected with HIV. *J Acquir Immune Defic Syndr.* **2004**;36:1011-1019.

Stern J, Lanes S, Love J, et al. Hepatic safety of nevirapine: results of the Boehringer Ingelheim Viramune hepatic safety project. In: Program and abstracts of the XIV International AIDS Conference; July 7-12, **2002**; Barcelona, Spain. Abstract LbOr15.

Sulkowski MS. Drug-induced liver injury associated with antiretroviral therapy that includes HIV-1 protease inhibitors. *Clin Infect Dis*. **2004**;38(suppl 2):S90-S97.

Sulkowski M, Mehta S, Moore R, et al. Population prevalence of hepatic steatosis among antiretroviral-experienced HCV/HIV co-infected adults with and without stavudine exposure. In: Program and abstracts of the 11th Conference on Retroviruses and Opportunistic Infections; February 8-11, **2004**; San Francisco, California. Abstract 72.

Sustiva (efavirenz) [prescribing information]. Princeton, NJ: Bristol-Myers Squibb. December **2004**.

van Leth F, Phanuphak P, Ruxrungtham K, et al. Comparison of first-line antiretroviral therapy with regimens including nevirapine, efavirenz, or both drugs, plus stavudine and lamivudine: a randomised open-label trial, the 2NN Study. *Lancet*. **2004**;363:1253-1263.

Verhelst D, Monge M, Rossert J, et al. Fanconi syndrome and renal failure induced by tenofovir: a first case report. *Am J Kidney Dis*. **2002**;40:1331-1333.

Videx EC (didanosine) [prescribing information]. Princeton, NJ: Bristol-Myers Squibb; January **2004**.

Viread (tenofovir) [prescribing information]. Foster City, Calif: Gilead Sciences; June **2004**.

Viramune (nevirapine) [prescribing information]. Ridgefield, Conn: Boehringer Ingelheim; January **2005**.

Wang S, Mulvey R, Elosua C, Flint OP, Parker RA. Association of HIV-protease inhibitors with insulin resistance is related to potency of inhibition of GLUT4 and GLUT1 activity in adipocytes and myocytes [abstract 47]. *Antiviral Ther.* **2003**;8:L36

Wit FW, Weverling GJ, Weel J, Jurriaans S, Lange JM. Incidence of and risk factors for severe hepatotoxicity associated with antiretroviral combination therapy. *J Infect Dis*. **2002**;186:23-31.

Zerit (stavudine) [prescribing information]. Princeton, NJ: Bristol-Myers Squibb; June **2004**.

(RLO-21)

IV.9. ANTIRETROVIRAL INTERACTIONS WITH NON-ANTIRETROVIRAL DRUGS

LEARNING OBJECTIVE: Identify the important drug-drug interactions that may be seen with current FDA-approved antiretroviral therapies and other medications.

Rifampin and Rifabutin

Rifampin and rifabutin are two antimycobacterial agents that induce the activity of CYP3A4 metabolic enzymes, which considerably decrease serum concentrations of protease inhibitors (PIs) and nonnucleoside reverse transcriptase inhibitors (NNRTIs) (CDC 2004). These two drugs differ in their effect on CYP3A4: Rifampin is a more potent inducer than rifabutin.

Rifabutin (unlike rifampin) is a substrate for CYP3A4, and its serum concentration is affected by the degree to which CYP3A4 is inhibited or induced by concurrent PIs and NNRTIs. Therefore, dose adjustment is required when used with antiretrovirals that affect CYP3A4 (CDC 2004).

The CDC has published specific dosing guidelines for rifampin or rifabutin and concurrent antiretrovirals (CDC 2004). When using rifampin, the only PIs recommended for coadministration are full-dose ritonavir (600 mg twice daily), lopinavir/ritonavir 400/100 mg plus additional ritonavir 300 mg twice daily, or efavirenz at an increased dose of 800 mg daily (CDC 2004). There is clinical experience using rifampin with nevirapine at its usual dose of 200 mg every 12 hours (Olivia et al. 2003), but the CDC recommends that "this combination should only be used when no other options are available and close clinical and virologic monitoring can be performed" (CDC 2004). No adjustments in the rifampin dose are required when used in these combinations.

Rifabutin can be used with PIs and NNRTIs, except for delavirdine and unboosted saquinavir, provided that the dose of rifabutin is reduced (CDC 2004). Rifabutin may be administered along with saquinavir only if ritonavir boosting is implemented to counteract the rifabutin-induced decrease in saquinavir levels. The two PIs requiring dose adjustment when used with rifabutin are indinavir (increase to 1000 mg every 8 hours) and nelfinavir (increase to 1000 mg every 8 hours). The rifabutin dose should be reduced to 150 mg daily (or 300 mg three times weekly) when given with amprenavir, fosamprenavir, indinavir or nelfinavir and reduced to 150 mg every other day (or 150 mg three times weekly) when given with atazanavir, ritonavir, lopinavir/ritonavir or any other ritonavir-boosted combination. Both efavirenz and nevirapine can be used with rifabutin at their usual doses. When given with nevirapine, rifabutin should be dosed at 300 mg daily or 300 mg three times weekly. As a CYP3A4 inducer, efavirenz can reduce concentrations of rifabutin, necessitating an increase in the dose of rifabutin to 450 mg daily or 600 mg three times weekly. Delavirdine should not be used with rifabutin.

Nucleoside reverse transcriptase inhibitors (NRTIs) and the fusion inhibitor enfuvirtide are not metabolized by CYP3A4, so rifampin or rifabutin dose adjustments are not required when coadministered with these antiretrovirals. (CDC 2004).

What's New

There are no interactions between rifampin and rifabutin and enfuvirtide. Significant interactions between antiretrovirals and SSRIs do not appear to be common. Proton-pump inhibitors should not be given with atazanavir. Protease inhibitors increase the levels of vardenafil and tadalafil, as they do with the first PDE5 inhibitor, sildenafil.

Key Points

- Caution must be exercised when combining protease inhibitors (PIs) or nonnucleoside reverse transcriptase inhibitors (NNRTIs) with other drugs metabolized by the P450 system.
- Rifabutin has fewer interactions with PIs and NNRTIs than does rifampin. Rifabutin can be used, after decreasing the dose, with all PIs except for unboosted saquinavir. Patients can take rifabutin with efavirenz, but they need a higher rifabutin dose.
- Patients taking amprenavir or fosamprenavir should not use hormonal contraceptives, which decrease amprenavir concentrations. Nelfinavir, ritonavir and nevirapine may decrease levels of hormonal contraceptives. Efavirenz, delavirdine and atazanavir may increase levels of hormonal contraceptives.
- Caution must be exercised when combining HMG-CoA reductase inhibitors (statins) with PIs. Pravastatin is not metabolized by the P450 system and is safe to combine with PIs.
- PIs and NNRTIs can decrease methadone levels, which may precipitate opiate withdrawal. Patients coadministered antiretrovirals and methadone require close monitoring for withdrawal symptoms during the first few weeks of therapy.

Key Points (cont.)

- There do not appear to be common, clinically relevant interactions between antiretrovirals and FDA-approved antidepressant medications, with the exception of ritonavir increasing levels of most antidepressants. St. John's wort, a commonly used herbal remedy for depression, is known to decrease NNRTI and PI levels.
- Reduced plasma concentrations of atazanavir are expected if it is given with agents that increase gastric pH. Proton-pump inhibitors should not be given with atazanavir.
- Drugs used for erectile dysfunction (PDE5 inhibitors) require lower and less frequent dosing when given to patients taking PIs.

Important warning: Ritonavir-boosted saquinavir should not be administered with rifampin at any time (Roche 2005). Significant hepatotoxicity occurred in a 28-day trial to assess ritonavir's corrective effect on saquinavir levels in the presence of rifampin. (Unboosted saquinavir is contraindicated with rifampin due to the reduction in the PI's plasma levels.)

Oral Contraceptives

Oral contraceptives can interact with some antiretrovirals, with package inserts indicating the following precautions. Patients taking amprenavir or fosamprenavir should be instructed not to use hormonal contraceptives because some birth control pills decrease amprenavir concentrations (DHHS 2004). Delavirdine and atazanavir may increase concentrations of hormonal contraceptives; although the clinical significance of the delavirdine interaction is not yet known, patients taking atazanavir are advised to take oral contraceptives at the lowest dose possible or to use alternative contraception methods (DHHS 2004). Patients taking lopinavir/ritonavir (Kaletra), nelfinavir, ritonavir, nevirapine or efavirenz should seek alternative or additional forms of contraception because these agents, too, may decrease or increase (efavirenz) concentrations of hormonal contraceptives (DHHS 2004).

Statins

As reviewed by Dubé and colleagues (2003), caution must be exercised when combining HMG-CoA reductase inhibitors (statins) with PIs, because the latter inhibit the P450 enzyme system in the liver. The P450 enzymes are responsible for the metabolism of most of the statin agents, so coadministration carries the risk of elevating statin blood levels with the possible consequence of rhabdomyolysis. Pravastatin (Pravachol) is not metabolized by the P450 enzyme system and is safe to combine with PIs, though higher doses of pravastatin may be needed when combined with ritonavir or other agents that induce enzymes responsible for metabolism of pravastatin. Atorvastatin (Lipitor) can probably be used at low doses (starting dose 10 mg daily) with PIs, with caution. Fluvastatin (Lescol) is also considered an acceptable alternative agent for coadministration with most PIs. Lovastatin (Mevacor) and simvastatin (Zocor) are extensively metabolized by the P450 enzyme system and are thus contraindicated with PIs. There appear to be few data available suggesting any significant interactions between the statins and NNRTIs. A recent study has shown efavirenz to be a significant inducer of simvastatin and atorvastatin metabolism, which may result in diminished antilipid efficacy (Gerber et al. 2004). Higher doses of these statins may be needed when used with efavirenz, but the potential for increased toxicity must be monitored. Delavirdine, a potent inhibitor of CYP3A4, may have interactions similar to but lesser than ritonavir when given with simvastatin (Zocor), lovastatin (Mevacor) or atorvastatin (Lipitor).

Methadone

Interactions between antiretroviral medications and methadone are complex, and there are relatively few studies on the clinical implications of using these drugs together (Gourevitch and Friedland 2000). In general, PIs and NNRTIs decrease methadone levels through induction of CYP3A4 (Gourevitch and Friedland 2000). Among the PIs, ritonavir, amprenavir, saquinavir, lopinavir and nelfinavir have been shown to decrease methadone levels, whereas indinavir appears to have no significant effect, and atazanavir does not appear to have any pharmacokinetic interactions with methadone (see package inserts for each medication and DHHS 2004). There are case reports of opiate withdrawal precipitated in patients on methadone after initiation of lopinavir/ritonavir (McCance-Katz et al. 2003) and nelfinavir (McCance-Katz et al. 2000). However, there have also been trials and case series showing a lack of withdrawal symptoms or dose alterations when lopinavir/ritonavir and methadone have been coadministered (Stevens et al. 2003; Clarke et al. 2002). Treatment with amprenavir and methadone together results not only in decreased methadone levels, but also in decreased amprenavir levels (Agenerase 2004; Lexiva 2004), and there are no suggestions for specific dose adjustments in this setting.

Both efavirenz and nevirapine decrease methadone levels (DHHS 2004; Stocker et al. 2004; Sustiva 2004; Viramune 2004; Clarke et al. 2001a,b; Otero et al. 1999), with a reduction in methadone area under the concentration time curve (AUC) by up to 57% with efavirenz (Clark et al. 2002b) and 70% with nevirapine (Stocker et al. 2004) .Clinical reports suggest that patients who are stabilized on methadone-maintenance therapy may experience opiate withdrawal symptoms when either efavirenz (Boffito et al. 2002) or nevirapine (Pinzani et al. 2000) is added to their HIV-regimen. Methadone-maintenance patients should be monitored for evidence of withdrawal, with the methadone dose adjusted accordingly (Clark et al. 2001a,b). In one series of patients, 9 of 11 experiencing opiate withdrawal symptoms after starting efavirenz required a mean increase in methadone dosage of 22% (Clarke 2001b). In another study of nevirapine and methadone, the median methadone dose increase was 15% (Stocker et al. 2004). Dose adjustments need to be individualized because of the extensive interpatient variability of this drug-drug interaction (Stocker et al. 2004; Calvo et al. 2002).

Patients who are on maintenance methadone when starting antiretroviral therapy with PIs or NNRTIs will need to be followed closely for symptoms of opiate withdrawal within the first few weeks after adding antiretrovirals (McCance-Katz et al. 2003; Clarke et al. 2001a,b). Measurements of serum methadone levels before and after the start of antiretroviral therapy can be used to guide dose adjustments (Gourevitch and Friedland 2000). It is also important to note that when patients are coadministered methadone with PIs or NNRTIs, special monitoring for methadone overdose is required when the antiretroviral therapy is stopped (Clarke et al. 2001b).

NRTIs do not appear to alter methadone levels, with the exception of abacavir, which can lower methadone levels by up to 22% (Ziagen 2004). Methadone, in turn, can increase zidovudine levels (Retrovir 2003; McCance-Katz et al. 1998) and decrease the levels of didanosine and stavudine (DHHS 2004; Rainey et al. 2000). Preliminary data indicate that methadone does not decrease didanosine levels when the enteric-coated formulation (Videx EC) is used (DHHS 2004; Friedland et al 2002). The clinical implications of these interactions are not known, and no specific dosing recommendations have been established. (For further details on methadone interactions, see Table 4 in Objective III.29 on Psychiatric Disorders in the AAHIVM 2003 Study Guide.)

Oxycodone (Roxicodone, OxyContin) is, in part, metabolized by CYP2D6 (OxyContin 2003). PIs are potent inhibitors of this enzyme, and therefore have the potential to increase oxycodone levels. The clinical implications of this interaction are unknown.

Sedatives, Antidepressants and Anticonvulsants

PIs may inhibit the metabolism of the sedative hypnotics midazolam (Versed) or triazolam (Halcion), leading to oversedation; these combinations are contraindicated (DHHS 2004; Antoniou and Tseng 2002). The interaction between midazolam and PIs needs to be communicated to physicians performing invasive procedures on patients in whom midazolam may be used for sedation. Lorazepam (Ativan) has minimal interactions with PIs, and these drugs can be given together with relative safety (Antoniou and Tseng 2002). The DHHS (2004) suggests temazepam (Restoril) as another alternative.

Some of the antidepressant drugs are metabolized by P450 cytochromes, and there are concerns for interactions with antiretrovirals. There are case reports of patients suffering from serotonin syndrome when given fluoxetine (Prozac) and NNRTIs and PIs (DeSilva et al. 2001), but this seems to be a very uncommon interaction. From limited clinical data, there do not appear to be any significant interactions between antiretrovirals and bupropion (Wellbutrin) (Pedrol et al. 2004). However, ritonavir increases levels of most antidepressants, including bupropion, nefazodone, selective serotonin reuptake inhibitors (SSRIs) and tricyclics (Norvir 2003). Drug levels should be monitored when these medications are given together.

There are extensive interactions between the older anticonvulsants (phenytoin [Dilantin], phenobarbital [Solfoton], and carbamazepine [Tegretol]) and antiretrovirals (DHHS 2004; Romanelli and Pomeroy 2003); delavirdine is contraindicated (DHHS 2004). Although blood levels of such anticonvulsants can be monitored to ensure therapeutic concentrations, these drugs may decrease the levels of concurrent PIs and NNRTIs. In general, the DHHS recommends monitoring drug levels, using with caution and/or considering alternative anticonvulsants. Newer anticonvulsants, such as gabapentin (Neurontin), tiagabine (Gabitril) or levetiracetam (Keppra), appear to have fewer interactions and may be preferred as alternatives to the older drugs (Romanelli and Pomeroy 2003).

Erectile Dysfunction Therapy

All of the drugs approved for treatment of erectile dysfunction (sildenafil, vardenafil and tadalafil) are PDE5 inhibitors, and are metabolized by CYP3A4, so levels are likely to be higher in patients receiving PIs (DHHS 2004; Cialis 2003; Levitra 2003; Viagra 2003; Merry 1999). Package inserts indicate that patients should start these drugs at a reduced dose, 25 mg for sildenafil (Viagra), 2.5 mg for vardenafil (Levitra) and 10 mg for tadalafil (Cialis), and should only take them once during a 48-hour (sildenafil) or 72-hour (vardenafil or tadalafil) period if they are also taking PIs (Cialis 2003; Levitra 2003; Viagra 2003).

Atazanavir

Many PIs are dependent upon the presence or absence of an acidic gastric environment for absorption. Atazanavir poses particular problems. The solubility of atazanavir decreases with higher gastric pH, and reduced plasma concentrations are expected if agents that increase gastric pH (e.g., antacids, buffered medications, H_2-receptor antagonists and proton-pump inhibitors) are administered along with this PI (Reyataz 2004). The prescribing information recommends that proton-pump inhibitors not be given with atazanavir and that H_2-receptor antagonists be dosed 12 hours from the time of atazanavir administration. Antacids and buffered medications, such as didanosine, should be given at least 2 hours before or one hour after atazanavir.

For atazanavir, in contradistinction to some other PIs, low-dose ritonavir may not circumvent an elevated pH. The results of a pharmacokinetic study showed substantial reductions (over 70%) in ritonavir-boosted atazanavir concentrations when given with the proton-pump inhibitor omeprazole (Prilosec), and these two drugs should not be used together (Agarwala et al. 2005; Bristol-Myers Squibb 2004). (Administering atazanavir with a cola soft drink in this study had no effect.) In addition, a retrospective study of medical records of 34 patients across 10 HIV clinics in Los Angeles found inadequate levels of ritonavir-boosted or unboosted atazanavir when given with a proton-pump inhibitor or an H2-receptor antagonist, prompting the investigators to recommend that the acid-control agents be stopped or the PI switched (Farthing and Khanlou 2004).

Prescribing information for atazanavir indicates that it has been associated with a twofold increase in plasma levels of the calcium-channel blocker diltiazem (Cardizem, Tiazac). This increase can cause prolongation of the cardiac PR interval (Reyataz 2004). The prescribing information also recommends that diltiazem doses be reduced by half when used in combination with atazanavir, and that routine ECG monitoring be performed. There are no data on interactions of atazanavir with other calcium-channel blockers, and these drugs should only be given concomitantly with careful and close monitoring. However, there is no apparent interaction between atazanavir and atenolol (Tenormin) (Reyataz 2004).

Recreational Drugs and Alternative Medicine

One fatal and one nearly fatal interaction have been reported in HIV-infected patients concurrently taking MDMA (ecstasy) respectively with or without GHB (gamma-hydroxybutyrate) (Harrington et al. 1999; Henry and Hill 1998). The 2 patients were previous users of these drugs who had begun taking ritonavir shortly before the incidents. Ritonavir inhibits the hepatic cytochrome P450 enzymes that metabolize MDMA. GHB is the subject of extensive first-pass hepatic metabolism. Other fatal or life-threatening cases involving ritonavir were not found in a 1999-2001 survey of U.S. medical examiners (Patel et al. 2004) or in a 2002 literature review (Antoniou and Tseng 2002).

The herb St. John's wort may decrease levels of NNRTIs and PIs, potentially leading to treatment failure. Patients on these antiretrovirals should avoid concomitant use of St. John's wort or preparations containing it. For more information please see Objective II.70 on Herbal Remedies in the AAHIVM 2003 Study Guide.

References

Agarwala S, Gray K, Wang Y, Grasela D. pharmacokinetic effect of omeprazole on atazanavir co-administered with ritonavir in healthy subjects. In: Program and abstracts of the 12th Conference on Retroviruses and Opportunistic Infections; February 22-25, **2005**; Boston, Massachusetts. Abstract 658.

Agenerase (amprenavir) [prescribing information]. Research Triangle Park, NC: GlaxoSmithKline; February **2004**.

Antoniou T, Tseng AL. Interactions between recreational drugs and antiretroviral agents. *Ann Pharmacother.* **2002**;36:1598-1613.

Boffito M, Rossati A, Reynolds HE, Hoggard PG, Back DJ, Di Perri G. Undefined duration of opiate withdrawal induced by efavirenz in drug users with HIV infection and undergoing chronic methadone treatment. *AIDS Res Human Retrovir.* **2002**;18:341-342.

Bristol-Myers Squibb. Reyataz® (atazanavir sulfate) with or without Norvir® (ritonavir) and proton pump inhibitors should not be coadministered: important new pharmacokinetic data. December **2004**. Available at: http://www.fda.gov/oashi/aids/listserv/2004/reyataz.pdf [accessed February 17, 2005].

Calvo R, Lukas JC, Rodriguez M, Carlos MA, Suarez E. Pharmacokinetics of methadone in HIV-positive patients receiving the non-nucleoside reverse transcriptase efavirenz [letter]. *Br J Clin Pharmacol.* **2002**;53:212-214.

Centers for Disease Control and Prevention (CDC). Updated guidelines for the use of rifamycins for the treatment of tuberculosis among HIV-infected patients taking protease inhibitors or nonnucleoside reverse transcriptase inhibitors. January 20, **2004**. Available at: http://www.cdc.gov/nchstp/tb/tb_hiv_drugs/toc.htm [accessed January 5, 2005].

Cialis (tadalafil) [prescribing information]. Indianapolis, Ind: Eli Lilly; November **2003**.

Clarke S. Mulcahy F. Bergin C. et al. Absence of opioid withdrawal symptoms in patients receiving methadone and the protease inhibitor lopinavir-ritonavir. *Clin Infect Dis.* **2002**;34:1143-1145.

Clarke SM, Mulcahy FM, Tjia J, et al. Pharmacokinetic interactions of nevirapine and methadone and guidelines for use of nevirapine to treat injection drug users. *Clin Infect Dis.* **2001a**;33:1595-1597.

Clarke SM, Mulcahy FM, Tjia J, et al. The pharmacokinetics of methadone in HIV-positive patients receiving the non-nucleoside reverse transcriptase inhibitor efavirenz. *Br J Clin Pharmacol.* **2001b**;51:213-217.

Department of Health and Human Services (DHHS). Guidelines for the use of antiretroviral agents in HIV-1-infected adults and adolescents. October 29, **2004**. Available at: http://aidsinfo.nih.gov/guidelines [accessed February 14, 2005].

DeSilva KE, Le Flore DB, Marston BJ, Rimland D. Serotonin syndrome in HIV-infected individuals receiving antiretroviral therapy and fluoxetine. *AIDS.* **2001**;15:1281-1285.

Dubé MP, Stein JH, Aberg JA, et al. Guidelines for the evaluation and management of dyslipidemia in human immunodeficiency virus (HIV) infected adults receiving antiretroviral therapy: recommendations of the HIV Medicine Association of the Infectious Disease Society of America and the Adult AIDS Clinical Trials Group. *Clin Infect Dis.* **2003**; 37:613-627.

Farthing C, Khanlou H. Co-administration of atazanavir with proton-pump inhibitors and h2-blockers. In: Program and abstracts of the 7th International Congress on Drug Therapy and HIV Infection; November 14-18, **2004**; Glasgow, United Kingdom. Abstract P289.

Friedland G, Rainey P, Jatlow P, Andrews L, Damle B, McCance-Katz E. Pharmacokinetics of didanosine from encapsulated enteric coated bead formulation (EC) vs chewable tablet formulation in patients on chronic methadone therapy. In: Program and abstracts of the XIV International AIDS Conference; July 7-12, **2002**; Barcelona, Spain. Abstract TuPeB4548.

Gerber JG, Fichtenbaum CJ, Rosenkranz S, et al. Efavirenz is a significant inducer of simvastatin and atorvastatin metabolism: results of ACTG A5108 study. In: Program and abstracts of the 11th Conference on Retroviruses and Opportunistic Infections; February 8-11, **2004**; San Francisco, California. Abstract 603.

Gourevitch MN, Friedland GH. Interactions between methadone and medications used to treat HIV infection: a review. *Mt Sinai J Med.* **2000**;67:429-436.

Harrington RD, Woodward JA, Hooton TM, Horn JR. Life-threatening interactions between HIV-1 protease inhibitors and the illicit drugs MDMA and gamma-hydroxybutyrate. *Arch Intern Med.* **1999**;159:2221-2224.

Henry JA, Hill IR. Fatal interaction between ritonavir and MDMA. *Lancet.* **1998**;352:1751-1752.

Levitra (vardenafil HCl) [prescribing information]. West Haven, Conn: Bayer Health Care; October **2004**.

Lexiva (fosamprenavir) [prescribing information]. Research Triangle Park, NC: GlaxoSmithKline; December **2004**.

McCance-Katz EF, Farber S, Selwyn PA, O'Connor A. Decrease in methadone levels with nelfinavir mesylate [letter]. *Am J Psych.* **2000**;157:481.

McCance-Katz EF, Rainey PM, Friedland G, Jatlow P. The protease inhibitor lopinavir-ritonavir may produce opiate withdrawal in methadone-maintained patients. *Clin Infect Dis.* **2003**;37:476-482.

McCance-Katz EF, Rainey PM, Jatlow P, Friedland G. Methadone effects on zidovudine disposition (AIDS Clinical Trials Group 262). *J Acquir Immune Defic Syndr Hum Retrovirol.* **1998**;18:435-443.

Merry C, Barry M, Ryan M, et al. Interaction of sildenafil and indinavir when co-administered to HIV-positive patients. *AIDS.* **1999**;13:F101-F107.

Norvir (ritonavir) [prescribing information]. Chicago: Abbott Laboratories; October **2003**.

Olivia J, Moreno S, Sanz J, et al. Co-administration of rifampin and nevirapine in HIV-infected patients with tuberculosis. *AIDS.* **2003**;17:637-638

Otero MJ, Fuertes A, Sanchez R, Luna G. Nevirapine-induced withdrawal symptoms in HIV patients on methadone maintenance programme: an alert [letter]. *AIDS.* **1999**;13:1004-1005.

OxyContin (oxycodone) [prescribing information]. Stamford, Conn: Purdue Pharma; July **2003**.

Patel MM, David W. Wright DW, Ratclif JJ, Miller MA. Shedding new light on the "safe" club drug: methylenedi oxymethamphetamine (ecstasy)-related fatalities. *Acad Emerg Med.* **2004**;11: 208-210 [followed by personal communication, March 2004].

Pedrol E, Ribell M, Vidal I, Garcia P, Deig E, Soler A. Concurrent use of bupropion with cytochrome p450 inhibitors: no outstanding clinical interactions. In: Program and abstracts of the XV International AIDS Conference, July 11-16, **2004**, Bangkok, Thailand. Abstract B11996.

Pinzani V, Faucherre V, Peyriere H, Blayac JP. Methadone withdrawal symptoms with nevirapine and efavirenz. *Ann Pharmacother.* **2000**;34:405-407.

Rainey PM, Friedland G, McCance-Katz EF, et al. Interaction of methadone with didanosine and stavudine. *J Acquir Immune Defic Syndr.* **2000**;24:241-248.

Retrovir (zidovudine) [prescribing information]. Research Triangle Park, NC: GlaxoSmithKline; April **2003**.

Reyataz (atazanavir) [prescribing information]. Princeton, NJ: Bristol-Myers Squibb; October **2004**.

Roche Pharmaceuticals. Important drug interaction warning: Drug-induced hepatitis with marked transaminase elevations has been observed in healthy volunteers receiving rifampin 600 mg once daily in combination with ritonavir 100 mg/saquinavir 1000 mg twice daily (ritonavir boosted saquinavir). [Dear Doctor Letter]. February 7, **2005**. Available at: http://www.fda.gov/medwatch/SAFETY/2005/Saquinavir-Rifampin_deardoc_Feb05.pdf [accessed February 18, 2005].

Romanelli F, Pomeroy C. Concurrent use of antiretrovirals and anticonvulsants in human immunodeficiency virus (HIV) seropositive patients. *Curr Pharm Des.* **2003**;9:1433-1439.

Stevens RC, Rapaport S, Maroldo-Connelly L, Patterson JB, Bertz R. Lack of methadone dose alterations or withdrawal symptoms during therapy with lopinavir/ritonavir [letter]. *J Acquir Immune Defic Syndr.* **2003**;33:650-651.

Stocker H, Kruse G, Kreckel P, et al. Nevirapine significantly reduces the levels of racemic methadone and (R)-methadone in human immunodeficiency virus-infected patients. *Antimicrob Agents Chemother.* **2004**;48:4148-4153.

Sustiva (efavirenz) [prescribing information]. Princeton, NJ: Bristol-Myers Squibb; December **2004**.

Viagra (sildenafil citrate) [prescribing information]. New York, NY: Pfizer; August **2003**.

Videx EC (didanosine, delayed-release) [prescribing information. Princeton, NJ: Bristol-Myers Squibb; January **2004**.

Viramune (nevirapine) [prescribing information]. Ridgefield, Conn: Boehringer Ingelheim; January **2005**.

Ziagen (abacavir sulfate) [prescribing information]. Research Triangle Park, NC: GlaxoSmithKline; August **2004**.

(RLO-22)

IV.10. RESISTANCE MUTATIONS

LEARNING OBJECTIVE: Identify the most important mutations and patterns of mutations associated with resistance to each of the currently FDA-approved antiretrovirals, and describe the concept of high and low genetic barriers to resistance.

Figures IV.10-1 through IV.10-3, reprinted from the International AIDS Society–USA Drug Resistance Mutations Group update (Johnson et al. 2004), detail the mutations that are associated with resistance to reverse transcriptase, protease and entry inhibitors in vivo. Main issues to note include the following:

- New information on resistance mutations accumulates quickly, and interpretation algorithms change. Refer to Web addresses below for frequently updated resistance interpretations:
    - Los Alamos HIV Sequence Database. Available at: http://hiv-web.lanl.gov
    - Stanford HIV RT and Protease Sequence Database. Available at: http://hivdb.stanford.edu/
    - HIVresistanceWeb. Available at: http://www.hivresistanceweb.com
    - The International AIDS Society-USA. Available at: http://www.iasusa.org
- Drugs for which a single mutation results in a large change in susceptibility are said to have a low "genetic barrier" to resistance. Examples of such drugs include lamivudine, emtricitabine and the entire NNRTI class of agents (nevirapine, delavirdine efavirenz). PIs, which are regarded as having a relatively high genetic barrier to resistance, require multiple mutations to confer substantially reduced drug susceptibility, and these mutations occur in a stepwise manner. Exceptions to this high genetic barrier include the PIs nelfinavir, atazanavir, amprenavir and saquinavir. Boosted PIs (blood levels increased by adding ritonavir) may still be active despite the presence of mutations that would reduce susceptibility to unboosted PIs (Hirsch et al. 2003).
- In 128,456 samples submitted for resistance testing from 1998 to 2004, there was a declining frequency of resistance-conferring mutations in the protease and reverse transcriptase genes. The emergence of previously undescribed mutation combinations seems to be occurring at a steady rate, but these remain rare (Rinehart 2005).
- There is a considerable degree of cross-resistance among several of the nucleoside reverse transcriptase inhibitors (NRTIs). Zidovudine and stavudine select for mutations at reverse transcriptase codons 41, 44, 67, 70, 118, 210, 215 and 219, which are referred to as NRTI-associated mutations (NAMs; previously referred to as thymidine analog mutations, TAMs). Exposure to other NRTIs is less likely to select for these mutations. The emergence of NAMs during treatment with such drugs as tenofovir and abacavir depends on previous and concurrent drugs and which mutations are already present. The presence of NAMs confers cross-resistance to members of the NRTI class.

What's New

Reports have described unexpected pathways to NNRTI, atazanavir and enfuvirtide resistance. There is also documentation of first-line lopinavir treatment failures, with and without development of resistance.

Key Points

- Drugs for which 1 mutation greatly changes susceptibility have a low "genetic barrier" to resistance.
- A considerable degree of cross-resistance exists among nucleoside reverse transcriptase inhibitors (NRTIs).
- NRTI-associated mutations (NAMs) on reverse transcriptase are capable of conferring resistance across the entire drug class. They are selected mainly by exposure to zidovudine and stavudine. Further NAM selection can occur during subsequent treatment with such drugs as tenofovir and abacavir.
- The 151 complex and the 69 insertion complex are associated with multi-NRTI resistance. Changes at both codons are generally accompanied by additional characteristic mutations that may play a critical role in broad NRTI cross-resistance.
- K65R, the 69 insertion complex or any 3 NAMs (inclusive of M41L or L210W) confer resistance to tenofovir. K65R contributes to resistance to most antiretroviral drugs except for zidovudine. However, K65R and the NAMs interfere with each other's mechanism for resistance.
- The codon M184V mutation conferring lamivudine resistance is associated with cross-resistance to emtricitabine and (with additional mutations) to abacavir and zalcitabine.

Key Points (cont.)

- Mutations at codons 103 and 188 cause high-level resistance to all currently FDA-approved nonnucleoside reverse transcriptase inhibitors (NNRTIs); a mutation at position 181 causes high-level resistance to nevirapine and may lead to rapid development of high-level resistance to the other approved NNRTIs.

- Protease inhibitors such as indinavir, ritonavir and lopinavir require multiple protease mutations for reduced drug susceptibility. Resistance to nelfinavir, atazanavir, amprenavir and saquinavir can occur with just 1 mutation. Accumulating multiple mutations is associated with cross-resistance in this class.

- The accumulation of 4 to 6 protease mutations has been associated with lopinavir/ritonavir resistance. Because the full spectrum of lopinavir/ritonavir mutations is not yet clearly defined, some authorities recommend phenotypic testing prior to initiating lopinavir/ritonavir in protease inhibitor-experienced patients.

- The 151 complex (Q151M plus mutations at codons 62, 75, 77 and 116) and the insertion mutation at codon 69 (T69S plus SS, SA SG, or, less commonly, 2 other amino acids) are associated with multi-NRTI resistance. The 69 insertion mutation can occur in conjunction with NAMs.

- Tenofovir resistance occurs in the presence of K65R, the 69 insertion complex, or at least 3 NAMs (inclusive of M41L or L210W). The 151 mutation complex does not appear to confer resistance to tenofovir independently of K65R (Wolf et al. 2003).

- The K65R mutation also contributes to resistance to all nucleoside analogs aside from zidovudine (Parikh et al. 2003). Along with M184V, K65R is common in the triple-NRTI regimen of abacavir/lamivudine/tenofovir (Landman et al. 2004).

- K65R interferes with the effect of NAMs, and vice versa (Parikh et al. 2003). The two are not usually seen together. Opposing conformational changes in reverse transcriptase cause this bi-directional antagonism. The NAMs facilitate the excision of nucleoside analogs after they have been put in place by reverse transcriptase. K65R prevents the incorporation of nucleoside analogs in the first place (White et al. 2004).

- The mutation at reverse transcriptase codon 184 that characterizes lamivudine resistance (M184V) is associated with cross-resistance to emtricitabine and (with additional mutations) to abacavir and zalcitabine. The M184V mutation does not affect didanosine activity (Winters et al. 2003; Molina 2003), but the presence of at least 3 NAMs substantially reduces susceptibility to this drug (Molina et al. 2003).

- Viral isolates containing the K65R, M184V, and K65R/M184V combination mutations have enhanced susceptibility to efavirenz, indicating that use of an NNRTI with a non-thymidine analog NRTI regimen is desirable (Coakley 2005b). However tenofovir should not be given with didanosine - see objective IV.18 on Not-Recommended Antiretroviral Combinations, in this Update.

- The L74V mutation alone causes decreased susceptibility to abacavir, didanosine and zalcitabine. When combined with M184V, it results in decreased phenotypic susceptibility to abacavir, didanosine, lamivudine and zalcitabine (Lanier et al. 2003) and increased susceptibility to tenofovir (Underwood 2005).

- The L74V/K65R double mutation, previously undetected in clinical specimens, was thought to diminish viral replication capacity to such an extent that it was nonviable. Although extremely rare (0.4% of patients in a 3,201 person Marseille database), the combined mutations can exist in the same HIV genome, and patients who harbor HIV possessing both L74V and K65R can exhibit high levels of viral replication (Colson 2005).

- Mutations at codons 103 and 188 lead to high-level resistance to all currently FDA-approved nonnucleoside reverse transcriptase inhibitors (NNRTIs). A mutation at position 181 leads to high-level resistance to nevirapine and subsequent rapid development of high-level resistance to the other 2 approved NNRTIs. Recent analysis of discordant NNRTI genotypic and phenotypic testing revealed that the K101P mutation and the combination of K103R plus V179D caused a greater than 10-fold phenotypic shift to at least 1 NNRTI (Petropoulos et al. 2003). The incidence of these mutations and their clinical relevance is currently unknown.

- Prior nonnucleoside experience appears to be a key determinant of subsequent treatment responses to NNRTI-containing highly active antiretroviral therapy (HAART) (Lecossier et al. 2005; Jourdain et al. 2004).

- Genotypic tests do not examine the genetic sequences determining the *gag* cleavage sites upon which protease acts. Interactions between protease and *gag* mutations can affect both resistance to PIs and clinical outcome (Hirsch et al. 2003). Mutated protease may be less efficient than the wild-type form, potentially leading to impaired replication capacity compared with wild type and lower plasma HIV RNA levels at least until compensatory mutations develop.

- Several protease mutations emerge during exposure to a variety of the protease inhibitors (PIs). The accumulation of 4 or more mutations at codons 10, 32, 46, 54, 82, 84 and 90 is associated with cross-resistance in this class. Some combinations of fewer than 4 mutations may also confer cross-resistance.

- The full extent of the mutations associated with reduced susceptibility to lopinavir/ritonavir has not been clearly established. To date, treatment failure of lopinavir/ritonavir-containing HAART has been rare in treatment-naive patients (Hicks et al. 2004; Molina et al. 2004). It has occurred without documented protease resistance, even when treatment-naive patients are on lopinavir/ritonavir without supporting drugs (Gathe 2004). Recently, though, a case of lopinavir resistance was detected in a patient taking lopinavir/ritonavir as first PI (Parkin et al. 2004). Genotypic analysis showed protease resistance mutations at positions V32I and I47A with a 38-fold reduction in lopinavir susceptibility on phenotypic testing. When lopinavir resistance is suspected because of prior PI experience or presence of protease mutations, some authorities recommend phenotypic testing. It should be noted that clinical data to support phenotypic testing in this circumstance are sparse. Although phenotype testing will pick up reduced susceptibility arising from previously uncharacterized mutations, it may miss resistance in isolates containing a mixture of wild-type and mutated protease. Also, standards for phenotypic resistance (clinical cutoffs) have only lately been defined (Bacheler et al. 2004). Some loss in susceptibility to lopinavir/ritonavir does not necessarily translate into worse clinical outcome.

- The new, ritonavir-boosted protease inhibitor tipranavir yields a better response in patients with HIV containing multiple resistance mutations than do other ritonavir-boosted protease inhibitors (Schapiro 2005). Clinical trial results indicate that tipranavir activity nonetheless is impaired by the standard key protease mutations at codons 33, 82, 84 and 90 (Cooper et al. 2003). With other protease mutations in the background, the presence of three of these key mutations will substantially reduce susceptibility to tipranavir whereas only one or two such mutations is sufficient to block other protease inhibitors. About 30% of highly treatment-experienced participants in phase II trials exhibited such loss of tipranavir activity (Cooper et al. 2003). More recent reports based on further analysis contest whether one of the common key mutations, L90M, is implicated in tipranavir resistance (Kohlbrenner 2004).

- Developing first PI failure while on an unboosted atazanavir regimen can arise from development of an I50L mutation (with or without A71V). The I50L mutation decreases atazanavir susceptibility while increasing in vitro susceptibility to other PIs. The clinical effects of I50L on subsequent PIs are unknown. Historically common protease resistance mutations (e.g., V82A, I84V and L90M) arise in treatment-experienced patients on ritonavir-boosted atazanavir and yield cross-resistance to other PIs (Reyataz 2004).

- The atazanavir associated resistance mutation N88S was observed for the first time emerging in a PI-naive patient receiving ritonavir-boosted atazanavir (Coakley 2005a). The patient had successfully taken a PI for a brief period and did not have phenotypic or genotypic PI resistance before starting boosted atazanavir. This single mutation resulted in high-level resistance and a reduced replicative capacity. N88S confers cross-resistance to nelfinavir and indinavir in clinical isolates.
- Several mutations in the gp41 envelope gene have been associated with resistance or reduced susceptibility to enfuvirtide. These are primarily at codons 36 through 45 of the first heptad repeat (HR1) region (Maroldo 2005). In one reported case, the V38E mutation emerged rapidly in a highly treatment-experienced patient who started a salvage regimen containing enfuvirtide. The result was high-level resistance to enfuvirtide. Enfuvirtide resistance can emerge rapidly in clinical practice. Testing for enfuvirtide resistance is not yet available commercially.

Figure IV.10-1. Mutations in the reverse transcriptase gene associated with resistance to reverse transcriptase inhibitors (Johnson et al. 2004). See also User Notes.

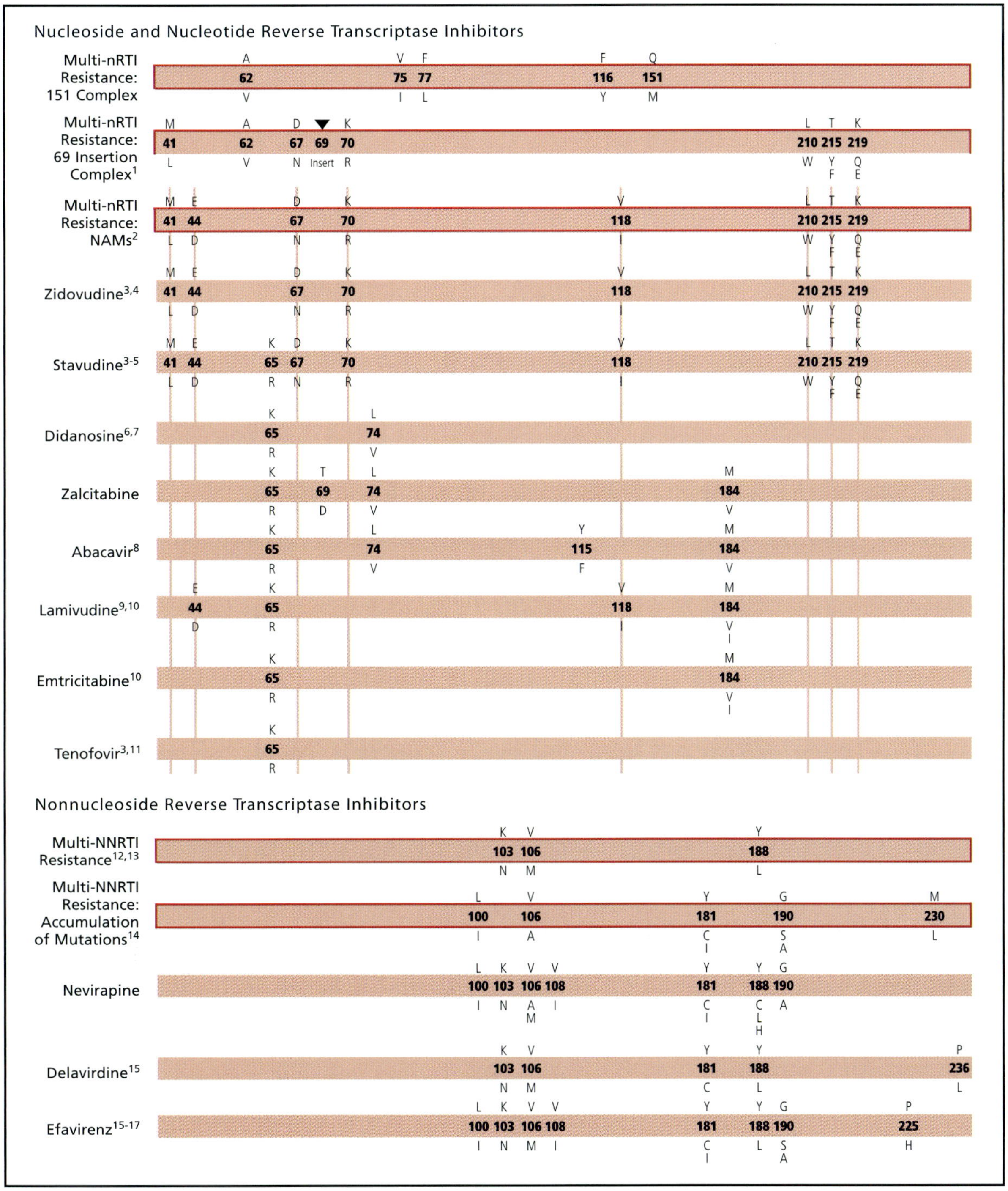

Reprinted with permission from the International AIDS Society-USA. Johnson VA, Brun-Vézinet F, Clotet B, et al. Update of the drug resistance mutations in HIV-1: 2004. *Topics in HIV Medicine*. **2004**;12(4):119-124. Updated information is available at www.iasusa.org.

Figure IV.10-2. Mutations in the protease gene associated with resistance to protease inhibitors (Johnson et al. 2004). See also User Notes.

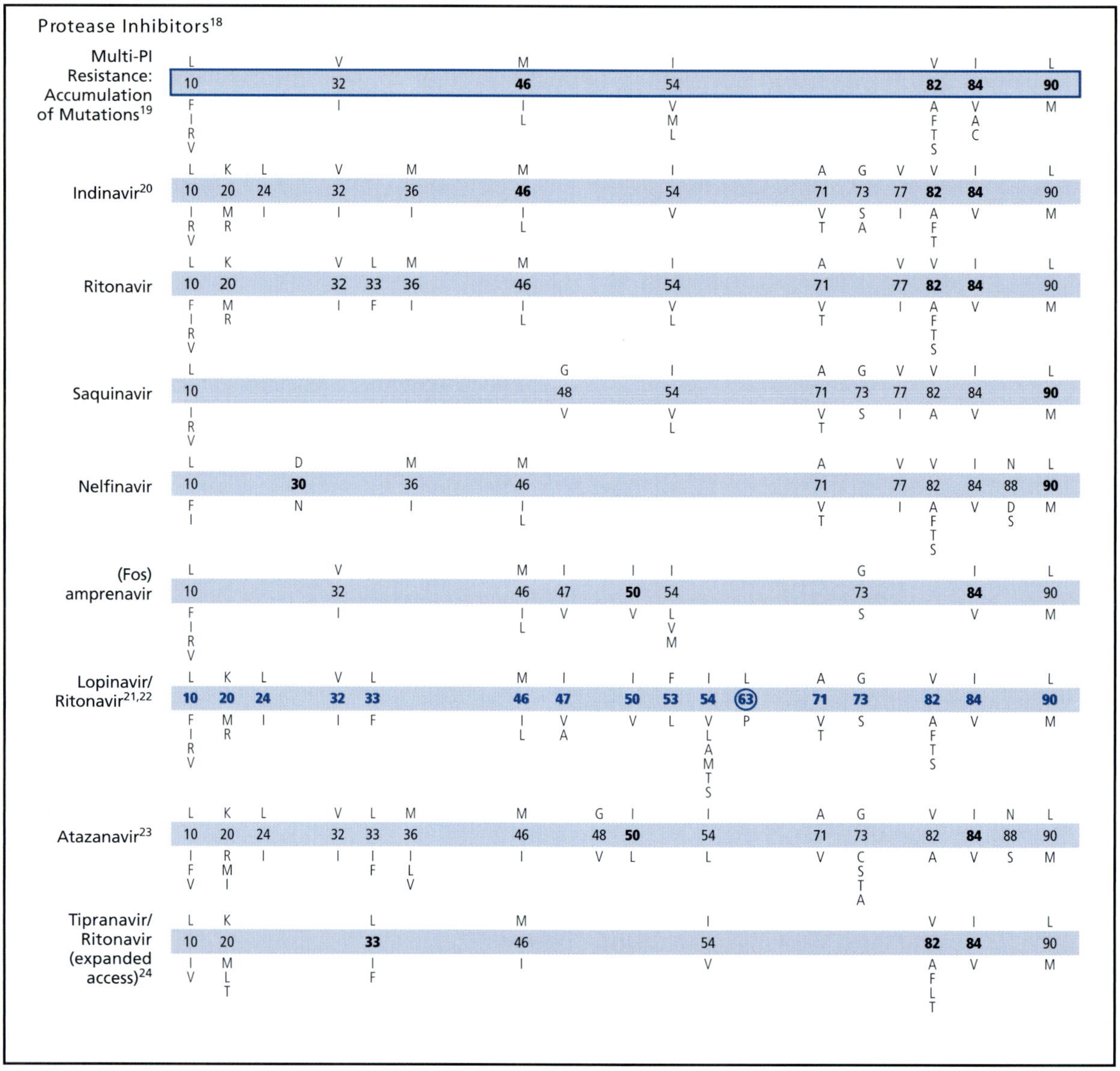

Reprinted with permission from the International AIDS Society-USA. Johnson VA, Brun-Vézinet F, Clotet B, et al. Update of the drug resistance mutations in HIV-1: 2004. *Topics in HIV Medicine*. 2004;12(4):119-124. Updated information is available at www.iasusa.org.

Figure IV.10-3. Mutations in the GP41 envelope gene associated with resistance to entry inhibitors (Johnson et al. 2004). See also User Notes.

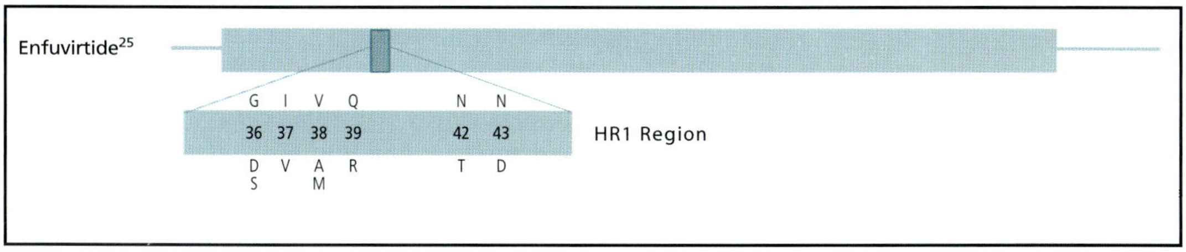

Reprinted with permission from the International AIDS Society-USA. Johnson VA, Brun-Vézinet F, Clotet B, et al. Update of the drug resistance mutations in HIV-1: 2004. *Topics in HIV Medicine*. 2004;12(4):119-124. Updated information is available at www.iasusa.org.

Key to Figures IV.10-1 through IV.10-3

For each amino acid residue, the letter above the bar indicates the amino acid associated with wild-type virus, and the letter(s) below indicate(s) the substitution(s) that confer(s) viral resistance. The number shows the position of the mutation in the protein. Mutations selected by protease inhibitors in Gag cleavage sites are not listed because their contribution to resistance is not yet fully defined.

HR1 indicates first heptad repeat; NAMs indicates nRTI-associated mutations; nRTI indicates nucleoside reverse transcriptase inhibitor; NNRTI indicates nonnucleoside reverse transcriptase inhibitor; PI indicates protease inhibitor.

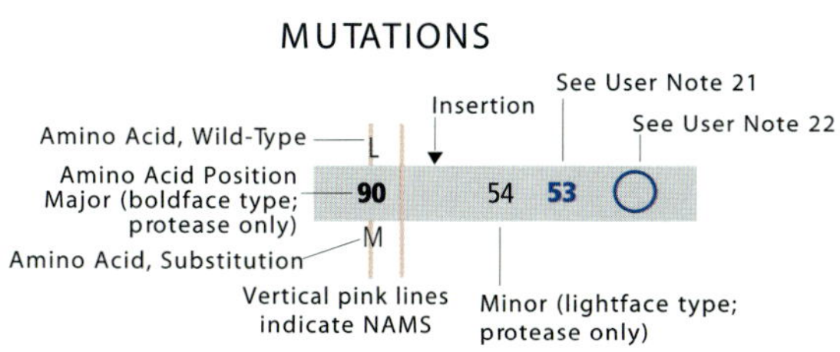

Amino acid abbreviations:

A, alanine; G, glycine; M, methionine; S, serine;
C, cysteine; H, histidine; N, asparagine; T, threonine;
D, aspartate; I, isoleucine; P, proline; V, valine;
E, glutamate; K, lysine; Q, glutamine; W, tryptophan;
F, phenylalanine; L, leucine; R, arginine; Y, tyrosine.

Reprinted with permission from the International AIDS Society-USA. Johnson VA, Brun-Vézinet F, Clotet B, et al. Update of the drug resistance mutations in HIV-1: 2004. *Topics in HIV Medicine*. 2004;12(4):119-124. Updated information is available at www.iasusa.org.

User Notes

Reprinted with permission from the International AIDS Society-USA. Johnson VA, Brun-Vézinet F, Clotet B, et al. Update of the drug resistance mutations in HIV-1: 2004. *Topics in HIV Medicine*. 2004;12(4):119-124. Updated information is available at www.iasusa.org.

The IAS–USA Drug Resistance Mutations Group reviews new data on HIV drug resistance in order to maintain a current list of mutations associated with clinical resistance to HIV. This list includes mutations that may contribute to a reduced virologic response to a drug. These mutations have been identified by 1 or more of the following criteria: (1) in vitro passage experiments or validation of contribution to resistance by using site-directed mutagenesis; (2) susceptibility testing of laboratory or clinical isolates; (3) genetic sequencing of viruses from patients in whom the drug is failing; (4) correlation studies between genotype at baseline and virologic response in patients exposed to the drug. Drugs that have been approved by the US Food and Drug Administration (FDA) or are available through-expanded access protocols are included. Additional information on the mutations is provided, where necessary, in these user notes.

1. The 69 insertion complex, consisting of a mutation at codon 69 (typically T69S) and followed by an insertion of 2 or more amino acids (S-S, S-A, S-G, or others), is associated with resistance to all FDA-approved nRTIs. The 69 insertion complex is often accompanied by mutations at other sites. Some other amino acid changes from the wild-type T in codon 69 without the insertion may also be associated with broad nRTI resistance.

2. The nRTI-associated mutations (NAMs), including M41L, E44D, D67N, K70R, V118I, L210W, T215Y/F, and K219Q/E, are associated with cross-resistance to nRTIs and are represented by vertical pink lines. Zidovudine and stavudine select for these mutations, and as such, the positions and mutations are indicated on the bars along with the pink lines. For other nRTIs, the NAMs are not commonly selected by those drugs, but the presence of the NAMs confers cross-resistance to the drugs. This is represented by pink lines only at the positions.

The E44D and V118I mutations are listed as NAMs. In a recent study, the E44D and V118I mutations were more common in virus from patients who had been on zidovudine and lamivudine, and were associated with higher-level resistance to zidovudine (Stoeckli et al, *Antimicrob Agents Chemother*, 2002). When present together with other NAMs, the E44D and V118I mutations confer resistance to lamivudine. Analysis from the AIDS Clinical Trials Group (ACTG) study 136 has shown that the V118I mutation is commonly selected by a zidovudine/didanosine regimen (Shafer et al, *J Infect Dis*, 1995). Findings from ACTG study 241 have shown that the E44D mutation is commonly selected by zidovudine/didanosine (Hanna et al, *J Infect Dis*, 2002) and that the E44D mutation is associated with a significantly worse response to treatment with zidovudine and didanosine, with or without nevirapine (Precious et al, *AIDS*, 2000). The significance of E44D or V118I when each occurs in isolation is unknown (Romano et al, *J Infect Dis*, 2002; Walter et al, *Antimicrob Agents Chemother*, 2002; Girouard et al, *Antivir Ther*, 2002).

3. The M184V mutation may enhance susceptibility to zidovudine, stavudine, or tenofovir. This effect may be overcome by an accumulation of NAMs or other mutations. The clinical significance of this effect is not known.

4. Data on revertant mutations in codon 215 indicate that the T215D/C/S/E/N/A/V substitutions confer increased risk of virologic failure of zidovudine and stavudine in antiretroviral-naive adults starting therapy with these drugs (Riva et al, *Antivir Ther*, 2002). In vitro studies and preliminary clinical studies suggest that the T215Y mutant may emerge quickly from these mutations in the presence of zidovudine or stavudine (Garcia-Lerma et al, *Proc Natl Acad Sci USA*, 2001; Lanier et al, *Antivir Ther*, 2002; Riva et al, *Antivir Ther*, 2002).

5. Mutations at codon 75 (V75T/M/S/A) have been observed in vitro and may confer a low-level change in susceptibility to stavudine (Lacey et al, *Antimicrob Agents Chemother*, 1994).

6. The K65R mutation or the L74V mutation, alone or in combination with the NAMs or T69D/N can lead to didanosine resistance.

7. Based on preliminary, yet-unpublished data, the M184V mutation does not appear to have a negative impact on in vivo responses to didanosine, even though the mutation reduces susceptibility in vitro (Winters et al, *Antivir Ther*, 2002; Eron et al, *Antivir Ther*, 2002; Pozniak et al, *Antivir Ther*, 2002).

8. When present with NAMs, the M184V mutation contributes to reduced susceptibility to abacavir and is associated with impaired response in vivo. However, when present alone, the M184V mutation does not appear to be associated with a reduced virologic response to abacavir in vivo (Harrigan et al, *J Infect Dis*, 2000).

9. The E44D and V118I mutations were reported to confer low-level resistance to lamivudine when accompanied by several other nRTI-associated mutations (M41L, D67N, L210W, T215Y/F, K219Q/E) in the absence of a concurrent M184V mutation (Hertogs et al, *Antimicrob Agents Chemother*, 2000). Data presented but not yet published (D'Arminio-Monforte et al, 8th CROI, 2001), reported no association over the short term between E44D or V118I and virologic response to a lamivudine-containing combination regimen. (See also user note 2.)

10. Emtricitabine and lamivudine have similar reverse transcriptase M184V/I patterns (Quinn et al, *ICAAC*, 2003). In addition, the K65R mutation can confer cross-resistance to emtricitabine and lamivudine (Miller et al, *ICAAC*, 2003; Miller et al, *Antivir Ther*, 2003; Miller et al, 10th CROI, 2003; Parikh et al, Antivir Ther, 2003; Ruane et al, *Antivir Ther*, 2003; McArthur et al, *Antivir Ther*, 2003). Additional mutations that confer resistance or cross-resistance to emtricitabine are possible, but are yet to be described.

11. The accumulation of NAMs (M41L, D67N, K70R, L210W, T215Y/F, K219Q/E [note: data here do not include E44D and V118I]) increases resistance to tenofovir. Mutations M41L and L210W contribute more than others. Therefore, the number and type of NAMs will determine the degree of reduced response. T69D/N/S may also contribute to a reduced response to tenofovir (Miller et al, *Antivir Ther*, 2002; Lu et al, *Antivir Ther*, 2002; Masquelier et al, *Antivir Ther*, 2002).

12. The K103N or Y188L mutation alone can substantially reduce the clinical utility of all currently approved NNRTIs.

13. The V106M mutation confers high-level resistance in vitro to nevirapine, delavirdine, and efavirenz (Brenner et al, *AIDS*, 2003). This mutation has been observed only in HIV clade C clinical isolates, although site-directed mutagenesis indicates that V106M confers cross-resistance to all NNRTIs in HIV clade B virus.

14. Accumulation of 2 or more of these mutations substantially reduces the clinical utility of all of the currently approved NNRTIs.

15. The prevalence of the Y318F mutation in clinical isolates along with mutations K103N, Y181C, or P236L was approximately 5%, 2%, and 15%, respectively (Kemp et al, *Antivir Ther*, 2001). In vitro this mutation confers resistance to nevirapine, delavirdine, and efavirenz.

16. The Y181C/I mutation is not selected by efavirenz, but its presence contributes to low-level cross-resistance to the drug. Clinical impact of this mutation may be overcome with a fully active antiretroviral combination regimen, although no clinical trial data yet address this question.

17. V108I and P225H each contribute to efavirenz resistance when present in combination with other NNRTI-associated mutations. Although V108I or P225H alone does not confer measurable resistance in laboratory strains of HIV-1, their presence in a clinical isolate may indicate prior selection for efavirenz-resistant variants.

18. Resistance mutations in the protease gene are classified as either "major" or "minor" (if known).

Major: In general, major mutations are either (1) selected first in the presence of the drug; or (2) shown at the biochemical or virologic level to lead to an alteration in drug binding or an inhibition of viral activity or viral replication. By themselves, major mutations have an effect on phenotype. In general, these mutations tend to be the major contact residues for drug binding.

Minor: In general, minor mutations appear later than major mutations, and by themselves do not have a significant effect on phenotype. In some cases, their effect may be to improve replicative fitness of virus carrying major mutations.

19. Accumulation of 4 or more of these mutations is likely to cause multi-PI resistance (Palmer et al, AIDS, 1999; Shafer et al, *Ann Intern Med*, 1998).

20. For indinavir, the mutations listed as major may not be the first mutations selected, but they are present in most clinical isolates in combination with other mutations.

21. Major and minor mutations have not been designated for lopinavir/ritonavir-associated resistance since currently there are no clear data defining degrees of influence with this drug combination. The accumulation of 6 or more of these mutations is associated with a diminished response to lopinavir/ritonavir. The product information states that accumulation of 7 or 8 mutations confers resistance to the drug. However, recent data suggest as few as 4 mutations can be associated with such high-level resistance (Prado et al, *AIDS*, 2002). Further clinical experience and research are needed to better define the mutations that affect the clinical effectiveness of lopinavir/ritonavir. It is reasonable to consider phenotyping to assess this in individual cases.

22. Protease mutation L63P is common in viruses that have never been exposed to PIs (Kozal et al, *Nat Med*, 1996) and may be more prevalent in viruses from patients in whom a PI-containing regimen has failed. However, by itself, L63P does not cause any appreciable increase in the IC_{50} for any PI. L63P is listed for lopinavir/ritonavir (and not any other PI) because studies have shown that this mutation, when present with multiple other mutations, is associated with clinical failure.

23. When administered to patients as the initial PI, atazanavir selects for the mutations I50L and A71V (Colonno et al, *Antivir Ther*, 2002). When used as a subsequent PI in combination with saquinavir, atazanavir selects for I54L and I84V (Colonno et al, *Antivir Ther*, 2002). In vitro, atazanavir selects for V32I, M46I, I84V, and N88S (Gong et al, *Antimicrob Agents Chemother*, 2000). Although other mutations, such as V82A and L90M, have not been selected for by atazanavir either in vitro or in vivo, these mutations have been shown to confer cross-resistance to atazanavir, particularly when present in combination with each other or with other known PI resistance mutations (Colonno et al, *Antivir Ther*, 2000). Recent data show the high impact of I84V (7- to 9-fold increase in IC_{50}) when in the background of A71V (Weinheimer at al, 11th CROI, 2004).

24. Tipranavir/ritonavir is currently available through an expanded-access protocol and is not approved by the FDA.

25. To date, resistance mutations in the gp41 envelope gene have been identified primarily at positions 36 to 45 of the first heptad repeat (HR1) region. These mutations have been identified in viruses from patients having been on enfuvirtide and have been shown to confer resistance or reduced susceptibility (Wei et al, *Antimicrob Agents Chemother.* 2002; Sista et al, *Antivir Ther*, 2002; Mink et al, *Antivir Ther*, 2002). It is important to note that wild-type viruses lacking any mutations in the depicted HR1 region vary 500-fold in susceptibility and such pretreatment susceptibility differences were not associated with differences in clinical response (Labrosse et al, J Virol, 2003; Greenberg et al, 10th CROI, 2003, Ab 141). Furthermore, it is possible that mutations and/or polymorphisms in other regions in the envelope (eg, the HR2 region or those yet to be identified) as well as coreceptor usage and density may affect susceptibility to enfuvirtide (Reeves et al, *PNAS*, 2002). Further research is needed to define the full spectrum of clinically relevant mutations conferring enfuvirtide resistance. Testing to detect only the depicted HR1 mutations may not be adequate for clinical management of suspected failure of regimens including enfuvirtide and must be interpreted in the context of resistance testing results for all other components of the regimen.

References

Bacheler L, Winters B, Harrigan PR, et al. Estimation of phenotypic clinical cutoffs for Virco TYPE through meta analyses of clinical trial and cohort data. In: Program and abstracts of the 44th Interscience Conference on Antimicrobial Agents and Chemotherapy; October 30-November 2, **2004**; Washington, DC. Abstract H-1133.

Coakley E, Mass M, Parkin N. Atazanavir resistance in a protease inhibitor-naive patient treated with atazanavir/ritonavir associated with development of high-level atazanavir resistance and the N88S mutation in protease. In: Program and abstracts of the 12th Conference on Retroviruses and Opportunistic Infections; February 22-25, **2005a**; Boston, Massachusetts. Abstract 716.

Coakley E, Parkin N. Contribution of non-thymidine analog nucleoside RT inhibitor associated mutations to phenotypic hypersusceptibility to efavirenz. In: Program and abstracts of the 12th Conference on Retroviruses and Opportunistic Infections; February 22-25, **2005b**; Boston, Massachusetts. Abstract 704.

Colson P, Henry M, Tourres C, Ravaux I, Poizot-Martin I, Tamalet C. Evidence by cloning analysis of the rare coexistence of the K65R/L74V mutant in the same HIV genome. In: Program and abstracts of the 12th Conference on Retroviruses and Opportunistic Infections, **2005**; Boston, Massachusetts. Abstract 701.

Cooper D, Hall D, Jayaweera D, et al. Baseline phenotypic susceptibility to tipranavir/ritonavir (TPV/r) is retained in isolates from patients with multiple–protease inhibitor (PI) experience (BI 1182.52). In: Program and abstracts of the 10th Conference on Retroviruses and Opportunistic Infections; February 10–14, **2003**; Boston, Massachusetts. Poster 596.

Gathe JC, Washington MY, Mayberry C, Piot D, Nemecek J. IMANI-1 TC3WP Single drug HAART- proof of concept study. Pilot study of the safety and efficacy of Kaletra (LPV/r) as single drug HAART in HIV + ARV-naive patients-interim analysis of subjects completing final 48 week data. In: Program and abstracts of the XV International Conference on AIDS; July 11-16, **2004**; Bangkok, Thailand. Abstract MoOrB1057.

Hicks C, da Silva B, Benson C, et al. Extensive resistance testing during 5 years of lopinavir/ritonavir treatment in antiretroviral-naive HIV infected patients: results from study m97-720. In: Program and abstracts of the XV International Conference on AIDS; July 11-16, **2004**; Bangkok, Thailand. Abstract WeOrB1291.

Hirsch MS, Brun-Vezinét F, Clotet B, et al. Antiretroviral drug resistance testing in adults infected with human immunodeficiency virus type 1: 2003 recommendations of an International AIDS Society-USA Panel. *Clin Infect Dis.* **2003**;37:113-128.

Johnson VA, Brun-Vézinet F, Clotet B, et al. Update on drug resistance mutations in HIV-1: 2004. *Top HIV Med.* **2004**;12:119-124. Available at: http://www.iasusa.org/pub/2004.html [accessed February 21, 2005].

Jourdain G, Ngo-Giang-Huong N, Le Coeur S, et al. Intrapartum exposure to nevirapine and subsequent maternal responses to nevirapine-based antiretroviral therapy. *N Engl J Med.* **2004**;351:229-240.

Kohlbrenner VM, Hall DB, Schapiro J, et al. Development of a tipranavir mutation score: analysis of protease mutations associated with phenotypic drug susceptibility and antiviral response in phase II clinical trials [abstract]. *Antivir Ther.* **2004**;9:S143.

Landman R, Peytavin G, Descamps D, et al. Low genetic barrier to resistance is a possible cause of early virologic failures in once-daily regimen of abacavir, lamivudine, and tenofovir: the TONUS study. In: Program and abstracts of the 11th Conference on Retroviruses and Opportunistic Infections; February 8-11, **2004**; San Francisco, California. Abstract 52.

Lanier ER, Irlbeck D, Ross L, et al. Prediction of NRTI options by linking reverse transcriptase genotype to phenotypic breakpoints. In: Program and abstracts of the 10th Conference on Retroviruses and Opportunistic Infections; February 10-14, **2003**; Boston, Massachusetts. Abstract 586.

Lecossier D, Shulman NS, Morand-Joubert L, et al. Detection of minority populations of HIV-1 expressing the K103N resistance mutation in patients failing nevirapine. *J Acquir Immune Defic Syndr.* **2005**;38:37-42.

Maroldo L, Coakley E, Chappey C, et al. Rapid selection of high-level resistance to enfuvirtide. In: Program and abstracts of the 12th Conference on Retroviruses and Opportunistic Infections; February 22-25, **2005**; Boston, Massachusetts. Abstract 717.

Molina JM, Gathe J, Lim PL, et al. Comprehensive resistance testing in antiretroviral naive patients treated with once-daily lopinavir/ritonavir plus tenofovir and emtricitabine: 48-week results from study 418. In: Program and abstracts of the XV International Conference on AIDS; July 11-16, **2004**; Bangkok, Thailand. Abstract WePeB5701.

Molina JM, Marcelin AG, Pavie J, et al. Didanosine (ddI) in treatment-experienced HIV-infected patients: results from a randomized double-blind study (AI454-176 Jaguar). In: Program and abstracts of the 43rd Interscience Conference on Antimicrobial Agents and Chemotherapy; September 14-17, **2003**; Chicago, Illinois. Abstract H-447.

Parikh U, Koontz D, Hammond J, et al. K65R: a multi-nucleoside resistance mutation of low but increasing frequency. *Antivir Ther.* **2003**;8:S152.

Parkin NT, Petropoulos CJ, Chappey C, et al. Isolated lopinavir resistance after virological rebound of a lopinavir/ritonavir-based regimen [abstract]. *Antivir Ther.* **2004**;9:S79.

Petropoulos CJ, Chappey C, Parkin NT. High-level resistance to HIV-1 non-nucleoside reverse transcriptase inhibitors (NNRTIs) in the absence of known resistance mutations. In: Program and abstracts of the 43rd Interscience Conference on Antimicrobial Agents and Chemotherapy; September 14-17, **2003**; Chicago, Illinois. Abstract H-451.

Reyataz (atazanavir) [prescribing information]. Princeton, NJ: Bristol-Myers Squibb; October **2004**.

Rinehart A, Lecocq P, Pattery T, Wasikowsi B, Bacheler L. Evolution in the diversity of HIV-1-resistance mutation patterns in over 128,000 clinical samples received for resistance analysis from 1998 to 2004. In: Program and abstracts of the 12th Conference on Retroviruses and Opportunistic Infections, **2005**; Boston, Massachusetts. Abstract 684.

Schapiro J, Cahn P, Trottier B, et al. Effect of baseline genotype on response to tipranavir/ritonavir (TPV/r) compared with standard-of-care comparator (CPI/r) in treatment-experienced patients: the phase 3 RESIST-1 and -2 trials. In: Program and abstracts of the 12th Conference on Retroviruses and Opportunistic Infections, **2005**; Boston, Massachusetts. Abstract 104.

Underwood M, St Clair M, Ross L, Gerondelis P, Parkin N, Lanier R. Cross-resistance of clinical samples with K65R, L74V, and M184V mutations. In: Program and abstracts of the 12th Conference on Retroviruses and Opportunistic Infections, **2005**; Boston, Massachusetts. Abstract 714.

White KL, Margot NA, Chen JM, et al. The HIV-1 K65R RT mutant utilizes a combination of decreased incorporation and decreased excision to evade NRTI. In: Program and abstracts of the 11th Conference on Retroviruses and Opportunistic Infections; February 8-11, **2004**; San Francisco, California. Abstract 55.

Winters MA, Bosch RJ, Albrecht MA, Katzenstein DA. Clinical impact of the M184V mutation on switching to didanosine or maintaining lamivudine treatment in nucleoside reverse-transcriptase inhibitor–experienced patients. *J Infect Dis*. **2003**;188:537-540.

Wolf K, Walter H, Beerenwinkel N, et al. Tenofovir resistance and resensitization. *Antimicrob Agents Chemother.* **2003**;47:3478-3484.

■

(RLO-23)

IV.11. ONCE-DAILY REGIMENS

LEARNING OBJECTIVE: Discuss the advantages and disadvantages of once-daily antiretroviral regimens, and identify agents with pharmacokinetics favorable to once-daily administration.

Although beneficial, combination antiretroviral therapy is often limited because of complex dosing schedules and frequent daily administration of many medications. Recent advances in antiretroviral therapy have included the development of newer agents with longer half-lives and the reevaluation of older agents using less frequent dosing intervals. Consequently, many agents and regimens are being evaluated for once-daily administration, and potential rewards and limitations to once-daily dosing have been found with all three classes of antiretroviral agents (Luber 2002). Furthermore, data are limited regarding improvements in patient adherence and clinical outcomes when agents and regimens are dosed once a day versus twice a day.

In order for an agent to be dosed once daily, sufficient concentrations of the agent (enough drug to inhibit the patient's viral isolate) should be present at the end of the dosing interval. Many factors influence the likelihood of sufficient drug exposure; these include maximum concentration of the agent following the dose, the half-life of the given agent, individual rates of metabolism or conversion to the active moiety (e.g., as with the nucleoside reverse transcriptase inhibitors [NRTIs]) and the amount of viral resistance. In general, for FDA-approved agents currently administered more than once daily, the goal is to reach equivalent total drug exposures (AUC; area under the concentration time curve) and minimum drug concentrations (C_{min}) that fall between standard and once-daily dosing. The amount of "buffer" that exists between the individual patient's drug exposure immediately before the next dose and the amount of drug that the individual patient's viral isolate requires for inhibition is referred to as the agent's "forgiveness factor." The greater the forgiveness factor, the lower the potential for viral breakthrough. Should extended periods of suboptimal drug levels occur, this could potentially accelerate the development of drug resistance; therefore, there is some concern that missed doses in once-daily regimens may have more serious consequences than those with twice- or three-times-daily regimens. However, if the pharmacokinetics are supportive, there is no reason to think a missed dose of a once-daily drug is more deleterious than that of a drug dosed multiple times per day.

Table IV.11-1 lists antiretroviral agents that could be used in once-daily regimens (DHHS 2004; Yeni et al. 2004). First, it lists single agents with pharmacokinetics that support once-daily dosing and that have been approved by the FDA for once-daily administration. Then the table lists two categories of agents that are not approved for once-daily dosing, but whose data appear to support the possibility: (a) other single agents with data that appear to support once-daily administration and (b) ritonavir-boosted protease inhibitors (PIs) that may be dosed once daily, although data is limited for some regimens.

What's New

New antiretroviral regimens approved for once-daily dosing include abacavir and the tenofovir/emtricitabine and abacavir/lamivudine combinations.

Key Points

- Although clinical data are limited, once-daily dosing may enhance short- and long-term adherence and thereby potentially improve virologic outcomes.
- Missed doses in once-daily regimens may have more serious consequences because of longer periods of lowered antiretroviral levels, and once-daily regimens may be complicated by varying food and fasting requirements of individuals agents.
- Antiretrovirals currently FDA-approved for once-daily dosing are the nonnucleoside reverse transcriptase inhibitor (NNRTI) efavirenz; nucleoside reverse transcriptase inhibitors (NRTIs) abacavir, didanosine, emtricitabine, lamivudine, stavudine (extended release) and tenofovir; the protease inhibitor (PI) atazanavir; and the boosted PIs amprenavir/ritonavir, fosamprenavir/ritonavir, and lapinavir/ritonavir (Kaletra). In addition, 2 recently marketed fixed-dose combinations have been approved for once-daily dosing: tenofovir/emtricitabine (Truvada) and abacavir/lamivudine (Epzicom).

Table IV.11-1. Antiretroviral agents that can be used in once-daily regimens.

Agent/Dose	Comment
FDA-approved for once-daily dosing	
Abacavir (600 mg)	Ziagen (2004)
Abacavir (600 mg)/lamivudine (300 mg)	Epzicom (2004)
Amprenavir (1200 mg)/ritonavir (200 mg)	Agenerase (2004)
Fosamprenavir (1400 mg)/ritonavir (200 mg)	Lexiva (2004); once-daily use in antiretroviral-naive subjects only
Atazanavir (400 mg)	Reyataz (2004); coadministration with nevirapine is not recommended; efavirenz reduces concentrations of coadministered, unboosted atazanavir; unboosted atazanavir should not be administered with tenofovir
Didanosine (400 mg as Videx EC or buffered tablets)	Videx EC (2004); coadministration with tenofovir may augment didanosine toxicity
Emtricitabine (200 mg)	Emtriva (2004)
Efavirenz (600 mg)	Sustiva (2004)
Lamivudine (300 mg)	Epivir (2004)
Lopinavir (800 mg)/ritonavir (200 mg)	Once-daily use in antiretroviral-naive subjects only; supported by pharmacokinetic and limited clinical data; greater interindividual drug level variability seen in the once-daily dosing arm (Bertz et al. 2002; Eron et al. 2002; Podczamer et al. 2003)
Stavudine (100-mg extended-release formulation)	Zerit XR (2005)
Tenofovir (300 mg)	Viread (2004); coadministration with didanosine may augment didanosine toxicity; coadministration with atazanavir reduces atazanavir levels – need to add ritonavir
Tenofovir (300 mg)/emtricitabine (200 mg)	Truvada (2005)
Not FDA-approved for once-daily dosing, but with data supporting the possibility	
Single agents	
Nevirapine (400 mg)	Supported by clinical and pharmacokinetic data; potential increase in liver-associated laboratory adverse events (Van Leth et al. 2003)
Ritonavir-boosted PIs	
Atazanavir (300 mg)/ritonavir (100 mg)	Badaro et al. (2003)
Atazanavir (400 mg)/saquinavir (1200-1600 mg)	Badaro et al. (2003); Haas et al. (2003) Also being evaluated in combination with low-dose ritonavir; this combination is not as potent in antiretroviral-experienced patients in comparison to atazanavir plus ritonavir or lopinavir/ritonavir (DeJesus 2004)
Indinavir (1200 mg)/ritonavir (100 mg)	Pharmacokinetics were more favorable when administered with 400 mg of ritonavir, but this is poorly tolerated (Hugen et al. 2000)
Saquinavir (2000 mg)/ritonavir (100 mg)	Supported by pharmacokinetic and clinical data (Boffito et al. 2003); saquinavir/ritonavir 1600/100 mg less effective than efavirenz in a clinical study (both combined with 2 NRTIs), primarily due to more discontinuations (Montaner et al. 2001)

Currently, atazanavir is the only FDA-approved PI that can be dosed once daily without pharmacokinetic boosting (Reyataz 2004). All of the PIs are metabolized to some degree via the cytochrome P450 enzyme system in the liver and small intestine (Piscitelli and Gallicano 2001). Inhibition of this enzyme system results in improved gastrointestinal absorption and/or decreased metabolism, thereby potentially allowing for once-daily dosing of many of the PIs. Ritonavir, a potent inhibitor of this enzyme system, has been evaluated in low doses (e.g., 100-400 mg) with most of the currently FDA-approved PIs (Cooper et al. 2003). As of May 2005, only amprenavir, fosamprenavir and lopinavir in combination with low-dose ritonavir have been FDA-approved for once-daily dosing. Note that fosamprenavir/ritonavir and lopinavir/ritonavir are approved only for once-daily use in antiretroviral-naive patients.

Clinical and pharmacokinetic data presented at the 9th Conference on Retroviruses and Opportunistic Infections (CROI) in Seattle and the 2nd European AIDS Clinical Society (EACS) Resistance and Pharmacology Workshop in Warsaw suggested that lopinavir/ritonavir (Kaletra) appears to be effective when administered once daily (Bertz et al. 2002; Eron et al. 2002; Podczamer et al. 2003). A study of once- versus twice-daily lopinavir/ritonavir (Kaletra) (400/100 mg twice daily versus 800/200 mg once daily) achieved similar 48-week results (Gathe et al. 2004). The trial combined lopinavir/ritonavir with once-daily emtricitabine and tenofovir for a complete once-daily regimen. In addition, saquinavir 2000 mg once daily combined with ritonavir 100 mg once daily also appears to be effective (Boffito et al. 2003).

With the NRTIs, plasma levels may not be critical. Rather, intracellular levels of the triphosphate form of the drug are the key to therapeutic success and toxicity (Anderson et al. 2003). However, measurement of antiviral intracellular triphosphates are not standardized or routinely assayed. The six NRTIs currently approved for once-daily dosing are abacavir, didanosine, emtricitabine, lamivudine, stavudine (extended release), and tenofovir. Notably, recent analyses of trials using once-daily regimens including didanosine and tenofovir have reported cases of early virologic failure and impaired CD4+ T cell responses (Videx 2004; Moyle et al. 2004; Barrios et al. 2004) as well as augmented didanosine toxicity (Videx 2004). (For details, see Objective IV.8 on Common Antiretroviral Toxicities in this Update.)

In August 2004, two fixed-dose combination nucleoside/nucleotide agents were approved for marketing. These are tenofovir/emtricitabine (Truvada) and abacavir/lamivudine (Epzicom). An interim, 24-week analysis of a 96-week trial suggested that antiviral, immunologic and adverse effects of tenofovir/emtricitabine and efavirenz once daily compare favorably with those of lamivudine/zidovudine twice daily plus efavirenz once daily (Arribas et al. 2004; Gazzard et al. 2004). In the intent-to-treat analysis, 87% of patients in the tenofovir-emtricitabine arm had achieved a viral load below 400 copies/mL, compared with 78% of patients in the zidovudine-lamivudine arm (P = .01); 73% of those receiving tenofovir-emtricitabine had reached viral loads below 50 copies/mL versus 65% of those in the zidovudine-lamivudine arm. In all, 3% of patients in the tenofovir-emtricitabine arm and 9% of those in the zidovudine-lamivudine arm dropped out of the study because of adverse drug effects.

References

Agenerase (amprenavir) [prescribing information]. Research Triangle Park, NC: GlaxoSmithKline; February **2004**.

Anderson PL, Kakuda TN, Kawle S, et al. Antiviral dynamics and sex differences of zidovudine and lamivudine triphosphate concentrations in HIV-infected individuals. *AIDS*. **2003**;17:2159-2168.

Arribas JR, DeJesus E , Campo R, et al. The combination of tenofovir DF (TDF), emtricitabine (FTC) and efavirenz (EFV) has significantly greater response vs fixed dose zidovudine/lamivudine (CBV) and EFV in antiretroviral naive patients: a 24-week preliminary analysis. In: Program and abstracts of the 7th International Congress on Drug Therapy in HIV Infection; November 14-18, **2004**; Glasgow, United Kingdom. Abstract PL14.2.

Badaro R, DeJesus E, Lazzarin A, et al. Efficacy and safety of atazanavir with ritonavir or saquinavir versus lopinavir/ritonavir in combination with tenofovir and one NRTI in patients who have experienced virologic failure to multiple HAART regimens: 16-week results from BMS AI424-045. In: Program and abstracts of the 2nd International AIDS Society conference on pathogenesis and treatment; July 13-16, **2003**; Paris, France. Abstract 118.

Barrios A, Negredo E, Rendon A, et al. Paradoxical CD4+ T cell decline in patients with complete virus suppression under tenofovir plus didanosine combinations. In: Program and abstracts of the 44th Interscience Conference of Antimicrobial Agents and Chemotherapy; October 30-November 2, **2004**; Washington, DC. Abstract H1132.

Bertz R, Foit C, Ye X, et al. Pharmacokinetics of once-daily vs twice-daily Kaletra (lopinavir/ritonavir) in HIV+ subjects. In: Program and abstracts of the 9th Conference on Retroviruses and Opportunistic Infections; February 24-28, **2002**; Seattle, Washington. Abstract 126.

Boffito M, Dickinson L, Hill A, et al. Pharmacokinetics (PK) of saquinavir/ritonavir (sqv/r) once daily (OD) in HIV+ subjects: Comparison with standard BD regimens. In: Program and abstracts of the 9th European AIDS Conference (EACS): 1st EACS Resistance & Pharmacology Workshop. October 25-29, **2003**, Warsaw, Poland. Abstract F2/3.

Cooper CL, van Heeswijk RPG, Gallicano K, et al. A review of low-dose ritonavir in protease inhibitor combination therapy. *Clin Infect Dis*. **2003**;36:1585-1592.

DeJesus E, Grinsztejn B, Rodriguez C, et al. Efficacy and safety of atazanavir with ritonavir or saquinavir vs lopinavir/ritonavir in patients who have experienced virologic failure on multiple HAART regimens: 48-week results from BMS A1424-045. In: Program and abstracts of the 11th Conference on Retroviruses and Opportunistic Infections; February 8-11, **2004**; San Francisco, California. Abstract 547.

Department of Health and Human Services (DHHS). Guidelines for the use of antiretroviral agents in HIV-1-infected adults and adolescents. October 29, **2004**. Available at: http://aidsinfo.nih.gov/guidelines [accessed February 9, 2005].

Emtriva (emtricitabine) [prescribing information]. Foster City, Calif: Gilead Sciences; September **2004**.

Epivir (lamivudine) [prescribing information]. Research Triangle Park, NC: GlaxoSmithKline; December **2004**.

Epzicom (abacavir sulfate and lamivudine) [prescribing information]. Research Triangle Park, NC: GlaxoSmithKline; August **2004**.

Eron JJ, Bernstein B, King M, et al. Once-daily vs twice-daily Kaletra (lopinavir/ritonavir) in antiretroviral-naïve HIV+ patients: 48-week follow-up. In: Program and abstracts of the 9th Conference on Retroviruses and Opportunistic Infections; February 24-28, **2002**; Seattle, Washington. Abstract 409.

Gathe J, Podzamczer D, Johnson M, et al. Once-daily vs twice-daily lopinavir/ritonavir in antiretroviral-naïve patients: 48-week results. In: Program and abstracts of the 11th Conference on Retroviruses and Opportunistic Infections; February 8-11, **2004**; San Francisco, California. Abstract 570.

Gazzard B, DeJesus E, Campo R, et al. The combinations of tenofovir DF (TDF), emtricitabine (FTC) and efavirenz (EFV) has significantly greater response vs fixed dose zidovudine/lamivudine (CBV) and EFV in antiretroviral naïve patients: a 24 week preliminary analysis. In: Program and abstracts of the 41st ICAAC; October 30-November 2, **2004**; Washington, DC. Abstract H-1137a.

Haas DW, Zala C, Schrader S, et al. Therapy with atazanavir plus saquinavir in patients failing highly active antiretroviral therapy: a randomized comparative pilot trial. *AIDS*. **2003**;17:1339-1349.

Hugen P, Burger D, ter Hofstede H, et al. Dose-finding study of a once-daily indinavir/ritonavir regimen. *J Acquir Immune Defic Syndr.* **2000**;25:236-245.

Lexiva (fosamprenavir calcium) [prescribing information]. Research Triangle Park, NC: GlaxoSmithKline; December **2004**.

Luber AD. The push for once-daily HAART: A call for caution (Letter to Editor). MedGenMed. **2002**;4(2). Available at: http://www.medscape.com/viewarticle/436567 [accessed February 22, 2005].

Montaner J, Saag M, Barylski C, Siemon-Hryczyk P. FOCUS study: saquinavir qd regimen versus efavirenz qd regimen 24 week analysis in HIV infected patients. In: Program and abstracts of the 41st Interscience Conference on Antimicrobial Agents and Chemotherapy; December 16-19, **2001**; Chicago, Illinois. Abstract 670.

Moyle G, Maitland D, Hand J, Mandalia S, Nelson M, Gazzard B. Early virological failure in persons with viral loads over 100,000 copies/mL and CD4 counts under 200/mm^3 receiving ddI/tenofovir/efavirenz as initial therapy: results from a randomised comparative trial. In: Program and abstracts of the 44th Interscience Conference of Antimicrobial Agents and Chemotherapy; October 30-November 2, **2004**; Washington, DC. Abstract H566.

Piscitelli SC and Gallicano KD. Interaction among drugs for HIV and opportunistic infections. *N Engl J Med.* **2001**;344:984-996.

Podczamer D, Gathe J, Johnson M, et al. Efficacy and safety of once-daily lopinavir/ritonavir vs. twice-daily lopinavir/ritonavir in antiretroviral-naïve patients: 24-week results. In: Program and abstracts of the 9th European AIDS Conference: 1st EACS Resistance and Pharmacology Workshop; October 25-29, **2003**; Warsaw, Poland. Abstract F1/3.

Reyataz (atazanavir sulfate) [prescribing information]. Princeton, NJ: Bristol-Myers Squibb; October **2004**.

Sustiva (efavirenz) [prescribing information]. Princeton, NJ: Bristol-Myers Squibb; December **2004**.

Truvada (emtricitabine and tenofovir disoproxil fumarate) [prescribing information]. Foster City, Calif: Gilead Sciences; January **2005**.

van Leth F, Hassink E, Phanuphak P, et al. Results of the 2NN study: a randomized comparative trial of first-line antiretroviral therapy with regimens containing either nevirapine alone, efavirenz alone or both drugs combined, together with stavudine and lamivudine. In: Program and abstracts of the 10th Conference on Retroviruses and Opportunistic Infections; February 10-14, **2003**; Boston, Massachusetts. Abstract 176.

Videx EC (didanosine) [prescribing information]. Princeton, NJ: Bristol-Myers Squibb; January **2004**.

Viread (tenofovir disoproxil fumarate) [prescribing information]. Foster City, Calif: Gilead Sciences; June **2004**.

Yeni PG, Hammer SM, Hirsch MS, et al. Treatment for adult HIV infection: 2004 recommendations of the International AIDS Society-USA Panel. *JAMA.* **2004**;292:251-265.

Zerit XR (stavudine) [NDA 21-453/S-004 approved labeling]. Princeton, NJ: Bristol-Myers Squibb Virology; January 19, **2005**. Available at: http://www.accessdata.fda.gov/scripts/cder/drugsatfda/ [accessed February 9, 2005].

Ziagen (abacavir sulfate) [prescribing information]. Research Triangle Park, NC: GlaxoSmithKline; August **2004**.

(RLO-24)

IV.12. REGIMEN SELECTION

LEARNING OBJECTIVE: Discuss the principles of how to combine antiretroviral medications, including reference to the U.S. Public Health Service and the International AIDS Society-USA guidelines for therapy, noting changes from previous guideline versions.

The high replication rate of HIV (Ho et al. 1995) means that viral progeny containing every possible single mutation occur at random every day in the average patient. This is the reason why resistance emerged relatively quickly when antiretroviral drugs were administered in monotherapy or dual-therapy regimens that were insufficiently potent to completely suppress viral replication. However, only very rarely will viral replication result in the simultaneous occurrence of mutations at several different points, as would be necessary to produce resistance to a multidrug antiretroviral regimen. Thus, combination therapy is said to present a genetic barrier to the development of resistance, protecting its efficacy and allowing sustained benefit.

Combination antiretroviral therapy is currently based on the use of three or more antiretroviral agents that individually may target the viral reverse transcriptase, protease or gp41 fusion protein in order to inhibit HIV replication. The use of combination regimens is required to assure suppression of viral replication and limit the chance for resistance to develop, thereby maximizing the likelihood of a sustained antiretroviral effect. Although 1-drug antiretroviral regimens are currently being evaluated (Arribas et al. 2004; Gathe et al. 2004; Kahlert et al. 2004), they are not recommended at this time. (See Objective IV.33 on Investigational Strategies Utilizing Approved Antiretroviral Agents in this Update.)

The following are the guiding principles for selecting a combination antiretroviral therapy regimen:

- The aim of therapy should be maximal suppression of viral replication to prevent the emergence of viral mutations resistant to 1 or more agents in the regimen
- Maximal suppression is currently described as maintenance of viral load below detectable levels, typically less than 50 copies/mL (DHHS 2004) by reverse transcriptase polymerase chain reaction (RT-PCR) or 75 copies/mL by bDNA assay
- Drugs should be used in combination to minimize the risk that resistance to a single agent will result in failure of the regimen
- The choice of individual agents may vary and should be individualized for the specific patient based on considerations of tolerability, prior experience and likelihood of adherence

Table IV.12-1 presents specific regimens recommended by the U.S. Public Health Service for the treatment of antiretroviral-naive adult and adolescent patients (DHHS 2004). Preferred regimens are listed along with the total number of pills per day; the preferred regimens have been selected by experts based on the totality of virologic, immunologic and toxicity data.

What's New

Abacavir plus lamivudine dosed once a day is an alternative nucleoside reverse transcriptase inhibitor (NRTI) backbone. Fosamprenavir may be boosted with ritonavir as an alternative protease inhibitor. Emtricitabine is an alternative to lamivudine.

Key Points

- Selection of antiretroviral agents for initial combination therapy should take into consideration sequencing/ resistance, tolerability and patient-specific issues.
- A key goal of therapy is to maintain maximal viral suppression when possible.
- Both the U.S. Public Health Service and the International AIDS Society-USA publish frequently updated guidelines on the general management and selection of antiretroviral therapies.

Table IV.12-1. Antiretroviral regimens recommended by the U.S. Public Health Service for initial treatment of established HIV infection in adults (DHHS 2004).

NNRTI Regimen		Pills/day
Preferred	Efavirenz + (lamivudine or emtricitabine) + (zidovudine or tenofovir)	2-3
Alternative	Efavirenz* + (lamivudine or emtricitabine) + (didanosine or abacavir or stavudine)	2-4
	Nevirapine† + (lamivudine or emtricitabine) + (zidovudine or stavudine or didanosine or abacavir or tenofovir)	3-6
PI-Based Regimen		**Pills/day**
Preferred	lopinavir/ritonavir (coformulation) + (lamivudine or emtricitabine) + zidovudine	8-9
Alternative	atazanavir + (lamivudine or emtricitabine) + (zidovudine or stavudine or abacavir or didanosine) or (tenofovir + ritonavir 100 mg/day)	3-6
	fosamprenavir + (lamivudine or emtricitabine) + (zidovudine or stavudine or abacavir or tenofovir or didanosine)	5-8
	fosamprenavir/ritonavir[a] + (lamivudine or emtricitabine) + (zidovudine or stavudine or abacavir or tenofovir or didanosine)	5-8
	indinavir/ritonavir[a] + (lamivudine or emtricitabine) + (zidovudine or stavudine or abacavir or tenofovir or didanosine)	7-12
	lopinavir/ritonavir + (lamivudine + emtricitabine) + (stavudine or abacavir or tenofovir or didanosine)	7-10
	nelfinavir + (lamivudine or emtricitabine) + (zidovudine or stavudine or abacavir or tenofovir or didanosine)	5-8
	saquinavir[b] /ritonavir[a] + (lamivudine or emtricitabine) + (zidovudine or stavudine or abacavir or tenofovir or didanosine)	13-16
Triple-NRTI Regimen‡		**Pills/day**
	abacavir + lamivudine + zidovudine	2

NNRTI, nonnucleoside reverse transcriptase inhibitor; NRTI, nucleoside reverse transcriptase inhibitor; PI, protease inhibitor.

[a] Low-dose (100–400 mg/day) ritonavir

[b] Soft gel or hard gel capsule

* Efavirenz should be avoided in women who are pregnant (first trimester), desiring to become pregnant or of childbearing potential and not using effective contraception. Efavirenz may be considered after the second trimester of pregnancy when no other antiretroviral options are available and the potential benefits outweigh the risks, and when adequate postpartum contraception can be assured (Perinatal HIV Guidelines Working Group 2004). (See Objective IV.35 on Antiretroviral Agent Toxicity and Contraindication in Pregnancy in this Update.)

† There is a high incidence of symptomatic hepatic events observed in women with pre-nevirapine CD4 counts above 250 cells/mm^3 (11%) and men with CD4 counts above 400 cells/mm^3 (6.3%). Use nevirapine with caution in these patients, with close clinical and laboratory monitoring, especially during the first 18 months of therapy.

‡ Use only when a preferred or an alternative NNRTI- or PI-based regimen cannot or should not be used.

When treating pregnant women with HIV-1, clinicians should refer to Recommendations for Use of Antiretroviral Drugs in Pregnant HIV-1-Infected Women for Maternal Health and

Interventions to Reduce Perinatal HIV-1 Transmission in the United States (Perinatal HIV Guidelines Working Group 2004).

The International AIDS Society-USA (IAS-USA) also provides treatment recommendations for selection of appropriate combination antiretroviral therapy for HIV-infected individuals (Yeni et al. 2004). The IAS-USA recommendations for therapy are very similar to the U.S. Public Health Service - Department of Health and Human Services (DHHS) guidelines. Some of the notable differences of the recommendations of the two groups include the IAS-USA selection of atazanavir boosted with ritonavir for use in treatment-naive patients despite the lack of published clinical data, and a wider choice of preferred NRTI backbone combinations: zidovudine plus lamivudine or emtricitabine, tenofovir plus lamivudine or emtricitabine; or emtricitabine plus didanosine (Yeni et al. 2004). The IAS-USA also lists tenofovir plus didanosine as an alternative NRTI backbone, though it notes the greater risk of pancreatitis and CD4+ T cell decline with these two drugs. After the IAS-USA developed its guidelines, new data on poor virologic response with tenofovir/didanosine/efavirenz have raised further concerns about combining tenofovir and didanosine (Podzamczer 2004). This combination should be avoided. (See also Chapter 38 on Specific Agents in the AAHIVM 2003 Study Guide; Objectives IV.6 to IV.11 for new information on specific agents in this Update; and Objective IV.18 on Not-Recommended Antiretroviral Combinations in this Update.)

Below is the rationale for the preferred use of specific NNRTI- and PI-containing regimens. For a brief discussion of triple NRTI regimens, see the section "Sequencing of Antiretroviral Regimens" below.

Rationale for Preferred NNRTI-Containing Regimens

Of the three NNRTIs currently marketed in the United States (delavirdine, efavirenz and nevirapine), delavirdine is not recommended for use in the initial regimen because it is the least potent of these agents.

Nevirapine has been compared with PI-based regimens in two small, randomized trials of antiretroviral-naive patients. The Atlantic trial (van Leeuwen et al. 2003) followed patients randomized to receive either indinavir, nevirapine or lamivudine in combination with didanosine and stavudine. At 96 weeks, 44% of patients in the indinavir arm, 55% of patients in the nevirapine arm and 28% of patients in the lamivudine arm achieved a viral load below 50 copies/mL. The Combine Study (Podzamczer et al. 2002) followed patients randomized to receive either nevirapine or nelfinavir in combination with zidovudine and lamivudine. At 12 months, 75% of the patients in the nevirapine group and 60% of the patients in the nelfinavir group achieved viral load levels below 200 copies/mL.

Efavirenz has been compared with PI-based regimens in antiretroviral-naive patients in two relatively large studies. The DuPont 006 trial randomized patients to receive efavirenz plus lamivudine and zidovudine, indinavir plus lamivudine and zidovudine, or efavirenz plus indinavir; 70% of patients assigned to the efavirenz plus lamivudine and zidovudine arm reached a viral load below 400 copies at 48 weeks, compared with 53% in the efavirenz-plus-indinavir arm and 48% of those in the indinavir-plus-lamivudine-and-zidovudine arm (Staszewski et al. 1999). The ACTG 384 trial randomized 310 patients to receive efavirenz and 310 patients to receive nelfinavir with 1 of 2 NRTI backbones (either zidovudine/lamivudine or stavudine/didanosine) (Robbins et al. 2003). Patients failing the initially assigned regimen were then switched to the other, complementary regimen. Overall, 132 patients (43%) assigned efavirenz and 140 (45%) assigned nelfinavir as the initial regimen experienced a primary endpoint (virologic failure on the second regimen; i.e., nelfinavir for those assigned to efavirenz and efavirenz for those assigned to nelfinavir; toxicity or intolerance; or premature study discontinuation for any reason). Data analysis revealed that all three-drug regimen comparisons favored efavirenz with the zidovudine/lamivudine backbone over the other combinations with nelfinavir or the stavudine/didanosine backbone. Thus, this study supports a combination of efavirenz, zidovudine and lamivudine as a useful starting regimen.

Efavirenz has also been compared with ritonavir-boosted PI regimens. The FOCUS trial compared efavirenz with boosted saquinavir (1600 mg soft-gel saquinavir plus 100 mg ritonavir once daily), each in combination with two NRTIs, in antiretroviral-naive patients, and demonstrated that 71% of patients in the efavirenz arm reached viral RNA load levels below 50 copies/mL at 48 weeks versus 51% in the saquinavir arm (Montaner et al. 2002). These data suggest that regimens containing NNRTIs are at least comparable to those containing PIs in treatment-naive patients.

The choice of efavirenz as the preferred NNRTI in nonpregnant adults is based on a combination of factors. The 2NN study compared patients randomized to receive either efavirenz 600 mg once daily, nevirapine 400 mg once daily, nevirapine 200 mg twice daily or nevirapine 400 mg plus efavirenz 800 mg both once daily, each along with a stavudine/lamivudine NRTI backbone (van Leth et al. 2004). There were no significant differences at 48 weeks between the once- or twice-daily nevirapine groups, the efavirenz group, and the nevirapine plus efavirenz group in terms of viral load below 50 copies (70.0%, 65.4%, 70.0%, and 62.7%, respectively) or CD4 cell increases (170, 160, 160, and 150 cells/mm^3, respectively). However, significantly more patients discontinued treatment because of an adverse event or virologic failure in the twice-daily and nevirapine/efavirenz combination groups than in the efavirenz group. Compared with those receiving efavirenz, more patients taking once- or twice-daily nevirapine experienced liver-associated laboratory adverse events. In addition, 2 patients in this study who received nevirapine died of complications ascribed to the drug.

Rationale for the Preferred PI-Containing Regimens

When used as the sole PI in a combination regimen, indinavir, saquinavir, ritonavir and nelfinavir all have been shown to be effective. But they also can be hard to tolerate at full dose, with inconvenient dosing schedules, large numbers of pills, and the possibility of significant gastrointestinal toxicities. The use of low-dose ritonavir to boost the levels of other PIs has resulted in several improvements in their tolerability and dosing (Cooper et al. 2003).

The fixed-dose combination of lopinavir/ritonavir appears to offer several advantages over other ritonavir-boosted combinations. A large trial involving 653 patients (Walmsley et al. 2002) demonstrated that lopinavir/ritonavir taken twice daily with an NRTI backbone was superior in maintaining a viral load below 400 copies/mL through 48 weeks compared with nelfinavir three times daily (75% versus 63%), with a comparable rate of adverse events. Data comparing lopinavir/ritonavir with other boosted regimens and efavirenz-containing regimens are limited, but DHHS guidelines recommend the lopinavir/ritonavir coformulation as the only preferred PI based on virologic potency, patient tolerance and pill burden (DHHS 2004). The IAS-USA guidelines list several boosted PIs regimens as preferred options, including not only the lopinavir/ritonavir coformulation but also boosted saquinavir, indinavir and atazanavir (Yeni et al. 2004). In a large retrospective study of three-drug regimens used as initial antiretroviral therapy, data was collected and evaluated from 49 studies comprising 85 treatment arms and over 13,000 patients (Bartlett et al. 2005). A central finding from this "systematic overview," which supports current treatment guidelines, was that regimens containing a boosted PI or an NNRTI plus a dual NRTI backbone had significantly better virologic responses compared with unboosted PI regimens or triple NRTI regimens.

Sequencing of Antiretroviral Regimens

One consideration in choosing the initial antiretroviral regimen is to preserve as many options as possible for future therapy. Resistance that develops to the drugs used in the initial regimen may result in cross-resistance to other antiretrovirals (Harrigan and Larder 2002), thus limiting the choices for any combination of medications that follow. Rational sequencing of antiretroviral agents may preserve future treatment options, thus possibly providing the patient a greater chance at prolonged viral suppression. However, sequencing is one of the many considerations in selecting the initial antiretroviral regimen. Because the initial regimen is the one most likely to lead to sustained virologic suppression, sequencing assumes less of a priority in the selection of a regimen when compared with efficacy and tolerability.

Failure of an NNRTI-based regimen should preserve PIs for future use, and vice versa, assuming that the patient was not infected with a resistant isolate. Although starting therapy with a triple-nucleoside combination would preserve both the PI and NNRTI classes for future use, the combination of abacavir/lamivudine/zidovudine is not a preferred initial therapy due to higher rates of virologic failure compared with efavirenz-containing regimens (see Table IV.12-1) (Gulick et al. 2004). Due to reports of high rates of early virologic failure, the triple NRTI-only regimens containing tenofovir/abacavir/lamivudine or tenofovir/didanosine/lamivudine should not be used at any time (DHHS 2004). Failure rates from these regimens are considerably higher than with the abacavir/lamivudine/zidovudine regimen. Among the available NNRTIs, there are no sequencing-based considerations since resistance to 1 NNRTI invariably leads to resistance to the others (DHHS 2004). Among PIs, however, there may be some sequencing considerations. When resistance has developed to initial regimens containing nelfinavir (Kemper et al. 2001), atazanavir (Reyataz 2004) or amprenavir (Paulsen et al. 2003), the resulting viral isolates have usually been sensitive in vitro to other PIs. Clinical data confirming that these isolates will be fully susceptible to other PIs in actual practice are relatively limited, especially for atazanavir and fosamprenavir. Several prospective studies of lopinavir/ritonavir (Hicks et al. 2004; Molina et al. 2004; Walmsley et al. 2002) and one of boosted fosamprenavir (MacManus et al. 2004) reported no phenotypic or genotypic resistance in subjects with virologic failure to these regimens. In addition, use of these boosted PI regimens also correlated with reduced frequency of resistance to the backbone NRTI drugs. The actual activity of an alternative PI after virologic failure with a boosted-PI-containing regimen is not known.

Enfuvirtide is an approved fusion inhibitor, a new class of antiretrovirals for use in treatment-experienced patients. It has not shown cross-resistance with the other three drug classes (Fuzeon 2004). Durability of response with the agent depends on the baseline characteristics of the patient, including HIV RNA level, CD4 count, number of prior drugs used and number of active available agents as determined by resistance testing (Clotet et al. 2004).

References

Arribas JR, Pulido F, Lorenzo A, et al. Simplification to lopinavir/r single-drug HAART: 24 weeks results of a randomized, controlled, open label, pilot clinical trial (OK Study). In: Program and abstracts of the XV International Conference on AIDS; July 11-16, **2004**; Bangkok, Thailand. Abstract TuPeB4486.

Bartlett J, Fath M, DeMasi R, et al. An updated systematic overview of triple combination therapy in antiretroviral-naive HIV-infected adults. In: Program and abstracts of the 12th Conference on Retroviruses and Opportunistic Infections; February 22-25, **2005**; Boston, Massachusetts. Poster 586.

Clotet B, Raffi F, Cooper D, et al. Clinical management of treatment-experienced, HIV-infected patients with the fusion inhibitor enfuvirtide: consensus recommendations. *AIDS*. **2004**;18:1137-1146.

Cooper CL, van Heeswijk RP, Gallicano K, Cameron DW. A review of low-dose ritonavir in protease inhibitor combination therapy. *Clin Infect Dis*. **2003**;36:1585-1592.

Department of Health and Human Services (DHHS). Guidelines for the use of antiretroviral agents in HIV-1-infected adults and adolescents. October 29, **2004**. Available at: http://www.aidsinfo.nih.gov/guidelines/adult/AA_102904.pdf [accessed February 22, 2005].

Fuzeon (enfuvirtide) [prescribing information]. Nutley, NJ: Roche Laboratories; March **2003**.

Gathe JC Jr, Washington MY, Mayberry C, Piot D, Nemecek J. IMANI-1 TC3WP single drug HAART proof of concept study. Pilot study of the safety and efficacy of Kaletra (LPV/r) as single drug HAART in HIV + ARV-naive patients-interim analysis of subjects completing final 48 week data. In: Program and abstracts of the XV International Conference on AIDS; July 11-16, **2004**; Bangkok, Thailand. Abstract MoOrB1057.

Gulick RM, Ribaudo HJ, Shikuma CM, et al. Triple-nucleoside regimens versus efavirenz-containing regimens for the initial treatment of HIV-1 infection. *N Engl J Med*. **2004**;350:1850-1861.

Harrigan PR, Larder BA. Extent of cross-resistance between agents used to treat human immunodeficiency virus type 1 infection in clinically derived isolates. *Antimicrob Agents Chemother.* **2002**;46:909-912.

Hicks C, King MS, Gulick RM, et al. Long-term safety and durable antiretroviral activity of lopinavir/ritonavir in treatment-naive patients: 4 year follow-up study. *AIDS*. **2004**;18:775-779.

Ho DD, Neumann AU, Perelson AS, et al. Rapid turnover of plasma virions and CD4+ lymphocytes in HIV-1 infection. *Nature*. **1995**;373:123-126.

Kahlert C, Hupfer M, Wagels T, et al. Ritonavir boosted indinavir treatment as a simplified maintenance mono"-therapy for HIV infection". *AIDS*. **2004**;18:955-957.

Kemper CA, Witt MD, Keiser PH, et al. Sequencing of protease inhibitor therapy: insights from an analysis of HIV phenotypic resistance in patients failing protease inhibitors. *AIDS*. **2001**;15:609–615.

MacManus S, Yates PJ, Elston RC, White S, Richards N, Snowden W. GW433908/ritonavir once daily in antiretroviral therapy-naive HIV-infected patients: absence of protease resistance at 48 weeks. *AIDS*. **2004**;18:651-656.

Molina JM, Gathe J, Lim PL, et al. Comprehensive resistance testing in antiretroviral naive patients treated with once-daily lopinavir/ritonavir plus tenofovir and emtricitabine: 48-week results from study 418. In: Program and abstracts of the XV International AIDS Conference; July 11-16, **2004**; Bangkok, Thailand. Abstract WePeB5701.

Montaner JSG, Saag MS, Barylski C, et al. FOCUS Study, Saquinavir QD regimen versus efavirenz QD regimen 48 week analysis in HIV infected patients. In: Program and abstracts of the 42nd Interscience Conference on Antimicrobial Agents and Chemotherapy. September **2002**, San Diego, California. Abstract H-167.

Paulsen D, Elston R, Snowden W, Tisdale M, Ross L. Differentiation of genotypic resistance profiles for amprenavir and lopinavir, a valuable aid for choice of therapy in protease inhibitor-experienced HIV-1-infected subjects. *J Antimicrob Chemother.* **2003**;52:319-323.

Perinatal HIV Guidelines Working Group. Recommendations for use of antiretroviral drugs in pregnant HIV-1-infected women for maternal health and interventions to reduce perinatal HIV-1 transmission in the United States. December 17, **2004**. Available at: www.AIDSinfo.nih.gov/guidelines [accessed February 16, 2005].

Podzamczer D, Ferrer E, Consiglio E, et al. A randomized clinical trial comparing nelfinavir or nevirapine associated to zidovudine/lamivudine in HIV-infected naïve patients (the Combine Study). *Antiviral Ther.* **2002**;7:81-90.

Podzamczer D, Ferrer E, Gatell JM, et al. Early virological failure and occurrence of resistance in naïve patients receiving tenofovir, didanosine and efavirenz. In: Program and abstracts of the 13th International HIV Drug Resistance Workshop; June 8-12 2004, Tenerife, Canary Islands, Spain; Abstract 156. *Antiviral Ther.* **2004**;9:S172.

Reyataz (atazanavir sulfate) [prescribing information]. Princeton, NJ: Bristol-Myers Squibb; October **2004**.

Robbins GK, De Gruttola V, Shafer RW, et al. Comparison of sequential three-drug regimens as initial therapy for HIV-1 infection. *N Engl J Med.* **2003**;349:2293-2303.

Staszewski S, Morales-Ramirez J, Tashima KT, et al. Efavirenz plus zidovudine and lamivudine, efavirenz plus indinavir, and indinavir plus zidovudine and lamivudine in the treatment of HIV-1 infection in adults. *N Engl J Med.* **1999**;341:1865-1873.

van Leeuwen R, Katlama C, Murphy RL, et al. A randomized trial to study first-line combination therapy with or without a protease inhibitor in HIV-1-infected patients. *AIDS.* **2003**;17:987-999.

van Leth F, Phanuphak P, Ruxrungtham K, et al. Comparison of first-line antiretroviral therapy with regimens including nevirapine, efavirenz, or both drugs, plus stavudine and lamivudine: a randomised open-label trial, the 2NN Study. *Lancet.* **2004**;363:1253-1263.

Walmsley S, Bernstein B, King M, et al. Lopinavir-ritonavir versus nelfinavir for the initial treatment of HIV infection. *N Engl J Med.* **2002**;346:2039-2046.

Yeni PG, Hammer SM, Hirsch MS, et al. Treatment for adult HIV infection: 2004 recommendations of the International AIDS Society-USA Panel. *JAMA.* **2004**;292:251-265.

(RLO-25)

IV.14. COFORMULATIONS

LEARNING OBJECTIVE: Name and describe all antiretroviral coformulated tablets and capsules available or soon to be available.

Coformulations in the United States

Currently 5 licensed antiretroviral preparations contain more than 1 medication within their formulation:

- **Combivir:** a combination tablet of zidovudine (300 mg) and lamivudine (150 mg). The usual adult dose is 1 tablet twice daily, with or without food.
- **Trizivir:** a combination tablet of zidovudine (300 mg), lamivudine (150 mg) and abacavir (300 mg). The usual adult dose is 1 tablet twice daily, with or without food.
- **Kaletra:** a combination capsule of lopinavir (133.3 mg) and ritonavir (33.3 mg). The usual adult dose is 3 capsules twice daily with food.
- **Truvada:** a combination tablet of emtricitabine (200 mg) and tenofovir (300 mg). The usual adult dose is 1 tablet once a day, with or without food.
- **Epzicom:** a combination tablet of abacavir (600 mg) and lamivudine (300 mg). The usual adult dose is 1 tablet once a day, with or without food.

International Generic Coformulations

Pharmaceutical companies outside the United States have begun to develop low-cost generic formulations of various U.S.-patented antiretroviral agents (WHO 2001). For example, Cipla in India currently manufactures generic indinavir, lamivudine, nevirapine, stavudine and zidovudine. In addition, it has coformulated stavudine plus lamivudine, zidovudine plus lamivudine, and stavudine/lamivudine plus nevirapine (Cipla 2005).

A number of studies of the Thai Government Pharmaceutical Organization's generic medication GPO-VIR, a combination of stavudine (30 mg), lamivudine (150 mg) and nevirapine (200 mg) in 1 pill, taken twice daily, have shown good results. In an assessment of quality, stability, uniformity and release profiles, the investigators judged that GPO-VIR tablets have acceptable product uniformity, dissolution profiles and stability under both typical and severe conditions, all at a cost of $30.00 U.S. per month (Srinarong et al. 2004). Clinical results have indicated a high level of efficacy in adults (Dettrairat et al. 2004; Jourdain et al. 2004; Ungkasrithongkul 2004). CD4 counts improved and viral loads decreased, with most patients reaching undetectable viral loads within 6 months. Failures and discontinuations due to intolerance were mainly in persons with advanced disease. There also were improvements in children (Phongsamart et al. 2004).

In both May and August of 2004, the World Health Organization (WHO) removed certain generic combination antiretroviral drugs manufactured in India from its prequalification list, the purpose of which is to help governments and others choose high-quality drugs for use in public health campaigns (WHO 2004). They were removed from the list because contract research organizations that had done bioequivalence studies on behalf of the manufacturers

What's New

Epzicom (abacavir/lamivudine) and Truvada (emtricitabine/tenofovir) have been approved. An all-in-one single-tablet combination of emtricitabine/tenofovir/efavirenz is in development. GPO-VIR, a generic stavudine/lamivudine/nevirapine combination drug, has been successfully used in Thailand. The FDA has approved a South African generic combination of lamivudine/zidovudine copackaged with generic nevirapine.

Key Points

Currently licensed antiretroviral coformulations:

- Combivir (zidovudine/lamivudine)
- Epzicom (abacavir/lamivudine)
- Kaletra (lopinavir/ritonavir)
- Trizivir (zidovudine/lamivudine/abacavir)
- Truvada (emtricitabine/tenofovir)

were found to be noncompliant with good clinical and laboratory practices. The WHO has pointed out that this does not mean that the drugs are not as effective as the originals on which they are based, but rather simply that bioequivalence has not been proved (Pincock 2004).

The FDA recently gave tentative approval the first internationally produced generic drug coformulation. A South African generic drug company received tentative approval for a generic lamivudine/zidovudine fixed dose combination that is co-packaged with generic nevirapine. Patent law forbids marketing or sale of this generic combination in the U.S., but the approval allows this coformulation to be purchased by President's Emergency Plan for AIDS Relief (PEPFAR) and used abroad (FDA 2005).

Under Development

Recent strides in the international scene have led the way to intercompany coformulations in the United States. In a joint venture, the manufacturers of efavirenz (Sustiva) and tenofovir/emtricitabine (Truvada) have begun work to coformulate a fixed-dose combination of these agents, to be taken once daily. The companies have announced that development of the coformulation will continue in 2005, with product availability likely by the second half of 2006 (Bristol-Myers Squibb and Gilead Sciences 2004). This novel approach could induce further collaborations between like-minded drug companies interested in improving the health of HIV-infected patients around the world.

References

Bristol-Myers Squibb, Gilead Sciences. Bristol-Myers Squibb and Gilead Sciences Establish U.S. Joint Venture to Develop and Commercialize Fixed-Dose Combination of Three HIV Medicines. New York and Foster City, CA. December 20, **2004**. Available at http://www.gilead.com/wt/sec/pr_656192 [accessed February 22, 2005].

Cipla Ltd. Product information. **2005**. Available at: http://www.cipla.com [accessed January 31, 2005].

Dettrairat S, Kunachiwa W, Leechanachai P, Leusaree T, Kohreanudom S. CD4 count and viral load monitoring of GPO-vir therapy in the access to care program in Northern Thailand. In: Program and abstracts of the XV International Conference on AIDS; July 11-14, **2004**; Bangkok, Thailand. Abstract MoPeB3150.

Food and Drug Administration (FDA). FDA grants the tentative approval to generic AIDS drug regimen for potential purchase under the president's emergency plan for AIDS relief. *FDA News*. January 25, **2005**. Available at: http://www.fda.gov/bbs/topics/news/2005/NEW01152.html [accessed March 8, 2005].

Jourdain G, Fregonese F, Kanabkaew C, et al. HIV medicine and HAART in community hospitals in Northern Thailand. In: Program and abstracts of the XV International Conference on AIDS; July 11-14, **2004**; Bangkok, Thailand. Abstract B12187.

Phongsamart W, Chearskul P, Lapphra K, et al. Safety and efficacy of GPO-VIR® in HIV-infected Thai children. In: Program and abstracts of the XV International Conference on AIDS; July 11-14, **2004**; Bangkok, Thailand. Abstract TuPeB4449.

Pincock S. AIDS drugs off WHO list. The Scientist Daily News. *Biomedcentral*. August 5, **2004**. Available at: http://www.biomedcentral.com/news/20040805/01/ [accessed February 22, 2005].

Srinarong P, Prayngam S, Chunhacha P, et al. Fixed-dose combination tablets of nevirapine, lamivudine, and stavudine. In: Program and abstracts of the XV International Conference on AIDS; July 11-14, **2004**; Bangkok, Thailand. Abstract WeOrA1240.

Ungkasrithongkul SK. Study on the outcome of GPO-VIR using at Bamrasnaradura institute. In: Program and abstracts of the XV International Conference on AIDS; July 11-14, **2004**; Bangkok, Thailand. Abstract B11148.

World Health Organization (WHO). Medicines for all, not just the rich. Bulletin of the World Health Organization. **2001**;79:377-378.

World Health Organization (WHO). Access to HIV/AIDS Drugs and Diagnostics of Acceptable Quality. 18th ed. August 9, **2004**. Available at: http://mednet3.who.int/prequal/ [accessed October 14, 2004].

(RLO-26)

IV.15. ANTIRETROVIRAL INTERACTIONS

LEARNING OBJECTIVE: Describe the known interactions that occur between antiretroviral medications, and describe the recommended antiretroviral dose adjustment.

The drug-drug interactions between nonnucleoside reverse transcriptase inhibitors (NNRTIs) and protease inhibitors (PIs) are complex. Two of the NNRTIs — nevirapine and efavirenz — induce the cytochrome P450 enzyme system, accelerating the metabolism of PIs and resulting in lower PI drug levels. Therefore, PI dosages may need to be increased and/or given with ritonavir boosting when given concurrently with either of these NNRTIs. By contrast, delavirdine modestly inhibits the P450 enzyme system, slows the metabolism of PIs and thus raises the levels of PIs.

Examples of dosing adjustments necessary when coadministering NNRTIs and PIs include the following:

- Drug levels of indinavir are significantly reduced when coadministered with efavirenz (Sustiva 2004; Aarnoutse et al. 2002). The optimal dose of indinavir, when given in combination with efavirenz, is not known. Increasing the indinavir dose to 1000 mg every 8 hours does not compensate for the increased metabolism due to efavirenz (Sustiva 2004). However, pharmacokinetic data in treatment-naive patients suggest that when indinavir 800 mg/ritonavir 100 mg twice daily is combined with efavirenz, drug levels are similar to those achieved with indinavir 800 mg 3 times daily (Aarnoutse et al. 2002).
- When fosamprenavir combined with low-dose ritonavir is coadministered with efavirenz, an additional 100 mg ritonavir is required for once daily dosing (fosamprenavir 1400 mg/300 mg ritonavir) but not twice daily dosing (fosamprenavir 700 mg/ritonavir 100 mg twice daily) (Lexiva 2004). A negative interaction has also been observed between fosamprenavir and nevirapine, resulting in reduced levels of the PI (DeJesus et al. 2004). It is inadvisable to use nevirapine together with fosamprenavir without ritonavir boosting (the standard 700/100 mg twice daily fosamprenavir-ritonavir combination proved sufficient).
- When lopinavir/ritonavir (400/100 mg) is coadministered with either efavirenz or nevirapine, it is recommended that the lopinavir/ritonavir be increased from 3 to 4 capsules twice daily (Kaletra 2004). Although not fully investigated, another option may be to add an extra 100-mg dose of ritonavir twice daily (Flexner et al. 2003). No data are currently available regarding the pharmacokinetics of once daily lopinavir/ritonavir with NNRTIs.
- Coadministration of NNRTIs such as efavirenz will reduce the concentration of atazanavir in the blood. The manufacturer recommends a dose of atazanavir 300 mg once daily boosted with 100 mg ritonavir if coadministered with efavirenz 600 mg in treatment-naive patients (Reyataz 2004). There are no dosage recommendations for treatment-experienced patients. When administered with efavirenz, ritonavir-boosted

What's New

Tenofovir-PI and NNRTI-PI drug interactions alter PI levels. Adjusting the dose of boosted PIs can counteract the latter.

Key Points

- Complex interactions occur between PIs and NNRTIs and among drugs in boosted PI regimens.
- When given with efavirenz or nevirapine, most PIs need ritonavir boosting and/or dosing modifications to overcome induction of metabolism.
- The dose of didanosine should be reduced when didanosine is coadministered with tenofovir. Also, there is an increasing consensus that tenofovir and didanosine should not be coadministered due to excessive virologic failure in treatment-naive patients.
- Some tenofovir-PI drug interactions result in tenofovir concentrations increasing by 20% to 30%. The clinical relevance of these interactions is currently unknown.

atazanavir concentrations resemble those seen with unboosted atazanavir 400 mg once daily given without efavirenz (Tackett et al. 2004). Atazanavir plus ritonavir without efavirenz results in considerably higher drug exposures (Reyataz 2004). The treatment-naive dosage with concomitant efavirenz may be insufficient for patients harboring protease-resistant viral isolates. Pharmacokinetic evaluation of atazanavir 400 mg/ritonavir 200 mg once daily in combination with efavirenz 600 mg once daily observed considerably higher atazanavir exposure (O'Mara et al. 2002), but clinical safety and efficacy of this regimen has not been evaluated.

- Coadministration of tenofovir and didanosine has resulted in a significant increase in didanosine drug exposures (Viread 2004). Pharmacokinetic drug-drug interaction studies have found that lower-dose didanosine EC (enteric coated, 250 mg) in combination with tenofovir (in a fasted or fed state) results in relatively similar drug exposures (AUC, area under the concentration-time curve) to those achieved with 400 mg didanosine alone in patients weighing over 60 kg (Viread 2004). Consequently, didanosine EC 250 mg is the recommended dose with tenofovir (Viread 2004). Data are not yet available regarding dose adjustments of didanosine when coadministered with tenofovir in patients weighing under 60 kg. Pharmacokinetic studies have shown that the increase in didanosine exposures is unrelated to decreases in didanosine renal elimination (Ray et al. 2004). Although not fully evaluated, it appears that tenofovir inhibits purine nucleoside phosphorylase (PNP), which is responsible for didanosine metabolism (Ray et al. 2004). Note that there are reports of excessive virologic failure using combinations of tenofovir, didanosine and efavirenz in treatment-naive patients. See Objective IV.18 on Not-Recommended Antiretroviral Combinations in this Update.

- In one small study, coadministration of tenofovir and with atazanavir/ritonavir (300/100 mg) correlated with lower atazanavir exposures and increases in tenofovir drug concentrations (Taburet et al. 2003). In another small study, coadministration of tenofovir 300 mg and atazanavir 400 mg resulted in lower atazanavir drug exposure and higher tenofovir drug exposure (Kaul et al. 2003). As a consequence, use of tenofovir and atazanavir is not recommended without low-dose ritonavir. The clinical significance of the increases in tenofovir exposures observed in these trials (roughly 20%-30% increases) is currently unknown.

- Tenofovir had no effect on efavirenz or indinavir concentrations when coadministered with these drugs (Flaherty 2001). When tenofovir was combined with lopinavir/ritonavir, no alterations in lopinavir concentrations occurred, but tenofovir AUC was increased by 32% (Kearney et al. 2003). The clinical relevance of this increase during chronic administration (e.g., increased risk for nephrotoxicity) is currently unknown. Investigators have proposed that PIs inhibit renal multidrug-resistant protein 2 (MRP2), a pump partially responsible for tenofovir renal elimination, resulting in increased tenofovir concentrations (Rollot et al. 2003).

- A recent small study found that addition of atazanavir to a ritonavir-boosted saquinavir hard-gel once-daily regimen significantly increased saquinavir concentrations (Boffito et al. 2004). This increase was predominantly observed in absorption and not in alterations in elimination (e.g., increases in half-life). A subsequent pharmacokinetic study comparing combinations of saquinavir and atazanavir (1600/400 mg once daily) with saquinavir/ritonavir (1600/100 mg once daily) in seronegative volunteers found that saquinavir did not affect atazanavir plasma concentrations whereas atazanavir had a weak boosting effect on saquinavir compared with ritonavir (Becker et al. 2005). Saquinavir/atazanavir at 2000/400 mg once daily appeared to be a pharmacologically acceptable combination. With all three combinations, women achieved considerably higher PI concentrations compared with the men in this study, even after adjusting for weight.

- Pharmacokinetic studies evaluating the concomitant administration of lopinavir/ritonavir and the amprenavir prodrug fosamprenavir found decreased blood levels of lopinavir and amprenavir (Kashuba et al. 2005; Wire et al. 2004). Adding efavirenz, a cytochrome P450 inducer, to the amprenavir/lopinavir/ritonavir combination did not exacerbate this problem (Pham et al. 2005). Separation of dosing by 4 and 12 hours did not correct this interaction (Corbett et al. 2004). Increasing the dose of each agent (to 533 mg/133 mg twice daily for lopinavir/ritonavir and 1400 mg twice daily for fosamprenavir) corrected lopinavir concentrations to levels observed when given without amprenavir (Wire et al. 2004). Blood concentrations of amprenavir increased, but remained significantly depressed. Adding 100 mg extra ritonavir to the normal dose regimen also corrected lopinavir levels, but amprenavir concentrations were lower than when the doses of all 3 agents were increased. Both of these regimens were poorly tolerated, provoking gastrointestinal symptoms in particular. No recommended dosing could be deduced.

- Nonpharmacokinetic evaluations from the Context trial suggest no negative effects on amprenavir trough concentrations when fosamprenavir is combined with tenofovir (Lexiva 2004). No data are available regarding fosamprenavir's effects on tenofovir concentrations.

- Coming soon is the issue of interactions between entry inhibitors and protease inhibitors. Coadministration of lopinavir/ritonavir caused an almost 8-fold increase in the AUC of the CCR5 antagonist 873140 (Adkison et al. 2005)

For interactions between PIs, see Objective IV.17 on Boosted Protease Inhibitors in this Update. Also, see Tables 21a and b of the U.S. Public Health Service guidelines (DHHS 2004) for dosing recommendations when PIs are administered concurrently with interacting second PIs or NNRTIs.

References

Aarnoutse RE, Grintjes KJ, Telgt DS, et al. The influence of efavirenz on the pharmacokinetics of a twice-daily combination of indinavir and low-dose ritonavir in healthy volunteers. *Clin Pharmacol Ther.* **2002**;71:57-67.

Adkison K, Shachoy-Clark A, Fang L et al. The pharmacokinetic interaction between the CCR5 antagonist 873140 and lopinavir/ritonavir in healthy subjects. In: Program and abstracts of the 12th Conference on Retroviruses and Opportunistic Infections; February 22-25, **2005**; Boston, Massachusetts. Abstract 664.

Becker S, Tse M, Sterman F, Kakuda T, Acosta E. Pharmacokinetics of once-daily saquinavir hard-gel capsule with low-dose ritonavir or full-dose atazanavir in seronegative volunteers: ASPIRE I. In: Program and abstracts of the 12th Conference on Retroviruses and Opportunistic Infections; February 22-25, **2005**; Boston, Massachusetts. Abstract 655.

Boffito M, Kurowski M, Kruse G, et al. Atazanavir enhances saquinavir hard gel concentrations in a ritonavir-boosted once-daily regimen. In: Program and abstracts of the 11th Conference on Retroviruses and Opportunistic Infections; February 8-11, **2004**; San Francisco, California. Abstract 607.

Corbett AH, Davidson L, Park JJ, et al. Dose separation strategies to overcome the pharmacokinetic interaction of a triple protease inhibitor regimen containing fosamprenavir lopinavir, and ritonavir. In: Program and abstracts of the 11th Conference on Retroviruses and Opportunistic Infections; February 8-11, **2004**; San Francisco, California. Abstract 611.

DeJesus E, Piliero P, Summers K, et al. Evaluation of the pharmacokinetic drug interaction between fosamprenavir (FPV), FPV plus ritonavir (RTV), and nevirapine (NVP) in HIV-infected patients (APV10014). In: Program and abstracts of the 44th Interscience Conference on Antimicrobial Agents and Chemotherapy; October 30-November 2, **2004**; Washington, DC. Abstract A447.

Department of Health and Human Services (DHHS). Guidelines for the use of antiretroviral agents in HIV-1-infected adults and adolescents, October 29, **2004**. Available at: http://www.aidsinfo.nih.gov [accessed February 22, 2005].

Flaherty J, Kearney B, Wolf J, Sayre J, Coakley D. A multiple-dose, randomized, crossover, drug interaction study between tenofovir DF and efavirenz, indinavir, or lopinavir/ritonavir. In: Program and abstracts of the 1st International AIDS Society Conference on Pathogenesis and Treatment; July 7-11, **2001**; Buenos Aires, Argentina. Abstract 336.

Flexner C, Chiu YL, Foit C, et al. Steady-state pharmacokinetics and short-term virologic response of two lopinavir/ritonavir high-dose regimens in multiple antiretroviral experienced subjects. In: Program and abstracts of the 2nd International AIDS Society Conference on Pathogenesis and Treatment; July 13-16, **2003**; Paris, France. Abstract 337.

Kaletra (lopinavir/ritonavir) [prescribing information]. North Chicago, IL: Abbott Laboratories; February **2004**.

Kashuba ADM, Tierney C, Downey GF, et al. Combining fosamprenavir with lopinavir/ritonavir substantially reduces amprenavir and lopinavir exposure: ACTG protocol A5143 results. *AIDS*. **2005**;19:145-152.

Kaul S, Bassi K, Damle B, et al. Pharmacokinetic (PK) evaluation of the combination of atazanavir (ATV), enteric coated didanosine (ddI-EC), and tenofovir disoproxil fumarate (TDF) for a once-daily antiretroviral regimen. In: Program and abstracts of the 43rd Annual Interscience Conference on Antimicrobial Agents and Chemotherapy; September 14-17, **2003**; Chicago, Illinois. Poster A-1616.

Kearney BP, Mittan A, Sayre J, et al. Pharmacokinetic drug interaction and long term safety profile of tenofovir DF and lopinavir/ritonavir. In: Program and abstracts of the 43rd Interscience Conference on Antimicrobial Agents and Chemotherapy; September 14-17, **2003**, Chicago, Illinois. Abstract 1617.

Lexiva (fosamprenavir) Tablets [prescribing information]. Research Triangle Park, NC: GlaxoSmithKline; December **2004**.

O'Mara E, Agarwala S, Randall D, Geraldes M, Stoltz R, Mummaneni V. Steady-state pharmacokinetic interaction study of atazanavir (ATV) with efavirenz (EFV) and ritonavir (RTV) in healthy subjects. In: Program and abstracts of the 9th Conference on Retroviruses and Opportunistic Infections; February 24-28, **2002**; Seattle, Washington. Abstract 444-W.

Pham P, Barditch-Crovo P, Redpath E, et al. Steady-state pharmacokinetics of amprenavir, lopinavir, and efavirenz combination in HIV-infected patients. In: Program and abstracts of the 12th Conference on Retroviruses and Opportunistic Infections; February 22-25, **2005**; Boston, Massachusetts. Abstract 79.

Ray AS, Olson L, Fridland A. Role of purine nucleoside phosphorylase in interactions between 2',3'-dideoxyinosine and allopurinol, ganciclovir, or tenofovir. Antimicrob Agents Chemother. **2004**;48:1089-1095.

Reyataz (atazanavir sulfate) Capsules [prescribing information]. Princeton, NJ: Bristol-Myers Squibb; October **2004**.

Rollot F, Nazal E-M, Chauvelot-Moachon L, et al. Tenofovir-related Fanconi syndrome with nephrogenic diabetes insipidus in a patient with acquired immunodeficiency syndrome: the role of lopinavir-ritonavir-didanosine. *Clin Infect Dis*. **2003**;37:e174-e176.

Sustiva (efavirenz) [prescribing information]. Princeton, NJ: Bristol-Myers Squibb; December **2004**.

Taburet AM, Piketty C, Gérard L, et al. Pharmacokinetic parameters of atazanavir/ritonavir when combined to tenofovir in HIV infected patients with multiple treatment failures: a sub-study of Puzzle2-ANRS 107 Trial. In: Program and abstracts of the 10th Conference on Retroviruses and Opportunistic Infections; February 10-14, **2003**; Boston, Massachusetts. Abstract 537.

Tackett D, Child M, Agarwala S, et al. Atazanavir: a summary of two pharmacokinetic drug interaction studies in healthy subjects. In: Program and abstracts of the 10th Conference on Retroviruses and Opportunistic Infections; February 10-14, **2003**; Boston, Massachusetts. Abstract 543.

Viread (tenofovir disoproxil fumarate) [prescribing information]. Foster City, Calif: Gilead Sciences; June **2004**.

Wire MB, Naderer OJ, Masterman AL, Lou Y, Stein DS. The pharmacokinetic interaction between GW433908 and lopinavir/ritonavir (APV10011 and APV10012). In: Program and abstracts of the 11th Conference on Retroviruses and Opportunistic Infections; February 8-11, **2004**; San Francisco, California. Abstract 612.

(RLO-27)

IV.17. BOOSTED PROTEASE INHIBITORS

LEARNING OBJECTIVE: Discuss the advantages and specific dosage recommendations when combining ritonavir with other protease inhibitors.

Despite being highly efficacious in combination antiretroviral therapy regimens, protease inhibitor (PI)-based therapies are often limited because of high pill burden, food restrictions and frequent daily administration. In situations in which PI-based therapy has failed, drug exposures of the PI may be insufficient to overcome the resistance that has developed. Because most PIs are metabolized to some extent by the cytochrome P450 enzyme system, inhibition of this enzyme may result in improved gastrointestinal absorption and/or delayed elimination (Becker and Hoetelmans 2002). This would enhance the pharmacokinetic profile of the other PIs, resulting in less frequent dosing, fewer food restrictions and higher trough levels. Raising trough levels reduces the likelihood that suboptimal drug levels will allow viral breakthrough and the development of drug resistance. For some patients, however, even low doses of ritonavir lead to increases in cholesterol/triglyceride levels and increased incidence of gastrointestinal side effects. Attempts are under way to find the lowest useful dose of ritonavir (Ruane et al. 2004).

Saquinavir/Ritonavir

Ritonavir is an inhibitor of the cytochrome P450 enzyme system (Norvir 2001) and is being investigated in combination with most of the currently available PIs (Table IV.17-1). Various dose combinations of saquinavir/ritonavir have been studied. These combinations remove the requirement that saquinavir be taken 3 times daily. The saquinavir/ritonavir 400 mg/400 mg dose provides therapeutic drug levels of 2 PIs (Cameron et al. 1999), with different resistance profiles (i.e., at this dose, ritonavir contributes to the antiretroviral activity of the regimen, rather than acting solely as a pharmacokinetic booster). This regimen, however, is often limited because of gastrointestinal side effects (Cameron et al. 1999). More recently, the U.S. Food and Drug Administration (FDA) has approved saquinavir/ritonavir 1000 mg/100 mg twice daily (Invirase 2003), which achieves rates of virologic suppression comparable to those of the 400 mg/400 mg regimen (O'Brien et al. 2002) or of lopinavir/ritonavir 400 mg/100 mg twice daily (Youle et al. 2003). Recent data indicate that when ritonavir is combined with saquinavir, similar saquinavir blood levels are achieved regardless of whether the hard-gel capsule (Invirase) or soft-gel capsule (Fortovase) formulation of saquinavir is used. The hard-gel capsule appears to be better tolerated with fewer gastrointestinal side effects (Kurowski et al. 2002; Plosker et al. 2003). Once-daily saquinavir/ritonavir combinations are currently under investigation (see Table IV.17-1). One limitation to using various saquinavir/ritonavir combinations has been the large saquinavir pill burden. The FDA has approved a new, more convenient 500-mg Invirase tablet.

What's New

Low-dose ritonavir enhances many PIs' pharmacokinetics. It also makes feasible once-daily lopinavir/ritonavir and once-daily fosamprenavir. Low-dose ritonavir plus atazanavir in combination with efavirenz or tenofovir also has been evaluated. Pharmacokinetic data for different triple-PI combinations are available.

Key Points

- Combination PI therapies with low-dose ritonavir (below 400 mg) improve overall PI drug exposures, lower total daily pill burdens and often remove the need for food restrictions.
- When combined with low-dose ritonavir, hard-gel saquinavir (Invirase) exhibits similar drug exposures and fewer gastrointestinal side effects than does soft-gel saquinavir (Fortovase).
- Results of a clinical study in treatment-naive patients suggest that the virologic efficacy of lopinavir/ritonavir is similar when given either once daily or twice daily, but the once-daily dose results in more frequent gastrointestinal side effects.
- Because of the high genetic barrier of boosted PIs, it appears that the development of protease resistance is significantly decreased or delayed. In addition, boosted PI regimens lower the incidence of nucleoside reverse transcriptase (NRTI) resistance.

Table IV.17-1. Dosing regimens for ritonavir combined with indinavir, saquinavir, amprenavir, fosamprenavir and atazanavir.

PI combination	Doses of each PI (respectively)
Indinavir/ritonavir	800 mg/100 mg twice daily 800 mg/200 mg twice daily 400 mg/400 mg twice daily 400-600 mg/100 mg twice daily (under investigation)
Saquinavir/ritonavir	400 mg/400 mg twice daily 1000 mg/100 mg twice daily 1600-2000 mg/100 mg once daily (under investigation)
Fosamprenavir/ritonavir	1400 mg/200 mg once daily (for PI-naive patients only) (100 mg ritonavir under investigation) 700 mg/100 mg twice daily
Atazanavir/ritonavir	300 mg/100 mg once daily

Indinavir/Ritonavir

Various combinations of indinavir/ritonavir have been investigated. Indinavir, at doses of 800 mg twice daily, have been combined with 100-200 mg ritonavir twice daily. In one trial, the regimen containing indinavir/ritonavir 800 mg/100 mg twice daily had comparable efficacy to the saquinavir/ritonavir 1000 mg/100 mg twice-daily arm (Dragsted et al. 2003). The indinavir/ritonavir recipients had a higher rate of adverse events, with 64% changing therapy due to adverse events. Lower-dose indinavir/ritonavir combinations — 600/100 mg and 400/100 mg, both twice daily — are undergoing testing. In Thai patients, indinavir trough levels proved just adequate at either dose to maintain viral suppression (Cressey et al. 2004). A European study compared the 800/100 mg twice daily combination with 400/100 mg twice daily in 107 treatment-naive patients, who also received 2 NRTIs (Konopnicki et al. 2005). Differences in virologic and immunologic response were not statistically significant, but the high-dose arm did have significantly more adverse events and discontinuations than the low-dose arm.

Lopinavir/Ritonavir

The recommended dose of lopinavir/ritonavir (coformulated as Kaletra) is 400 /100 mg twice daily (Kaletra 2004). This coformulation is listed in the U.S. Department of Health and Human Services (DHHS) guidelines as a preferred agent for use in combination antiretroviral therapy regimens in treatment-naive patients (DHHS 2004). In addition, among patients with extensive treatment histories, treatment with lopinavir/ritonavir-containing antiretroviral therapy regimens may offer improved virologic outcomes (Kaletra 2004). Lopinavir/ritonavir-containing antiretroviral therapy regimens have performed well against other boosted PI combinations, including saquinavir/ritonavir (MaxCmin1 study) (Dragsted et al. 2003; Youle et al. 2003), fosamprenavir/ritonavir (APV30003 study) (Lexiva 2004) and atazanavir/ritonavir (BMS 045 study) (Badaro et al. 2003). However, lopinavir/ritonavir treatment can trigger large increases in total cholesterol and triglyceride levels (Kaletra 2004). Pharmacokinetic studies of once-daily lopinavir/ritonavir have observed steady-state plasma concentrations that, after 24 hours, are still sufficient to suppress wild-type viral isolates (Eron et al. 2004). Because these trough levels are roughly 50% of those seen with standard twice daily dosing, investigations of once daily lopinavir/ritonavir are focusing on treatment-naive patients. A recent 48-week study comparing once-daily (800/200 mg) versus twice-daily (400/100 mg) lopinavir/ritonavir in treatment-naive HIV-infected patients showed that both regimens have similar virologic efficacy, although there was a higher rate of discontinuations due to adverse events (mostly diarrhea) with the once-daily dose (11% versus 5%) (Gathe et al. 2004a).

Recent data from small observational trials have evaluated the use of lopinavir/ritonavir twice daily as monotherapy (without other antiretroviral agents), either initially (Gathe et al. 2004b) or as maintenance therapy following induction with standard highly active antiretroviral therapy (HAART) (Arribas et al. 2004). Data from these small trials have been promising, and larger controlled studies are under way. (See also Objective IV.33 on Investigational Antiretroviral Treatment Strategies Using Approved Agents, in this Update.)

Amprenavir/Ritonavir and Fosamprenavir

The clinical use of amprenavir has often been limited by the high pill burden required to administer the appropriate amount of drug per dose. The development of the prodrug formulation of amprenavir, fosamprenavir, results in a significant reduction in overall total pill burden (from 16 per day to 2 tablets per day) (Agenerase 2004; Lexiva 2004). Clinical trials of boosted fosamprenavir have shown fosamprenavir to be a potential alternative to lopinavir/ritonavir-containing antiretroviral therapy regimens for treatment-experienced patients (Lexiva 2004) and as once-daily dosing among treatment-naive patients as compared with nelfinavir-containing antiretroviral therapy regimens (Gathe et al. 2004c). Fosamprenavir is currently FDA-approved for once-daily and twice-daily dosing in treatment-naive patients and twice-daily dosing in PI-experienced patients (Lexiva 2004). Given the increased rates of gastrointestinal side effects and increased lipid levels that can occur with even small doses of ritonavir, there is interest in using 100 mg daily ritonavir for boosting fosamprenavir. In one study, ritonavir 100 mg with fosamprenavir 1400 mg once daily produced lower amprenavir trough concentrations (38% lower) than those observed with fosamprenavir 1400 mg/ritonavir 200 mg once daily, but these concentrations were still well in excess of wild-type IC_{50} values (Ruane et al. 2004). In addition, dosing with 100 mg ritonavir resulted in a lower incidence of gastrointestinal adverse drug events.

Atazanavir/Ritonavir

Clinical trials have also evaluated pharmacokinetically enhanced atazanavir. One study demonstrated at week 48 that combination antiretroviral therapy regimens including once-daily atazanavir 300 mg combined with once-daily ritonavir 100 mg among highly treatment-experienced patients produced good virologic response rates compared with a lopinavir/ritonavir-containing antiretroviral therapy regimen (DeJesus et al. 2004). Furthermore, patients in this study who were treated with atazanavir/ritonavir experienced fewer elevations in total cholesterol and triglycerides from baseline compared with patients who received lopinavir/ritonavir. To date, limited data exist on the safety, efficacy and lipid profiles of atazanavir/ritonavir-containing regimens among treatment-naive patients.

Atazanavir is a modest P450 inhibitor and has been shown to boost levels of saquinavir (Haas et al. 2003) but far less than ritonavir does (Becker et al. 2005). Among treatment-experienced patients, atazanavir (400 mg once daily) combined with saquinavir (1200 mg once daily) and nucleoside analogues performed more poorly than lopinavir/ritonavir- and atazanavir/ritonavir-containing antiretroviral therapy regimens (Badaro et al. 2003). More effective dosing recommendations for saquinavir/atazanavir have not been established (Reyataz 2004). The poor results may be partially due to decreased atazanavir concentrations arising from a negative drug-drug interaction with tenofovir (all patients received tenofovir in this study).

Negative drug-drug interactions occur when atazanavir is combined with either tenofovir or efavirenz. When unboosted atazanavir is combined with tenofovir, atazanavir total drug exposures and minimum drug concentrations decrease by 25% and 40% (Bristol-Myers Squibb 2003). If boosted with ritonavir, these values decrease by 25% and 23%. To ensure sufficient drug levels, ritonavir boosting (100 mg once daily) is recommended when prescribing atazanavir with concurrent tenofovir. When combined with efavirenz, atazanavir total drug exposure (AUC; area under the concentration time curve) declined by 21% (Tackett et al. 2003). Consequently, when combined with efavirenz, atazanavir should be pharmacokinetically enhanced with ritonavir 100 mg once daily (Tackett et al. 2003). It should be appreciated that even when combined with low-dose ritonavir, atazanavir concentrations in the presence of efavirenz are roughly equivalent to those seen with unboosted atazanavir without efavirenz (Tackett et al. 2003) and may be insufficient for patients with resistant virus.

Resistance and Boosted PIs

Resistance data from clinical trials among treatment-naive patients receiving lopinavir/ritonavir or fosamprenavir/ritonavir have not indicated development of detectable PI resistance upon virologic failure (Gathe et al. 2004c; Hicks et al. 2004; Kempf et al. 2004; MacManus et al. 2004). Regimens containing these boosted PIs lead to decreased development of reverse transcriptase mutations. It appears that high genetic barriers prevent development of resistance (Kempf et al. 2004; MacManus et al. 2004). This finding has not yet been fully evaluated, and it is unclear at this time whether it will be applicable to other boosted-PI combinations (e.g., atazanavir/ritonavir or saquinavir/ritonavir).

Triple-PI Regimens

Triple-PI regimens (i.e., 2 PIs in combination with low-dose ritonavir) are now being used by many clinicians, particularly in patients with extensive NRTI resistance or intolerance. It should be recognized that these triple-PI regimens have not been fully evaluated. They often result in complex drug-drug interactions, and limited pharmacokinetic and clinical data exist to evaluate the safety and efficacy of these regimens. There are a number of potential pharmacologic reasons for using double-boosted-PI regimens (Luber 2004):

1. To provide additive to synergistic antiviral activity against HIV
2. To combine agents with counteracting or conflicting resistance mutations so as to inhibit resistance from emerging
3. To achieve high plasma levels of 2 different PIs so that each PI can remain active against isolates that are resistant to the other

Pharmacokinetic data on the various double-boosted-PI regimens that have been studied are listed below in Table IV.17-2 (Luber 2004).

Table IV.17-2. Drug-drug interactions in double-boosted PI regimens (Luber 2004).

Combination	Impact on Drug Levels		Dosing recommendation*
LPV/r/FPV	↔LPV	↓APV	533 mg LPV/133 mg RTV/1400 mg FPV twice daily
LPV/r/SQV	↔LPV	↔SQV	400 mg LPV/100 mg RTV/1000 mg SQV twice daily
LPV/r/NFV	↓LPV	↔NFV	400 mg LPV/100 mg RTV/1000 mg NFV twice daily (LPV dose adjustments may be necessary)
LPV/r/IDV	↔LPV	↔IDV	400 mg LPV/100 mg RTV/600 mg IDV twice daily
ATV/r/SQV-hgc	↔ATV	↑SQV	300 mg ATV/100 mg RTV/1600 mg SQV-hgc once daily
FPV/r/SQV-hgc	↔FPV	↔SQV (↓SQV with 100 mg RTV)	700 mg FPV/200 mg RTV/1000 mg SQV-hgc twice daily

APV, amprenavir; ATV, atazanavir; FPV, fosamprenavir; IDV, indinavir; LPV, lopinavir; NFV, nelfinavir; RTV (or "/r/"), ritonavir; SQV-hgc, saquinavir hard-gel capsules.

*Data are limited evaluating the safety and efficacy for many of these regimens.

In general, the majority of the studies to date have been small, prospective, proof-of-concept studies that lack a comparator arm (Schapiro 2004; Staszewski 2004). The concomitant administration of lopinavir/ritonavir and fosamprenavir results in decreased lopinavir and amprenavir concentrations (Kashuba et al. 2003). Separation of dosing by 4 and 12 hours did not correct the amprenavir levels (Corbett et al. 2004). Increasing the dose of each agent (to 533 mg/133 mg twice daily for lopinavir/ritonavir and 1400 mg twice daily for fosamprenavir) corrected lopinavir concentrations to those observed when given without amprenavir (Wire et al. 2004). Blood concentrations of amprenavir increased but were still significantly depressed. Alternatively, an extra 100 mg ritonavir added to the standard dosing also corrected lopinavir levels, but amprenavir concentrations were even lower than with the regimen that used higher doses of all three drugs. Both of these regimens were poorly tolerated, provoking gastrointestinal symptoms in particular. No recommended dosing could be deduced.

Boosted Tipranavir With a Second PI

Tipranavir is a potent inducer of the cytochrome P450 enzyme CYP3A4 and thus speeds metabolism of many other drugs, including other HIV PIs. A recent clinical study of ritonavir-boosted tipranavir in combination with saquinavir, amprenavir or lopinavir found substantial declines in total drug exposure as well as minimum and maximum drug concentrations of the concomitant PI (Walmsley et al. 2004). Trial participants in this study had highly advanced disease and extensive PI resistance. Adding tipranavir effected a transient viral load reduction of about 1.2 $\log_{10}$ copies/mL (Clinical Care Options for HIV 2004). The eventual virologic failure is probably due to several factors: the lack of active NRTIs or other support drugs as well as the negative drug-drug interactions of tipranavir on the other PIs.

See also Objective IV.14 on Ritonavir Plus Other PIs and IV.16 on Pharmacodynamics and Pharmacokinetic Enhancement in the AAHIVM 2003 Study Guide.

References

Agenerase (amprenavir) [prescribing information]. Research Triangle Park, NC. GlaxoSmithKline. February **2004**.

Arribas JR, Pulido F, Lorenzo A, et al. Simplification to lopinavir/r single-drug HAART: 24 weeks results of a randomized, controlled, open label, pilot clinical trial (OK Study). In: Program and abstracts of the 15th International Conference on AIDS; July 11-16, **2004**; Bangkok, Thailand. Abstract TuPeB4486.

Badaro R, DeJesus E, Lazzarin A, et al. Efficacy and safety of atazanavir (ATV) with ritonavir (RTV) or saquinavir (SQV) versus lopinavir/ritonavir (LPV/RTV) in combination with tenofovir (TFV) and one NRTI in patients who have experienced virologic failure to multiple HAART regimens. In: Program and abstracts of the 2nd IAS Conference on HIV Treatment and Pathogenesis. July 13-16, **2003**; Paris, France. Abstract 118.

Becker S, Hoetelmans RMW. Exploiting pharmacokinetics to optimize antiretroviral therapy. Medscape HIV/AIDS Clinical Management Series. April **2002**. Available at: http://www.medscape.com/viewprogram/703 [accessed February 23, 2005].

Becker S, Tse M, Sterman F, Kakuda T, Acosta E. Pharmacokinetics of once-daily saquinavir hard-gel capsule with low-dose ritonavir or full-dose atazanavir in seronegative volunteers: ASPIRE I. In: Program and abstracts of the 9th Conference on Retroviruses and Opportunistic Infections; February 22-25, **2004**; Boston, Massachusetts. Abstract 79.

Bristol-Myers Squibb. Dear Doctor Letter. August 8, **2003**. Available at: http://www.medadvocates.org/drugs/ataz/Reyataz%20Dear%20Healthcare%20Provider%20Letter%20080803.pdf [accessed February 23, 2005].

Cameron DW, Japour AJ, Xu Y, et al. Ritonavir and saquinavir combination therapy for the treatment of HIV infection. *AIDS*. **1999**;13:213-224.

Clinical Care Options for HIV. PK Interactions and Antiviral Activity of Tipranavir/Ritonavir in Patients with PI Resistance. In: Coverage of the XV International AIDS Conference. July **2004**. Available at: http://www.clinicaloptions.com/hiv/conf/iac2004/cs/1236.asp [accessed February 10, 2005].

Corbett AH, Davidson L, Park JJ, et al. Dose separation strategies to overcome the pharmacokinetic interaction of a triple protease inhibitor regimen containing fosamprenavir lopinavir, and ritonavir. In: Program and abstracts of the 11th Conference on Retroviruses and Opportunistic Infections; February 8-11, **2004**; San Francisco, California. Abstract 611.

Cressey TR, Leenasirimakul P, Sukrakanchana P, et al. Pharmacokinetic studies comparing 600/100 IDV/RTV vs. 400/100 IDV/RTV as part of highly active antiretroviral therapy in HIV-infected Thai patients. In: Program and abstracts of the 15th International AIDS Conference; July 11-16, **2004**; Bangkok, Thailand. Abstract TuPeB4637.

DeJesus E, Grinsztejn B, Rodriguez C, et al. Efficacy and safety of atazanavir with ritonavir or saquinavir vs lopinavir/ritonavir in patients who have experienced virologic failure on multiple HAART regimens: 48-week results from BMS A1424-045. In: Program and abstracts of the 11th Conference on Retroviruses and Opportunistic Infections; February 8-11, **2004**; San Francisco, California. Abstract 547.

Department of Health and Human Services (DHHS). Guidelines for the use of antiretroviral agents in HIV-1-infected adults and adolescents October 29, **2004**. Available at: http://www.aidsinfo.nih.gov [accessed February 23, 2005].

Dragsted UB, Gerstoft J, Pedersen C, et al. Randomized trial to evaluate indinavir/ritonavir versus saquinavir/ritonavir in human immunodeficiency virus type 1-infected patients: the MaxCmin1 Trial. *J Infect Dis*. **2003**;188:635-642.

Eron JJ, Feinberg J, Kessler HA, et al. Once-daily versus twice-daily lopinavir/ritonavir in antiretroviral-naive HIV-positive patients: a 48-week randomized clinical trial. *J Infect Dis*. **2004**;189:265-272.

Gathe J, Podzamczer D, Johnson M, et al. Once-daily vs. twice-daily lopinavir/ritonavir in antiretroviral-naïve patients: 48-week results. In: Program and abstracts of the 11th Conference on Retroviruses and Opportunistic Infections; February 8-11, **2004a**; San Francisco, California. Abstract 570.

Gathe JC, Washington MY, Mayberry C, Piot D, Nemecek J. IMANI-1 TC3WP single drug HAART- proof of concept study. Pilot study of the safety and efficacy of Kaletra (LPV/r) as single drug HAART in HIV + ARV-naive patients-interim analysis of subjects completing final 48 week data. In: Program and abstracts of the 15th International Conference on AIDS; July 11-16, **2004b**; Bangkok, Thailand. Abstract MoOrB1057.

Gathe JC Jr, Ive P, Wood R, et al. SOLO: 48-week efficacy and safety comparison of once-daily fosamprenavir/ritonavir versus twice-daily nelfinavir in naive HIV-1-infected patients. *AIDS*. **2004c**;18:1529-1537.

Haas DW, Zala C, Schrader S, et al. Therapy with atazanavir plus saquinavir in patients failing highly active antiretroviral therapy: a randomized comparative pilot trial. *AIDS*. **2003**;17:1339-1349.

Hicks C, da Silva B, Benson C, et al. Extensive resistance testing during 5 years of lopinavir/ritonavir treatment in antiretroviral-naive HIV infected patients: results from study m97-720. In: Program and abstracts of the 15th International Conference on AIDS; July 11-16, **2004**; Bangkok, Thailand. Abstract WeOrB1291.

Invirase (saquinavir mesylate) [prescribing information]. Nutley, NJ: Roche Laboratories, Inc. December **2004**.

Kaletra (lopinavir/ritonavir) [prescribing information]. North Chicago, Illinois: Abbott Laboratories; February **2004**.

Kashuba ADM, Tierney C, Downey GF, et al. Combining GW433908 (fosamprenavir; 908) with lopinavir/ritonavir (LPV/R) in HIV-1 infected adults results in substantial reductions in amprenavir (APV) and LPV concentrations: pharmacokinetic (PK) results from Adult ACTG Protocol A5143. In: Program and abstracts of the 43rd Annual Interscience Conference on Antimicrobial Agents and Chemotherapy; September 14-17, **2003**; Chicago, Illinois. Abstract H-855a.

Kempf DJ, King MS, Bernstein B, et al. Incidence of resistance in a double-blind study comparing lopinavir/ritonavir plus stavudine and lamivudine to nelfinavir plus stavudine and lamivudine. *J Infect Dis*. **2004**;189:51-60.

Konopnicki D, De Wit S, Poll B, Crommentuyn K, Huitema A, Clumeck N. Indinavir/ritonavir-based therapy in HIV-1-infected antiretroviral therapy-naive patients: comparison of 800/100 mg and 400/100 mg twice daily. *HIV Med*. **2005**;6:1-6.

Kurowski M, Sternfeld T, Sawyer A, Hill A, Mocklinghoff C. Pharmacokinetic and tolerability profile of twice-daily saquinavir hard gelatin capsules and saquinavir soft gelatin capsules boosted with ritonavir in healthy volunteers. *HIV Med*. **2003**;4:94-100.

Lexiva (fosamprenavir calcium) [prescribing information]. Research Triangle Park, NC: GlaxoSmithKline; December **2004**.

Luber AD. Double-boosted protease inhibitor regimens: a pharmacologic and pharmacokinetic perspective [Clinical Care Options for HIV]. **2004**. Available at: http://www.clinicaloptions.com/hiv/manage/doubleboost/ [accessed November 4, 2004].

Norvir (ritonavir) [prescribing information]. North Chicago, Ill: Abbott Laboratories; October **2003**.

MacManus S, Yates PJ, Elston RC, White S, Richards N, Snowden W. GW433908/ritonavir once daily in antiretroviral therapy-naive HIV-infected patients: absence of protease resistance at 48 weeks. *AIDS*. **2004**;18:651-655.

O'Brien WA, Rojo D, Acosta E, et al. Switch of saquinavir 400 mg/ritonavir 400 mg to saquinavir 1000 mg/ritonavir 100 mg during BID four drug antiretroviral therapy in patients with viral load less than 200 copies/mL. In: Program and abstracts of the 14th International AIDS Conference; July 7-12, **2002**; Barcelona, Spain. Abstract WeOrB1263.

Plosker GL, Scott LJ. Saquinavir: a review of its use in boosted regimens for treating HIV infection. *Drugs*. **2003**;63:1299-1324.

Reyataz (atazanavir) [prescribing information]. Princeton, NJ: Bristol-Myers Squibb Company; October **2004**.

Ruane P, Wire M, Shelton M, Lou Y, Lancaster C, Pappa K. Plasma amprenavir (APV) pharmacokinetics (PK) and safety following co-administration of fosamprenavir (FPV) with a reduced ritonavir (RTV) dose once daily (QD) (COL10053). In: Program and abstracts of the 44th Interscience Conference on Antimicrobial Agents and Chemotherapy; October 30-November 2, **2004**; Washington, DC. Abstract A-449.

Schapiro JM. Clinical data on double-boosted protease inhibitor regimens [Clinical Care Options for HIV]. **2004**. Available at: http://www.clinicaloptions.com/hiv/manage/doubleboost/ [accessed February 24, 2005].

Staszewski S. Potential therapeutic strategies using double-boosted protease inhibitor regimens [Clinical Care Options for HIV]. **2004**. Available at: http://www.clinicaloptions.com/hiv/manage/doubleboost/ [accessed February 24, 2005].

Tackett D, Child M, Agarwala S, et al. Atazanavir: A summary of two pharmacokinetic drug interaction studies in healthy subjects. In: Program and abstracts of the 10th Conference on Retroviruses and Opportunistic Infections; February 10-14, **2003**; Boston, Massachusetts. Abstract 543.

Walmsley S, Leith J, Katlama C, et al. Pharmacokinetics and safety of tipranavir/ritonavir (TPV/r) alone or in combination with saquinavir (SQV), amprenavir (APV), or lopinavir (LPV): interim analysis of BI1182.51. In: Program and abstracts of the 15th International Conference on AIDS; July 11-16, **2004**; Bangkok, Thailand. Abstract WeOrB1236.

Wire MB, Naderer OJ, Masterman AL, Lou Y, Stein DS. The pharmacokinetic interaction between GW433908 and lopinavir/ritonavir (APV10011 and APV10012). In: Program and abstracts of the 11th Conference on Retroviruses and Opportunistic Infections; February 8-11, **2004**; San Francisco, California. Abstract 612.

Youle M, Gerstoft Z, Fox M, et al. The final week 48 analysis of a phase IV, randomised, open-label, multi-centre trial to evaluate safety and efficacy of lopinavir/ritonavir (400/100 mg bid) versus saquinavir/ritonavir (1000/100): the MaxCMin2 study. In: Program and abstracts of the 2nd IAS Conference on HIV Pathogenesis and Treatment, July 13-16, **2003**; Paris, France. Abstract LB23.

(RLO-28)

IV.18. NOT-RECOMMENDED ANTIRETROVIRAL COMBINATIONS

LEARNING OBJECTIVE: Discuss which antiretroviral combinations are contraindicated and those that should be coadministered with caution, and why.

Table IV.18-1 lists reasons for avoiding antiretroviral treatments that are contraindicated or should be coadministered with caution.

Table IV.18-1. Antiretroviral regimens that should be contraindicated or coadministered with caution (DHHS 2004).

Treatment	Reason for contraindication
Dual- (or single-) NRTI therapy alone	High rates of virologic failure with development of resistance
Amprenavir with fosamprenavir	No additional benefit, and potential additive toxicities
Amprenavir oral solution with ritonavir oral solution	The propylene glycol in the amprenavir formulation and the alcohol in the ritonavir formulation compete for the same elimination pathway; accumulation of either has risk of toxicity.
Amprenavir oral solution in pregnant women, young children, patients with hepatic or renal failure or those taking metronidazole or disulfiram	The propylene glycol in the formulation is especially toxic to these groups
Atazanavir with indinavir	Potential for additive hyperbilirubinemia
Didanosine with stavudine	Overlapping toxicity profiles (pancreatitis, peripheral neuropathy, elevated lactic acid); among pregnant women, increased risk for lactic acidosis with hepatic steatosis with or without pancreatitis
Efavirenz in first trimester of pregnancy or in women likely to become pregnant	Teratogenic in primates and likely to be so in humans
Emtricitabine with lamivudine	Similar resistance profile; no additional benefit
Saquinavir hard-gel capsules (without ritonavir boosting) in any regimen	Poor oral availability inferior efficacy
Saquinavir (without ritonavir-boosting) as only PI with efavirenz or nevirapine	Negative drug interaction with efavirenz and nevirapine lowers saquinavir concentrations
Tenofovir and lamivudine (or emtricitabine) with abacavir or didanosine	High rate of virologic failure in treatment-naive patients (see below for other combinations of tenofovir and didanosine)
Zalcitabine with didanosine or stavudine	Overlapping toxicity profiles (peripheral neuropathy)
Zalcitabine with lamivudine	Antagonistic effect
Zidovudine with stavudine	Antagonistic effect

NRTI, nucleoside reverse transcriptase inhibitor

What's New

Tenofovir and didanosine have a complicated drug interaction. There is a high rate of virologic failure with tenofovir/didanosine/efavirenz when used as initial HAART.

Key Points

- Contraindicated or coadministered with caution:
  - Dual NRTI therapy alone
  - Didanosine and stavudine
  - Saquinavir (unboosted) and efavirenz
  - Saquinavir (unboosted) and nevirapine
  - Tenofovir, lamivudine and abacavir
  - Tenofovir, lamivudine and didanosine
  - Tenofovir, didanosine, and abacavir
  - Tenofovir, didanosine, and efavirenz (or nevirapine) as initial therapy
  - Tipranavir (boosted) with saquinavir, amprenavir or lopinavir
  - Zidovudine and stavudine

Tenofovir Combinations

Reports from clinical studies note that once-a-day regimens containing tenofovir, abacavir and lamivudine (Gallant et al. 2004; Farthing et al. 2003) or tenofovir, didanosine and lamivudine (Jemsek et al. 2004) result in early virologic nonresponse and/or treatment failure. The exact cause of these failures is unknown but a number of potential causes have been suggested, including: (1) a low genetic barrier to resistance, in particular the potential for the K65R mutation to reduce activity of all 3 drugs in the regimen; (2) a potential drug-drug interaction between abacavir and tenofovir; and (3) a pharmacokinetic limitation of abacavir and lamivudine when taken once a day (Ruane and Luber 2003).

Regarding interaction between abacavir and tenofovir, one study found that tenofovir did not significantly affect abacavir plasma pharmacokinetics (Kearney et al. 2003). An intracellular pharmacokinetic study also found no negative drug-drug interaction between tenofovir and abacavir (Hawkins et al. 2004). Given that once-daily administration of abacavir and lamivudine in combination with efavirenz resulted in little to no virologic failure (Gazzard et al. 2003) and that the intracellular pharmacokinetic evaluations of both lamivudine and abacavir suggest sufficient drug exposures when taken once daily (Epivir 2003; Piliero et al. 2003), this potential etiology for treatment failures appears to be minimal.

These treatment failures could be a direct result of a low genetic barrier to resistance. Abacavir, lamivudine and tenofovir all demonstrate reduced susceptibility to K65R (Farthing et al. 2003; Gallant et al. 2003). In addition, recent reports of treatment failures with similar genotypic mutational patterns (M184V with or without K65R) occurred among patients receiving didanosine plus lamivudine and tenofovir (Gilead 2003) as well as didanosine plus abacavir and tenofovir (K65R mutation only) (Winston et al. 2003). One limitation to this theory is that not all patients initially fail with K65R. Further genotypic and phenotypic evaluations are ongoing to determine the precise cause of failure. Recently reported results of several studies show that the rapid failure of once-daily triple-nucleoside regimens containing tenofovir and lamivudine plus didanosine or abacavir seems to be related to the inadequate potency of the regimen to suppress viral replication and to a low genetic barrier for development of the M184V and K65R resistance mutations (Elion et al. 2004; Jemsek et al. 2004; Landman et al. 2004). The previously rare K65R mutation appears to be increasing in prevalence (Parikh et al. 2004) and may be due to the increasing use of regimens that do not include the thymidine analogues, zidovudine and stavudine.

It may be that the presence of zidovudine severely inhibits the pathway to K65R-based resistance (see Objectives IV.10 on Resistance Mutations and IV.26 on Antiretroviral Cross-Resistance in this Update). Administering zidovudine with nucleoside analogue combinations that select for the K65R mutation will likely prevent this mutation from emerging (Parikh et al. 2004). The poor virologic response to the once-daily regimen of tenofovir/lamivudine/abacavir was not observed when zidovudine was added, even when dosed once daily (Elion et al. 2004). In addition, the virologic failure rate of the triple-NRTI combination abacavir, zidovudine and lamivudine (Trizivir) is considerably lower than in these newer regimens (Gallant et al. 2004). Finally, the triple NRTI combination of zidovudine, lamivudine and tenofovir produced acceptable results in a recent small trial, with 90% of participants having viral loads under 50 copies/mL after 6 months (on-treatment analysis) (Rey et al. 2005).

Whatever the cause of early virologic failure, caution is clearly needed when prescribing tenofovir, particularly in simplified, non-thymidine-containing NRTI-based regimens. For treatment-naive patients, the combination of tenofovir, lamivudine and efavirenz has been found to provide virologic benefit comparable to a regimen of stavudine, lamivudine and efavirenz (Miller et al. 2003). Combinations of tenofovir with a protease inhibitor (PI)-based regimen are expected to result in similar efficacy, as was found in Abbott 418, a trial of once- versus twice-daily lopinavir/ritonavir in which all participants also received tenofovir and emtricitabine (Gathe et al. 2004).

The combination of tenofovir, didanosine and efavirenz theoretically appeared to be a convenient once-a-day combination. Preliminary data showed this regimen to maintain viral suppression upon treatment switches among patients with well-controlled HIV infection (Barrios et al. 2004). However, when used as initial therapy for treatment-naive patients, this regimen resulted in a high virologic failure rate (Leon et al. 2005; Moyle et al. 2004; Podzamczer et al. 2004), especially among patients with low CD4 counts and high viral loads (Podzamczer et al. 2004; Moyle et al. 2004). Tenofovir, didanosine and nevirapine likewise produced high failure rates (Leon et al. 2005). These high rates of virologic failure add to a body of data showing impaired CD4 responses even when virologic suppression occurs with regimens containing tenofovir/didanosine (Barrios et al. 2005; Negredo et al. 2004a). CD4 count recovery was poor when the didanosine dose was subsequently reduced (Negredo et al. 2004b). Not all studies have reported poor results: A Swiss Cohort analysis of 194 patients on regimens containing tenofovir plus reduced dose didanosine (250 mg/day) found immunologic responses (CD4 count improvements) comparable with those of patients on tenofovir-containing regimens that did not include didanosine (Karrer et al. 2005). Nonetheless, the tenofovir-ddI combination should be avoided as part of initial therapy, and likely entirely until further studies are done.

A number of PI-PI drug-drug interactions exist with and without tipranavir. Some have significant negative impact on PI exposure. Recent pharmacokinetic evaluations of boosted tipranavir in combination with saquinavir, amprenavir or lopinavir have shown substantial declines in total drug exposure and minimum and maximum drug concentrations of the concomitant PI (Walmsley et al. 2004). See Objective IV.17 on Boosted Protease Inhibitors in this Update.

References

Barrios A, Negredo E, Rendon A, et al. Paradoxical CD4+ T-cell decline in patients with complete virus suppression under tenofovir plus didanosine combinations. In: Program and abstracts of the 44th Interscience Conference on Antimicrobial Agents and Chemotherapy; October 30-November 2, **2004**; Washington, DC. Abstract H-1132.

Barrios A, Negredo E, Vilaró-Rodríguez J, et al. Safety and efficacy of a QD simplification regimen. In: Program and abstract of the 11th Conference of Retroviruses and Opportunistic Infections; February 8-11, **2004**; San Francisco, California. Abstract 566.

Department of Health and Human Services (DHHS). Guidelines for the use of antiretroviral agents in HIV-1-infected adults and adolescents. October 29, **2004**. Available at: http://www.aidsinfo.nih.gov [accessed January 5, 2005].

Elion R, Cohen C, DeJesus E, et al. COL40263: resistance and efficacy of once-daily Trizivir and tenofovir DF in antiretroviral-naïve patients. In: Program and abstracts of the 11th Conference on Retroviruses and Opportunistic Infections; February 8-11, **2004**; San Francisco, California. Abstract 53.

Epivir (lamivudine) [prescribing information]. Research Triangle Park, NC: GlaxoSmithKline; December **2004**.

Farthing C, Khanlou H, Yeh V, et al. Early virologic failure in a pilot study evaluating the efficacy of abacavir, lamivudine and tenofovir in treatment-naive HIV-infected patients. In: Program and abstracts of the 2nd International AIDS Society Conference on Pathogenesis and Treatment; July 13-16, **2003**; Paris, France. Abstract 43.

Gallant JE, Rodriguez A, Weinberg W, et al. Early non-response to tenofovir DF (TDF) + abacavir (ABC) and lamivudine (3TC) in a randomized trial compared to efavirenz (EFV) + ABC and 3TC: ESS30009 unplanned interim analysis. In: Program and abstracts of the 43rd Interscience Conference on Antimicrobial Agents and Chemotherapy; September 14-17, **2003**; Chicago, Illinois. Abstract 1722a.

Gallant JE, Vibhagool A, Staszewski S, et al. Comparison of tenofovir (TDF) + abacavir (ABC) + lamivudine (3TC) virologic non-response rate reported in ESS30009 with virologic non-response rates observed in studies evaluating other triple nucleoside regimens containing ABC + 3TC. In: Program and abstracts of the XV International Conference on AIDS; July 11-16, **2004**; Bangkok, Thailand. Abstract TuPeB4502.

Gathe J, Podzamczer D, Johnson M, et al. Once-daily vs. twice-daily lopinavir/ritonavir in antiretroviral-naïve patients: 48-week results. In: Program and abstracts of the 11th Conference on Retroviruses and Opportunistic Infections; February 8-11, **2004**; San Francisco, California. Abstract 570.

Gazzard B, DeJesus E, Cahn P, et al. Abacavir (ABC) once daily (OAD) plus lamivudine (3TC) OAD I combination with efavirenz (EFV) OAD is well-tolerated and effective in the treatment of antiretroviral therapy (ART) naive adults with HIV-1 infection; Zodiac study, CNA30021. In: Program and abstracts of the 43rd Interscience Conference on Antimicrobial Agents and Chemotherapy; September 14-17, **2003**; Chicago, Illinois. Abstract H-1722b.

Gilead. Healthcare provider important drug warning letter. October 14, **2003**. Available at: http://www.fda.gov/medwatch/SAFETY/2003/viread_deardoc.pdf [accessed February 24, 2005].

Hawkins T, Veikley W, St.Claire R, Hey A, Guyer B, Kearney BP. Intracellular pharmacokinetics of tenofovir-DP and Carbovir-TP in patients receiving triple nucleoside regimens. In: Program and abstracts of the 5th International Workshop on Clinical Pharmacology of HIV Therapy; April 1-3, **2004**; Rome, Italy. Abstract 6.

Jemsek J, Hutcherson P, Harper E. Poor virologic responses and early emergence of resistance in treatment naïve, HIV-infected patients receiving a once-daily triple nucleoside regimen of didanosine, lamivudine and tenofovir DF. In: Program and abstracts of the 11th Conference on Retroviruses and Opportunistic Infections; February 8-11, **2004**; San Francisco, California. Abstract 51.

Karrer U, Ledergerber B, Weber R, et al. No evidence for poor immunologic response in patients treated with a combination of tenofovir and didanosine at 250 mg daily. In: Program and abstracts of the 12th Conference on Retroviruses and Opportunistic Infections; February 22-25, **2005**; Boston, Massachusetts. Abstract 588.

Kearney BP, Isaacson E, Sayre J, et al. The pharmacokinetics of abacavir, a purine nucleoside analogue, are not affected by Tenofovir DF. In: Program and abstracts of the 43rd Annual Interscience Conference on Antimicrobial Agents and Chemotherapy; September 14-17, **2003**; Chicago, Illinois. Poster #A-1615.

Landman R, Peytavin G, Descamps D, et al. Low genetic barrier to resistance is a possible cause of early virologic failures in once daily regimen of abacavir, lamivudine, and tenofovir: the Tonus study. In: Program and abstracts of the 11th Conference on Retroviruses and Opportunistic Infections; February 8-11, **2004**; San Francisco, California. Abstract 52.

Leon A, Martinez E, Mallolas J, et al. Early virological failure in treatment-naive HIV-infected adults receiving didanosine and tenofovir plus efavirenz or nevirapine [research letter]. *AIDS*. **2005**;19:213-215.

Miller M, Margot N, McColl D, et al. Characterization of virologic failure through 96 weeks among treatment naïve patients taking tenofovir DF (TDF) or stavudine (d4T) in combination with lamivudine (3TC) and efavirenz (EFV). In: Program and abstracts of the 2nd International AIDS Society Conference on Pathogenesis and Treatment; July 13-16, **2003**; Paris, France. Abstract 553.

Moyle G, Maitland D, Hand J, Mandalia S, Nelson M, Gazzard B. Early virological failure in persons with viral loads >100,000 cps/ml and CD4 counts <200/mm^3 receiving ddI/tenofovir/efavirenz as initial therapy: Results from a randomised comparative trial. In: Program and abstracts of the 44th Interscience Conference on Antimicrobial Agents and Chemotherapy; October 30-November 2, **2004**; Washington, DC. Abstract H-566.

Negredo E, Moltó J, Burger D, et al. Unexpected CD4 cell count decline in patients receiving didanosine and tenofovir-based regimens despite undetectable viral load. *AIDS*. **2004a**;18:459–463.

Negredo E, Puig J, Masmitja E, Moltó J, Ruiz L, Clotet B. CD4 cell count changes after reduction of didanosine dosage in patients receiving standard doses of didanosine and tenofovir-based regimens. In: Program and abstracts of the 44th Interscience Conference on Antimicrobial Agents and Chemotherapy; October 30-November 2, **2004b**; Washington, DC. Abstract H-561.

Parikh U, Koontz D, Sluis-Cremer N, et al. K65R: a multinucleoside resistance mutation of increasing prevalence exhibits bidirectional phenotypic antagonism with TAM. In: Program and abstracts of the 11th Conference on Retroviruses and Opportunistic Infections; February 8-11, **2004**; San Francisco, California. Abstract 54.

Piliero P, Shachoy-Clark AD, Para M, et al. A study examining the pharmacokinetics of abacavir and the intracellular carbovir triphosphate (GSK protocol CNA 10905). In: Program and abstracts of the 43rd Interscience Conference on Antimicrobial Agents and Chemotherapy; September 14-17, **2003**; Chicago, Illinois. Abstract 1797.

Podzamczer D, Ferrer E, Gatell JM, et al. Early virological failure and occurrence of resistance in naive patients receiving tenofovir, didanosine and efavirenz [abstract]. *Antivir Ther.* **2004**;9:S172.

Rey D, Krebs M, Partisani M, et al. Early virologic response at 1-month and 8-month median follow-up of a new triple NUC combination (zidovudine, lamivudine, and tenofovir) in 36 antiretroviral-naive, HIV-1-infected patients. In: Program and abstracts of the 12th Conference on Retroviruses and Opportunistic Infections; February 22-25, **2005**; Boston, Massachusetts. Abstract 599.

Ruane P, Luber A. Possible causes of early treatment failure with a novel ARV regimen. Medscape HIV/AIDS. **2003**;9(2). Available at: http://www.medscape.com/viewarticle/460673 [accessed February 24, 2005].

Walmsley S, Leith J, Katlama C, et al. Pharmacokinetics and safety of tipranavir/ritonavir (TPV/r) alone or in combination with saquinavir (SQV), amprenavir (APV), or lopinavir (LPV): interim analysis of BI1182.51. In: Program and abstracts of the XV International Conference on AIDS; July 11-16, **2004**; Bangkok, Thailand. Abstract WeOrB1236.

Winston A, Pozniak A, Gazzard B, et al. Which nucleoside and nucleotide backbone combinations select for the K65R mutation in HIV-1 reverse transcriptase? In: Program and abstracts of the 12th International HIV Drug Resistance Workshop; June 10-14, **2003**; Los Cabos, Mexico. Abstract 137.

(RLO-29)

IV.20. RESISTANCE TESTING

LEARNING OBJECTIVE: Discuss the following aspects of genotypic, phenotypic and virtual phenotypic resistance tests:

- **(a) Evaluation of currently available resistance assays, including proper use, strengths and limitations, as well as interpretation and management of discordant phenotype and genotype resistance testing;**
- **(b) The role of resistance testing in selecting a drug regimen for a treatment-naive patient;**
- **(c) The role of resistance testing in selecting a drug regimen for a patient whose regimen is failing (in contrast to empiric selection of antiretroviral therapy based on the patient's treatment history).**

The acquisition of resistant virus can occur through 1 of 3 distinct ways: (1) via error-prone viral replication; (2) via transmission of a resistant viral isolate from a source case to a newly infected patient; or (3) through selective pressure from inadequate drug exposures in the presence of replicating virus (either through pharmacokinetic limitations or from patient nonadherence).

Drug resistance quickly becomes widespread after the introduction of antiretroviral agents. In 1998, the HIV Cost and Service Utilization Survey (HCSUS) study obtained blood specimens from 1797 patients, a representative national sample of those who received HIV care in 1996 and survived until 1998 (Richman et al. 2004). Within this population, 63% had viral loads over 500 copies/mL, and among these viremic patients, 76% had HIV with drug resistance to at least 1 antiretroviral. Resistance to nucleoside reverse transcriptase inhibitors (NRTIs), nonnucleoside reverse transcriptase inhibitors (NNRTIs) and protease inhibitors (PIs) was respectively 71%, 25% and 41%. Thirteen percent had triple-class resistance. The odds of resistance increased with current antiretroviral drug use, lower current viral load and low nadir CD4 count. A British Columbia prospective study of 1191 treatment-initiating patients more exactly determined the correlations with drug-resistance (Harrigan et al. 2005). Drug resistance of any kind appeared in 25% of this cohort during the first 30 months of antiretroviral therapy. Lower initial CD4 count and higher initial viral load were important factors, as was adherence. Suboptimal, but not negligible, drug levels promoted resistance: Patients with moderate-to-good adherence were more likely to develop drug-resistant HIV than were those with poor or excellent adherence. However, those with excellent adherence still had a high probability of drug resistance if drug concentrations in their blood were paradoxically low.

Drug resistance may be detected in treatment-naive individuals at the time of diagnosis. The Centers for Disease Control and Prevention evaluated the occurrence of HIV resistance mutations among 1082 treatment-naive HIV-infected patients (Weinstock et al. 2004).The Centers found the prevalence of these mutations to be almost 12% among men who have sex with men and 6% among women. Fifteen percent of patients whose partners took antiretroviral medications had drug-resistant HIV.

What's New

Rates of transmission of resistance virus to newly infected patients elicit still more controversy. Baseline resistance is a key predictor of virologic failure to new HAART regimens. Companies have established new clinical cutoffs to define resistance in their phenotype and virtual phenotype assays.

Key Points

- Using genotyping and phenotyping to guide antiretroviral choice in a second-line regimen appears to be better than using "standard of care."
- Genotyping detects specific mutations in the genome of a patient's isolate that are associated with antiretroviral resistance. An algorithm is developed relating the specific mutations to resistance to specific drugs.
- Phenotyping assesses how well recombinant virus grows in vitro with different concentrations of antiretroviral drugs.
- Virtual phenotyping uses a genotype to predict the phenotype by referencing a database of matched genotypes and corresponding phenotypes. It has high predictive value for most drugs. The major exceptions are newer agents or unusual genotypes that do not yet have extensive representation in the database.
- Phenotyping may be more useful than genotyping in complex cases with multiple resistance mutations in which it is very difficult to predict the outcome of the interaction of multiple resistance mutations.

Key Points (cont.)

- Resistance testing can be unreliable when only a small proportion of virus is resistant, with plasma viral loads below 500-1000 copies/mL, or when the patient tested is has discontinued therapy. However, even when patients are no longer on therapy, detected resistance mutations may provide useful information for selection of the next regimen.
- Resistance testing is recommended for acute or recent (less than 12 months) HIV infection and before initiation of antiretrovirals in chronic HIV infection. (The latest data show persistence of detectable resistance mutations for over 3 years after acute infection.) Resistance testing before therapy is particularly important if the index case is treatment-experienced, HIV was acquired in a community with greater than 5% resistance; regimen failure, or the patient is pregnant.

The impact of resistance on treatment options can be observed from a number of studies. Of the 546 treatment-naive patients who had genotypic testing in FTC 301A , a phase III trial that compared emtricitabine/didanosine/efavirenz with stavudine/didanosine/efavirenz, 90 (16%) had NRTI or NNRTI resistance mutations at baseline (Borroto-Esoda et al. 2004). These baseline resistance mutations, especially those associated with NNRTI resistance, were a key predictor of virologic failure. In the Jaguar study, 168 patients were on stable highly active antiretroviral therapy (HAART) but had viral loads between 1000 and 100,000 copies/mL (Molina et al. 2003). They were randomized to add didanosine EC (enteric-coated) or placebo to their previous regimen. Significant viral load decreases were observed if fewer than 3 thymidine analogue mutations were present at baseline. Among patients with previous treatment with PIs and receiving either lopinavir/ritonavir or fosamprenavir/ritonavir in the CONTEXT trial, response to either agent could be predicted from the baseline protease mutations (Elston et al. 2004). Those patients who harbored the D30N mutation had high rates of virologic response to both regimens; those with baseline M46I/L or L90M had roughly only a 50% chance of achieving viral loads below 400 copies/mL. Finally, the presence or absence of previous NNRTI resistance mutations appears to be a key determinant of subsequent treatment responses to NNRTI-containing HAART (Jourdain et al. 2004; Mellors et al. 2004).

Evaluation of Resistance Assays

Genotype testing involves the detection of specific mutations that are known to be associated with antiretroviral resistance in the genome of a patient's isolate. A laboratory may perform genotype testing using either 1 of 2 kits approved by the U.S. Food and Drug Administration (FDA), or a "homegrown" assay (not under FDA purview). Phenotype testing, currently performed commercially by only a few companies, is an in vitro assessment of the degree of growth of a recombinant virus (prepared using the reverse transcriptase and protease portions of the genome of the patient's viral isolate) in the presence of different concentrations of antiretroviral drugs. Table IV. 20-1 compares the 2 types of resistance tests.

Most commercial phenotype and genotype assays require that patients have plasma viral loads of at least 500-1000 copies/mL (Hirsch et al. 2003). Otherwise, there is insufficient virus present to ensure that the test result will correctly characterize the viral population.

Resistance tests of either type fail to detect minority drug resistant quasispecies (less than 10% to 20% of the total viral population) (DHHS 2004). The test result may report that the virus population is drug-sensitive. Nevertheless, treatment chosen on the basis of that test result may fail rapidly as the resistant minor quasispecies becomes the predominant quasispecies (Mellors et al. 2004; Hirsch et al. 2003; Albrecht et al. 2002).

When patients are off medications, some resistance mutations will disappear from the majority species, with reversion on the resistance test to "wild type." This is a misleading result because drug-resistant viruses are often less fit than wild-type viruses and soon become minor quasispecies (DHHS 2004). For this reason, a resistance test cannot always accurately determine the absence of resistance to a class of drugs that the patient has taken in the past. Consider, for example, a patient who formerly took a regimen containing an NNRTI but is now on a different type of combination. Even years after stopping the NNRTI regimen, a negative resistance test will not guarantee susceptibility to NNRTIs (Palmer et al. 2004). However, detected resistance when patients are off therapy is valuable clinical information. Although it is optimal to obtain resistance tests when patients are on a failing regimen, it is still worthwhile within 4 weeks after discontinuing therapy (DHHS 2004).

Table IV.20-1. Summary of advantages and disadvantages of genotype and phenotype resistance tests.

Resistance test	Advantages	Disadvantages
Genotype	• May improve virologic outcome • Cheaper • Rapid turnaround	• May not detect minority subpopulations • Unreliable if viral load below 1000 copies/mL • Indirect measure of resistance; detects only mutations that have been characterized • Results subject to mistaken interpretation
Phenotype	• May improve virologic outcome • Direct measure of resistance and cross-resistance • More information for newer drugs	• May not measure minority subpopulations • Unreliable if viral load below 1000 copies/mL • More expensive • Slower turnaround

Phenotypic testing has the advantage of being a direct measure of resistance and cross-resistance. However, it usually does not take into account the fact that different levels of drug can be achieved in different patients. There can be large interpersonal variations in drugs levels, which are also subject to manipulation by such strategies as ritonavir-boosting. It may be possible to achieve suppression of a virus that is reported to display phenotypic resistance to a certain drug if sufficiently high levels of that drug can be achieved (Luber 2000).

This issue goes to the heart of the "cutoff" issue. Originally, phenotypic resistance was considered present if the test detected a 4-fold loss of susceptibility compared to the assay's standard HIV isolate (as measured by the increase in a drug's 50% inhibitory concentration [IC_{50}], the level at which the drug reduces viral replication by half). This threshold arose out of the variability of the test (reproducibility cutoff). It was not a medical judgment call. Drugs may still be active despite increases above this level (Hirsch et al. 2003; Kempf et al. 2002). The contrary is also true: Stavudine, for example, has been found to fail with little more than a 1-fold loss in susceptibility (Shulman et al. 2002).

Labs next began using "biologic cutoffs" based on the average susceptibility to each drug in wild-type patient isolates. The more predictive indicators of resistance are "clinical cutoffs," which are becoming available for a number of drugs, including ritonavir-boosted protease inhibitors (Bacheler 2004; Szumiloski et al. 2002). These originate in clinical data that show a loss in viral suppression in patients with a certain amount of phenotypic resistance to a particular drug. They reflect the previous drug experience of the test population and the resulting background mutations (Shulman et al. 2002).

A major problem with clinical cutoffs is that they are sensitive to the drug concentration achieved in a patient's body. The impact of individualized pharmacokinetics represents a crucial variable. If a high drug concentration is reached, either because of natural interpersonal variability or through ritonavir-boosting, then the in vitro cutoff point of a phenotype test may not be relevant (Hirsch et al. 2003). A relatively large in vitro increase in IC_{50} may be countered by drug levels that far surpass the necessary level. The converse is also true. For individuals in whom a certain drug has marginal PK, very small changes in phenotypic resistance can result in drug failure. A common situation is the intermediate one: Resistance is detected, but the drug continues to have some effect at the drug concentrations achieved, and the treatment regimen remains viable (Hirsch et al. 2003).

Unlike the graduated results of phenotypic testing, those of genotypic testing are a simple binary yes-no deduced from a viral isolate's genetic sequence. Clinical outcome is expressed in a genotype test's interpretive algorithm rather than in measurements above and below the cutoff level. Genotypes may therefore be subject to mistakes in the interpretation of the clinical significance of specific resistance mutations.

Genotype tests are perhaps better at detecting evolving resistance because they may be more sensitive to mutations that survive in a minority subpopulation (Hirsch et al. 2003). They also can detect "transitional" mutations – those that do not change phenotype by themselves but can quickly lead to resistant HIV after introducing a particular drug to the treatment regimen. Unlike phenotyping, genotyping has the ability to detect "back mutations," successors of past resistance mutations that can re-emerge rapidly during treatment with the relevant drug (Zolopa 2002). However, genotyping may fail to account for the conflicting effects of concurrent mutations that impart phenotypic susceptibility to drugs despite the detectable presence of resistance-conferring genetic changes. Genotyping also will not flag mutations whose resistance properties have not been established. To be reliable, interpretive algorithms for genotypes should be derived from a large database correlating HIV gene sequences with treatment outcomes or, at least, phenotype (Norton et al. 2004). Reliability is also increased when genotype algorithms weight mutations differently when analyzing each drug. Frequent updating of the algorithm – to take account of new information – is also important (Servais et al. 2001).

For these reasons, phenotyping is advantageous in complex cases with multiple resistance mutations (Hirsch et al. 2003; Norton et al. 2004). Nonetheless, the reverse of resistance – hypersusceptibility – has been difficult to cope with. It can cause a better response than that predicted by the resistance test's assessment of the individual drugs in the treatment regimen. This issue has arisen concerning NNRTIs, in which hypersusceptibility correlates with the presence of various NRTI-associated mutations (NAMs) (Bosch et al 2003). In three large clinical trials involving efavirenz, a 2.5-fold decrease in susceptibility in this NNRTI's IC_{50} was the threshold for a significantly improved response rate. Further investigation to sort out mutational and drug interactions is necessary before hypersusceptibility can have a role in patient management.

A virtual phenotype is an extrapolation from a genotype of a current patient's specimen. The interpretation algorithm is based on a database of viruses that have been subject to both genotypic and phenotypic testing in the past. A computerized search identifies viruses from the database with the same genotypic resistance pattern as the test virus. The average phenotypic resistance properties of the matched viruses are reported as the "virtual phenotype." This match is based on certain specific mutations, not the entire sequence. The mutations used for each drug are proprietary information not subject to independent evaluation. The limitations of virtual phenotypes relate to the size of the database, especially concerning newer drugs and less common genotypes. There is also considerable uncertainty in relating genotypic findings to actual clinical response to particular drugs. Experts do not always agree with database interpretations of genotype data (Zolopa et al. 2002), and high variability in laboratory genotype results may lead to inaccurate interpretations (Wensing et al. 2001).

Still, by correlating genotypic results closely with phenotypic results, virtual phenotype considerably strengthens the predictive power of genotyping. It has also transformed genotyping into a graduated assay. One company has gone to the lengths of establishing clinical cutoffs for its virtual phenotype analysis (Bacheler 2004). The company's survey estimated phenotypic resistance from the HIV genotypes in about 3100 patients who were switching regimens. It linked the predicted phenotype with these patients' virologic outcomes. Modeling data suggest that the lower and higher cutoff values be defined as the fold-change associated with an expected 20% and 80% loss of activity of a drug within the regimen (Winters et al. 2004). For 5 NRTIs, the clinical cutoffs for 80% reduced response ranged from an estimated 2.2-fold predicted increase in IC50 above wild-type HIV (tenofovir) to 12.7-fold (zidovudine) (Bacheler 2004). For 4 unboosted PIs, the range was 1.7-fold higher than wild type (saquinavir) to 3.1-fold (indinavir). The 80% cutoffs for ritonavir-boosted PIs were higher: 10.8-fold above wild type for amprenavir/ritonavir and 77.5-fold for lopinavir/ritonavir. Flagging active drugs in a regimen according to the virtual phenotype clinical cutoffs resulted in a trend toward improved ability to predict treatment response compared with the older biologic cutoffs.

Genotype and phenotype tests frequently disagree in their assessment of a patient's drug resistance profile (Zolopa 2003). In one comparative study, discordant results occurred for at least one antiretroviral in 83% of 1150 patient samples (Parkin et al. 2002). Genotype predicting sensitivity to a certain drug, coupled with phenotype results indicating resistance, were mainly due to the absence of recognized key resistance mutations. Resistance emerged instead through alternative mutational pathways. Such alternatives can involve rather complicated mutational patterns arising from exposure to other drugs (e.g., the presence of multiple NAMs – see Objective IV.26 on Cross-Resistance in this Update). The opposite sort of discordance – resistant genotype result with sensitive phenotype – was largely the result of interactions between mutations, in which one modulated the resistance conferred by the other (e.g., M184V counteracts resistance conferred by NAMs). Discordance in PIs frequently resulted when genotypes categorized an HIV isolate as saquinavir- or indinavir-resistant because the key protease resistance mutations at codons 90 and 82 were present. Resistance to PIs requires supplementary mutations (Servais et al. 2001) that were not present in these cases, leading to PI-sensitive results in the phenotype assay (Parkin et al. 2002).

Mixed populations that include minority drug-resistant quasispecies may cause misreading of either genotype or phenotype, depending on the sensitivity of each assay. Most often, as noted above, the genotype signaled the presence of a resistant genetic sequence, but the size of the resistant population is not high enough to raise the phenotypic measurement above the resistance cutoff (Parkin et al. 2002).

Newer, more sensitive genotypic assays, such as single genome sequencing (Kearney et al. 2004) and clonal analysis (Dykes et al. 2004), may allow for detection of minority species that standard genotypic tests often miss. Currently, these tests are available for research purposes only, and their application to clinical practice remains undefined.

The Role of Resistance Testing in Treatment-Naive Patients

Both the International AIDS Society-USA (IAS-USA) (Hirsch et al. 2003) and the Department of Health and Human Services (DHHS 2004) recommend resistance testing when initiating treatment in patients who present with primary or early HIV infection (less than 12 months but possibly as long as 2 years after infection). If therapy must begin immediately, before the resistance results are available, clinicians can later adjust therapy as indicated by the test results (Hirsch et al. 2003). Genotype testing will give faster results and may be preferable for this reason (DHHS 2004).

Accumulating data suggest that transmitted resistant virus is genetically homogenous and that it would have to progressively mutate to revert back to wild type (Brenner et al. 2002). Transmitted resistance virus may persist in newly infected persons (Hanna et al. 2003). Investigators in one study reported that PI- and NNRTI-associated mutations persisted in 11 untreated, newly infected individuals during a follow-up period of 82 to 1346 days after acquiring HIV (Little et al. 2004). Complete reversion to wild type occurred in only 1 patient, at 1019 days post-infection. Elsewhere, multidrug-resistant viruses containing primary protease mutations have been reported to persist for between 36 weeks and 5 years (Brenner et al. 2002). Nucleoside analogue resistance mutations can persist for at least 2 years (Trabaud et al. 2000), and the M184V mutation associated with lamivudine has been reported to persist for 36 to 250 weeks (Brenner et al. 2002).

Modeling has suggested that genotypic testing before starting therapy in chronically infected treatment-naive patients is cost-effective at resistance prevalence rates above 5% (Weinstein et al. 2001). This is a level already achieved in developed countries. (Cost-effectiveness was defined here as less than $69,000 cost per quality-adjusted life-year saved.) Testing is particularly worthwhile if there is reason to believe that the patient was infected by someone receiving antiretroviral therapy (DHHS 2004). Despite the above-mentioned data, drug-resistant HIV may not remain detectable over the long term. As in the patient with a remote history of prior treatment, lack of detectable of resistance does not guarantee that it is not present as a minor quasispecies. Even if therapy is not initiated immediately, it may be useful to test for drug resistance as soon as possible after infection to facilitate planning future treatment (Hirsch et al. 2003).

The Role of Resistance Testing in Patients Whose Regimen Is Failing

The guidelines from both the DHHS and the IAS-USA recommend that resistance testing should be considered after any treatment failure, whether in the case of either viral rebound or inability after 8 to 12 weeks to suppress viral load to undetectable levels (DHHS 2004; Hirsch et al. 2003). Both groups cited evidence that resistance testing improved the choice of new drugs in the regimen, at least as far as short-term outcome is concerned. (See Table IV.20-2 for a summary of the 2004 DHHS recommendations on the clinical application of resistance testing.)

Table IV.20-2. Recommendations for the use of drug-resistance assays (DHHS 2004; Hirsch et al. 2003).

Clinical setting/recommendation	Rationale
Drug-resistance assay recommended	
Virologic failure during combination antiretroviral therapy	Determine the role of resistance in drug failure and maximize the number of active drugs in the new regimen, if indicated.
Suboptimal suppression of viral load after antiretroviral therapy initiation	Determine the role of resistance and maximize the number of active drugs in the new regimen, if indicated.
Acute HIV infection, if decision is made to initiate therapy	Determine whether drug-resistant virus was transmitted and change regimen accordingly.
Chronic HIV infection prior to first treatment, if infection was acquired less than 2 years ago and possibly longer*	Determine whether drug-resistant virus was transmitted and choose regimen accordingly.*
Drug-resistance assay should be considered	
Chronic HIV infection before therapy initiation	Available assays might not detect minor drug-resistant species; however, should consider using if significant probability that patient was infected with drug-resistant virus (i.e., if the patient is thought to have been infected by a person receiving antiretroviral drugs).
Consider testing for any HIV infection if community has greater than 5% prevalence of resistance in acute infection, or history suggests acquisition from drug-treated patients.*	Detect prior transmission of drug-resistant HIV, although this may not always be possible with current tests.*
Drug resistance assay not usually recommended	
After discontinuation of drugs	Drug-resistance mutations might become minor species in the absence of selective drug pressure, and available assays might not detect minor drug-resistant species; if testing is performed in this setting, the detection of drug resistance may be of value, but its absence does not rule out the presence of minor drug-resistant species.
Plasma viral load below 1000 HIV RNA copies/mL	Resistance assays cannot be consistently performed because of low copy number of HIV RNA; patients/providers may incur charges and not receive results.

*From IAS-USA guidelines in Hirsch et al. 2003. The remainder is taken from DHHS 2004.

Clinical trials conducted among patients failing an antiretroviral regimen have shown that the use of either genotypic or phenotypic resistance testing to guide the choice of antiretroviral agents in a rescue regimen is associated with better short-term virologic response rates, compared with the selection of a rescue regimen based on the patient's treatment history alone (Tural et al. 2002; Cohen et al. 2000; Baxter et al. 2000; Durant et al. 1999). Other clinical trials evaluating the benefit of these resistance tests have shown less favorable results (Meynard et al. 2002; De Luca et al. 2001; Haubrich et al. 2001), and a meta-analysis of 10 trials concluded that the evidence for resistance tests' benefit was "sparse" (Panidou et al. 2004). Some additional viral suppression appeared in genotyped patients (compared with untested ones); less benefit was found for virtual phenotyping and none at all for standard phenotyping. (See Table IV.20-3.)

Treatment failure in the absence of detectable pretreatment resistance may be due to poor adherence on the patient's part (Hirsch et al. 2003) but that is not the only explanation. A review of possible pharmacokinetic problems should also be undertaken. Other possible mechanisms are under study, including the preexistence of minor, undetectable subpopulations of resistant virus.

If poor adherence and inadequate drug levels are excluded, genotypic testing after treatment failure will allow clinicians to exclude specific drugs from a new regimen (Hirsch et al. 2003). Phenotyping may help patients with complex resistance patterns, but studies have not shown that phenotyping is superior overall to genotyping in selecting a regimen. (See Table IV.20-3 for a summary of clinical studies on the use of genotyping and phenotyping.) The CERT study observed no advantage to phenotyping over genotyping in NNRTI-experienced patients (Wegner et al. 2002). The VIHRES study observed that regimens selected by either genotyping or phenotyping were associated with a similar degree of viral suppression in patients experiencing failure of a second regimen (Blanco et al. 2002). Most recently, the ERA study reported that adding phenotyping to genotyping does not improve outcome in patients with very limited treatment options (Loveday et al. 2003).

The NARVAL trial found that neither resistance test significantly improved clinicians' ability to choose successful successor regimens (Meynard et al. 2002). The only exception was that genotyping improved the results in patients who had required only 1 previous PI. In another report, expert advice and rules-based genotype interpretation independently improved physicians' success rates when prescribing salvage therapy (Tural et al. 2002). The benefit from expert advice was concentrated in those failing their second regimen as compared with those with only 1 treatment failure (fewer resistance mutations) or 3 (more mutations and greater chance of further failure) (Tural et al. 2003).

Resistance testing has yet to prove useful when starting an entry inhibitor (enfuvirtide) as part of salvage therapy. Differences in enfuvirtide's baseline IC50 have not predicted virologic response at week 24 (Sista et al. 2003). However, characteristic genotypic mutations in the gene encoding gp41 and phenotypic resistance have emerged in patients with viremia on enfuvirtide-containing regimens (Greenberg et al. 2003).

Table IV.20-3. Summary of clinical studies on the use of genotyping and phenotyping.

	Population	Study arms	Effect on treatment response
VIRADAPT (Durant et al. 1999)	1st PI failure	G vs. SOC	Benefit from G
GART (CPCRA 046) (Baxter et al. 2000)	1st PI failure	G + Exp vs. SOC	Benefit from G
VIRA 3001 (Cohen et al. 2000)	1st PI failure	P vs. SOC	Benefit from P
KAISER (Melnick et al. 2000)	Mixed	P vs. SOC	P improved selection of active drugs but no benefit from P at wk 16
CCTG 575 (Haubrich et al. 2001)	Mixed	P vs. SOC	No benefit from P overall, but benefit if more than 3 resistant PIs
NARVAL (Meynard et al. 2002)	Mixed	G vs. P vs. SOC	Overall, no difference between G, P and SOC, but benefit from G in patients with most limited PI experience
HAVANA (Tural et al. 2002)	Multiple failure	G vs. G + Exp vs. SOC vs. SOC + Exp	Benefit from G, and from Exp at 2nd failure
CERT (Wegner et al. 2002)	Mixed	G vs. P vs. SOC	Benefit from G or P
ARGENTA (Cingolani et al. 2002)	Mixed	G vs. SOC	Benefit from G at wk 12, but lost by wk 24 in pts with 1st or 2nd failure
VIHRES (Blanco et al. 2002)	Multiple failure	G + Exp vs. P + Exp	No difference
CREST (Emery et al. 2002)	Mixed	G vs. G + VP	No difference
ERA (Loveday et al. 2003)	Multiple failure	G vs. G + P	No added benefit from P

Exp, expert advice; G, genotyping; P, phenotyping; SOC, standard of care (i.e., no resistance testing); VP, virtual phenotyping.

References

Albrecht D, Zollner B, Feucht HH, et al. Reappearance of HIV multidrug-resistance in plasma and circulating lymphocytes after reintroduction of antiretroviral therapy. *J Clin Virol.* **2002**;24:93-98.

Bacheler L. Clinical cut-offs: a new standard for interpreting phenotypic resistance information. In: Program of the 7th International Conference on Drug Therapy in HIV Infection. Nov. 14-18, **2004**; Glasgow, UK. Presentation CW 3.2. Available at: http://www.conferencecapture.com/cc/HIV04C1/pdf_presentation_2.pdf [accessed March 30, 2005].

Baxter JD, Mayers DL, Wentworth DN, et al. A randomized study of antiretroviral management based on plasma genotypic antiretroviral resistance testing in patients failing therapy. CPCRA 046 Study Team for the Terry Beirn Community Programs for Clinical Research on AIDS. *AIDS.* **2000**;14:F83-F93.

Blanco JL, Valdecillos G, Arroyo JR, et al. A prospective randomized study on the usefulness of genotypic resistance tests versus real phenotypic resistance tests in heavily pretreated patients with virological failure (VIHRES Study). In: Program and abstracts of the 14th International AIDS Conference; July 7-12, **2002**; Barcelona, Spain. Abstract TuPeB4624.

Borroto-Esoda K, Harris J, Waters J, et al. Baseline Genotype as a predictor of virological failure in patients receiving emtricitabine once daily or stavudine twice daily in combination with didanosine and efavirenz. In: Program and abstracts of the 11th Conference on Retroviruses and Opportunistic Infections; February 8-11, **2004**; San Francisco, California. Abstract 672.

Bosch RJ, Downey GF, Katzenstein DA, Hellmann N, Bacheler L, Albrecht MA. Evaluation of cutpoints for phenotypic hypersusceptibility to efavirenz [Research Letter]. *AIDS.* **2003**;17:2395-6.

Brenner BG, Routy J-P, Petrella M, et al. Persistence and fitness of multidrug-resistant human immunodeficiency virus type 1 acquired in primary infection. *J Virol*. **2002**;76:1753-1761.

Cingolani A, Antinori A, Rizzo MG, et al. Usefulness of monitoring HIV drug resistance and adherence in individuals failing highly active antiretroviral therapy: a randomized study (ARGENTA). *AIDS*. **2002**;16:369-379.

Cohen C, Kessler H, Hunt S, et al. Phenotypic resistance testing significantly improves response to therapy: final analysis of a randomized trial (VIRA3001) [abstract]. *Antivir Ther.* **2000**;5(suppl 3):67.

De Luca A, Antinori A, Cingolani A, et al. A prospective, randomized study on the usefulness of genotypic resistance testing and the assessment of patient-reported adherence in unselected patients failing potent HIV therapy (ARGENTA): final 6-month results. In: Program and abstracts of the 8th Conference on Retroviruses and Opportunistic Infections; February 4-8, **2001**; Chicago, Illinois. Abstract 433.

Department of Health and Human Services (DHHS). Guidelines for the Use of Antiretroviral Agents in HIV-1-Infected Adults and Adolescents. October 29, **2004**. Available at: http://aidsinfo.nih.gov/guidelines/ [accessed February 21, 2005].

Durant J, Clevenbergh P, Halfon P, et al. Drug-resistance genotyping in HIV-1 therapy: the VIRADAPT randomised controlled trial. *Lancet*. **1999**;353:2195-2199.

Dykes C, Najjar J, Bosch RJ, et al. Detection of drug-resistant minority variants of HIV-1 during virologic failure of indinavir, lamivudine, and zidovudine. *Infect Dis*. **2004**;189:1091-1096.

Elston RC, Yates P, Tisdale M, Richards N, White S, DeJesus E. GW433908 (908)/ritonavir (r): 48 week results in PI-experienced subjects: a retrospective analysis of virological response based on baseline genotype and phenotype. In: Program and abstracts of the XV International Conference on AIDS; July 11-16, **2004**; Bangkok, Thailand. Abstract MoOrB1055.

Emery S, Birch C, Crowe S, et al. CREST—a randomised comparison of two resistance test platforms: genotype and genotype plus VirtualPhenotype™: interim results [abstract]. *Antivir Ther.* **2002**;7:S116.

Greenberg ML, Melby T, Sista P, et al. Baseline and on-treatment susceptibility to enfuvirtide seen in TORO 1 and TORO 2 to 24 weeks. In: Program and abstracts of the 10th Conference on Retroviruses and Opportunistic Infections; February 10-14, **2003**; Boston, Massachusetts. Abstract 141.

Hanna GJ, Balaguera HU, Freedberg KA, et al. Drug-selected resistance mutations and non-B subtypes in antiretroviral-naïve adults with established human immunodeficiency virus infection. *J Infect Dis*. **2003**;188: 986-991.

Haubrich R, Keiser P, Kemper C, et al. CCTG 575: a randomized, prospective study of phenotype testing versus standard of care for patients failing antiretroviral therapy [abstract]. *Antivir Ther.* **2001**;6(suppl 1):63.

Harrigan PR, Hogg RS, Dong WW, et al. Predictors of HIV drug-resistance mutations in a large antiretroviral-naive cohort initiating triple antiretroviral therapy. *J Infect Dis*. **2005**;191:339-347.

Hirsch MS, Brun-Vezinet F, Clotet B, et al. Antiretroviral drug resistance testing in adults infected with human immunodeficiency virus type 1: 2003 recommendations of an International AIDS Society-USA Panel. *Clin Infect Dis*. **2003**;37:113-128.

Jourdain G, Ngo-Giang-Huong N, Tungyai P, et al. Exposure to Intrapartum Single-dose Nevirapine and Subsequent Maternal 6-Month Response to NNRTI-based Regimens. In: Program and abstracts of the 11th Conference on Retroviruses and Opportunistic Infections; February 8-11, **2004**; San Francisco, California. Abstract 41LB.

Kearney M, Palmer S, Maldarelli F, et al. Single-genome sequencing is more sensitive than standard genotype analysis for detection of HIV-1 drug-resistance mutations. In: Program and abstracts of the 11th Conference on Retroviruses and Opportunistic Infections; February 8-11, **2004**; San Francisco, California. Abstract 695.

Kempf DJ, Isaacson JD, King MS, et al. Analysis of the virological response with respect to baseline viral phenotype and genotype in protease inhibitor-experienced HIV-1-infected patients receiving lopinavir/ritonavir therapy. *Antivir Ther.* **2002**;7:165-174.

Little SJ, Koelsch KK, Ignacio CC, et al. Persistence of transmitted drug-resistant virus among subjects with primary HIV infection deferring antiretroviral therapy. In: Program and abstracts of the 11th Conference on Retroviruses and Opportunistic Infections; February 8-11, **2004**; San Francisco, California. Abstract 36LB.

Loveday C, Dunn DT, Green H, Rinehart A, McKenna P. A 1-year randomized controlled trial of genotypic versus genotypic plus phenotypic resistance testing to guide antiretroviral therapy (the ERA Trial). *Antiviral Ther.* **2003**;8:S165.

Luber AD. To ABT or not to ABT—a re-evaluation of pharmacokinetics in HIV clinical practice [expert column]. Medscape HIV/AIDS. **2000**;6(6). Available at: http://www.medscape.com/viewarticle/408274 [accessed February 21, 2005].

Mellors J, Palmer S, Nissley D, et al. Low-frequency NNRTI-resistant variants contribute to failure of efavirenz-containing regimens. In: Program and abstracts of the 11th Conference on Retroviruses and Opportunistic Infections; February 8-11, **2004**; San Francisco, California. Abstract 39.

Melnick D, Rosenthal J, Cameron M, et al. Impact of phenotypic antiretroviral drug resistance testing on the response to salvage antiretroviral therapy (ART) in heavily experienced patients. In: Program and abstracts of the 7th Conference on Retroviruses and Opportunistic Infections; January 30-February 2, **2000**; San Francisco, California. Abstract 786.

Meynard JL, Vray M, Morand-Joubert L, et al. Phenotypic or genotypic resistance testing for choosing antiretroviral therapy after treatment failure: a randomized trial. *AIDS.* **2002**;16:727-736.

Molina J, Marcelin AG, Pavie J, et al. Didanosine (ddI) in treatment-experienced HIV-infected patients: results from a randomized double-blind study (AI454-176 Jaguar). In: Program and abstracts of the 43rd Interscience Conference on Antimicrobial Agents and Chemotherapy; September 14-17, **2003**; Chicago, Illinois. Abstract H-447.

Norton M, Kempf D, Brun S, Omachi J, Cernohous P, King M. Genotypic algorithms specific to lopinavir/ritonavir outperform nonspecific lists of PI mutations in predicting virological response to lopinavir/ritonavir in PI-experienced patients [Poster 117]. *Antivir Ther.* **2004**;9:S131.

Palmer S, Boltz V, Maldarelli F, et al. Emergence and long-term persistence of NNRTI-resistant variants in patients starting and stopping NNRTI-containing regimens. In: Program and abstracts of the 11th Conference on Retroviruses and Opportunistic Infections; February 8-11, **2004**; San Francisco, California. Abstract 37.

Panidou ET, Trikalinos TA, Ioannidis JPA. Limited benefit of antiretroviral resistance testing in treatment-experienced patients: a meta-analysis. *AIDS.* **2004**;18:2153-2161.

Parkin N, Chappey C, Maroldo L, Bates M, Hellmann NS, Petropoulos CJ. Phenotypic and genotypic HIV-1 drug resistance assays provide complementary information. *J Acquir Immune Defic Syndr.* **2002**;31:128-136.

Richman DD, Morton SC, Wrin T, et al. The prevalence of antiretroviral drug resistance in the United States. *AIDS.* **2004**;18:1393-1401.

Servais J, Plesséria JM, Lambert C, et al. Genotypic correlates of resistance to HIV-1 protease inhibitors on longitudinal data: the role of secondary mutations. *Antivir Ther.* **2001**;6:239-248.

Shulman NS, Hughes MD, Winters MA, et al. Subtle decreases in stavudine phenotypic susceptibility predict poor virologic response to stavudine monotherapy in zidovudine-experienced patients. *J Acquir Immune Defic Syndr.* **2002**;31:121-127.

Sista P, Melby T, Greenberg ML, et al. Subgroup analysis of baseline susceptibility and early virological response to enfuvirtide in the combined TORO studies [abstract]. *Antiviral Ther.* **2003**;8:S60.

Szumiloski J, Wilson H, Jensen E, et al. Relationships between indinavir resistance and virologic responses to indinavir-ritonavir-containing regimens in patients with previous protease inhibitor failure. *Antivir Ther.* **2002**;7(Suppl 1):S127

Trabaud MA, Leriche-Guerin K, Regis C, et al. Prevalence of primary resistance to zidovudine and lamivudine in drug-naïve human immunodeficiency virus type-1 infected patients: high proportion of reverse transcriptase codon 215 mutant in circulating lymphocytes and free virus. *J Med Virol.* **2000**;61:352-359.

Tural C, Ruiz L, Holtzer C, et al. Clinical utility of HIV-1 genotyping and expert advice: the Havana trial. *AIDS.* **2002**;16:209-218.

Wegner SA, Wallace M, Aronson N, et al. Long-term clinical efficacy of resistance testing: results of the CERT trial. In: Program and abstracts of the 14th International Conference on AIDS; July 7-12, **2002**; Barcelona, Spain. Abstract ThOrB1389.

Weinstein MC, Goldie SJ, Losina E, et al. Use of genotypic resistance testing to guide HIV therapy: clinical impact and cost-effectiveness. *Ann Intern Med.* **2001**;134:440-450.

Weinstock HS, Zaidi I, Heneine W, et al. The epidemiology of antiretroviral drug resistance among drug-naive HIV-1–infected persons in 10 US cities. *J Infect Dis.* **2004**;189:2174-2180.

Wensing AM, Keulen W, Buimer M, Brambilla D, Schuurman R, Boucher C. Analysis of the world-wide evaluation study on HIV-1 genotype interpretation: ENVA-3 [abstract]. *Antivir Ther.* **2001**;6(suppl 1):101.

Winters B, Bacheler LT, Nauwelaers D, et al. Evaluation of different approaches for the definition of clinically relevant breakpoints for phenotypic resistance data [abstract]. *Antivir Ther.* **2004**;9:S127.

Zolopa AR. Genotype-phenotype discordance: the evolution in our understanding HIV-1 drug resistance. *AIDS.* **2003**;17:1077-1078.

Zolopa AR, Lazzeroni LC, Rinehart A, Kuritzkes D. Accuracy, precision and consistency of expert HIV-1 genotype interpretation: an international comparison (the GUESS study) [abstract]. *Antivir Ther.* **2002**;7:S97.

(RLO-30)

IV.23. REGIMEN FAILURE/INTOLERABILITY

LEARNING OBJECTIVE: Define failure of an antiretroviral regimen, discuss possible etiologies and discuss the significance of viral load "blips."

Determination of Regimen Failure and Guidelines for Changing Therapy

The definition of success or failure of an antiretroviral regimen depends on the circumstances of a given patient and the objectives of therapy for that individual. In the case of patients on their first antiretroviral regimen, the objectives of therapy may be more ambitious than in highly treatment-experienced patients. In such first-line treatment, complete viral suppression (below 50 copies/mL) and increased CD4 counts would be the usual goal. As patients become more treatment-experienced with fewer therapy options, therapeutic goals may shift from high-level viral suppression to protection against clinical events by maintaining the CD4 count at the highest level possible. Thus, regimen failure would simply be defined by the inability to achieve or to continue meeting these goals, according to the specific guidelines listed below. Current U.S. Public Health Service guidelines on antiretroviral use in adults and adolescents (DHHS 2004) offer the following guidelines for defining regimen failure, which should lead to considering a change of therapy:

- Virologic failure on treatment is defined as a confirmed HIV viral load over 400 copies/mL after 24 weeks, over 50 copies/mL at 48 weeks or repeated viral loads over 400 copies/mL after prior suppression of viremia to under 400 copies/mL. Repeated detection of HIV RNA after virologic suppression signifies virologic rebound.
- Immunologic failure can be defined as a failure to increase the CD4 count by 25-50 cells/mm^3 above baseline during the first year of therapy or a decrease in the CD4 cell count to below baseline levels while on therapy.
- Clinical progression can be defined as the occurrence or recurrence of HIV-related events (after over 3 months on combination antiretroviral therapy), excluding immune reconstitution syndromes.

It should be noted that in highly treatment-experienced patients, a regimen that is failing virologically may continue to offer immunologic benefit for a considerable period (Deeks et al. 2002), possibly due to reduced viral fitness (see Objective IV.28 on Viral Fitness and Replication Capacity in this Update). The degree of initial HIV suppression and the change in viral loads from the pretreatment baseline predict the likelihood of subsequent immunologic failure when a failing regimen continues to be used (Deeks et al. 2002).

Etiologies of Regimen Failure

Possible causes of treatment failure include prior use of suboptimal therapies, including nucleoside analog monotherapy or dual therapy used in the pre-HAART era (Phillips et al. 2002), poor adherence, poor tolerability or drug toxicity, individual variation in drug pharmacokinetics, negative drug-drug interactions, inadequate potency and drug resistance (DHHS 2004). It is necessary to understand the attributes and features of a successful regimen for a given patient in order to define regimen failure and understand its causes. As discussed above, the criteria for successful therapy will vary depending on the stage of treatment and the treatment options that are available for the patient.

What's New

Resistance testing, when possible, is important for patients on therapy who maintain consistently low but quantifiable viral loads and stable CD4 counts. Mutations associated with resistance to drugs in the antiretroviral regimen can emerge even with low-level viremia and affect future regimen choices.

Key Points

- The definition of "regimen failure" depends on the phase of antiretroviral treatment (first-line, second-line, salvage) and the associated therapeutic objectives.
- Detailed guidelines help define treatment failure and considerations for changing regimens.
- Possible etiologies for regimen failure include poor adherence, drug toxicity, unfavorable drug pharmacokinetics, inadequate antiviral potency, negative drug-drug interactions and drug resistance. The last of these may arise from either prior suboptimal therapy or initial infection with resistant virus.
- Intermittent low-level viremia (viral "blips" from a previously undetectable viral load) is not uncommon and does not necessarily predict emergence of resistant virus or failure of therapy.
- Recurrent viral blips and/or rebounds to higher viral loads are more likely to lead to virologic failure.
- In highly treatment-experienced patients, a regimen that fails to fully suppress viral replication may continue to offer immunologic benefit for a considerable period of time.

In initial therapy, a successful regimen should suppress the viral load to below the limits of detection and be well tolerated. Virologic success usually requires high levels of adherence (see Objective IV.39 on Principles of Adherence in this update) and the use of a potent regimen with a reasonable barrier to resistance. In one study, patients with stable CD4 counts and low-level but detectable viremia (50-1000 copies/mL) developed resistance mutations because of ongoing viral replication (Lafeuillade et al. 2004). In 47 treatment-experienced patients with stable low level viremia for over 60 weeks (mean of 802 days), genotypic testing revealed limited emergence of resistance mutations (mean of less than 1 new mutation for both reverse transcriptase and protease genes) (Morse 2005). The same study found that the HIV in 15 patients with low-level but rising viremia accumulated mutations at a higher rate. No analysis of statistical significance was provided, nor did the investigators seek to detect the existence of small minority viral subpopulations with new mutations. Two studies have recommended genotypic resistance testing for patients with low-level viremia so that their treatment regimens can be modified before overt failure occurs (Nettles et al. 2004; Parra-Ruiz et al. 2004).

Commercially available resistance tests usually require viral loads of at least 500-1000 copies/mL. Waiting for the viral load to reach that level may lead to the accumulation of important resistance mutations, especially with regimens that include drugs for which a single mutation results in significant resistance (e.g., NNRTIs, lamivudine, emtricitabine, didanosine, tenofovir DF and abacavir). This raises the question of whether regimens should be "intensified" with early failure. In one study of patients with undetectable viral loads (below 50 copies/mL), no evolution of drug resistance virus occurred (Kieffer et al. 2004). This reinforces the goal of maintaining an undetectable viral load when this is reasonable.

Data from one uncontrolled study suggest that poor adherence increases the risk of resistance more with NNRTI-based therapy than with protease inhibitor (PI)-based regimens (Bangsberg et al. 2004). Results from the APROVIR study examined the mechanisms of early virologic failure among treatment-naive subjects initiating a PI-based regimen (Masquelier et al. 2002). The mechanisms of early virologic failure and development of PI resistance differed by type of PI and were dependent on PI levels.

However, with many regimens in current use, failure does not stem from inability to maintain viral suppression, but rather from tolerability or adherence issues. In fact, the majority of patients who switch from an initial regimen do so because of intolerance to one or more of the agents (Mocroft et al. 2001). Murri and colleagues (2003) reported that women are less tolerant of antiretrovirals and more likely to discontinue at least one drug in a regimen because of toxicity.

Regimen failure can thus be caused by patient factors (adherence behavior), medication factors (potency, pharmacokinetics, genetic barrier to resistance and tolerability, which includes short- and long-term toxicity, pill burden and dosing complexity) and disease state factors (i.e., CD4 count, viral load, and preexisting resistance) (DHHS 2004). Thus, the possible etiologies for regimen failure may spring from any of the features outlined above and span the spectrum from lack of regimen potency in an adherent patient to unacceptable side effects in an otherwise potent regimen.

Significance of Viral Load Blips

Episodes of intermittent low-level viral load ("blips") are not uncommon among patients receiving antiretroviral therapy after initially achieving optimal HIV suppression; they have been reported in up to 40% of patients. In a recent study, blips were detected in 9 of 10 closely monitored patients (Nettles et al. 2005).

In another analysis of the clinical significance of blips in 114 patients with virologic suppression to below 50 copies/mL, Havlir and colleagues (2001) reported that frequent occurrence of intermittent low-level viremia was not predictive of subsequent virologic failure. With use of an ultrasensitive assay that allowed detection of HIV viral loads as low as 2.5 copies/mL, they did find that a higher viral load was associated with intermittent viremia, but this observation was not statistically significant. Interpretation of these results was compromised by the small number of patients and the unique study design.

A much larger study of 1730 patients, the Dutch ATHENA cohort, has reported that patients who experienced blips had similar clinical outcomes to those who maintained viral loads below 50 copies/mL through 3 years of treatment (Valkengoed 2005), but a still larger study contradicts this finding. Greub and colleagues (2002) examined data on 2055 patients with optimal HIV suppression (at least two consecutive values below 50 copies/mL within a 24-week interval) after the initiation of antiretroviral therapy. A "blip" was defined as a low-level viral rebound (between 51 and 500 copies/mL) followed by a return to viral load value below 50 copies/mL. Blips occurred in 70% of patients. After a median follow-up of 18 months, patients with at least one blip were twice as likely to experience confirmed virologic failure as those with no blips (Greub et al. 2002). In another report from the CDC-sponsored HOPS study, blips were seen in 27% of subjects achieving two consecutive viral loads below 50 copies/mL, while only 13% of those with viral blips later developed persistent viremia (over 50 copies/mL) (Sklar et al. 2002).

Possible explanations for low-level viral rebound include lapses in adherence, intercurrent infections, vaccination, limitations of viral load measurements at the limits of detection and laboratory contamination. According to a study at Northwestern Memorial Hospital, the switch from ethylenediaminetetraacetic acid (EDTA) tubes to Plasma Preparation Tubes (PPT) for specimen collection could also cause apparent blips (Murphy 2005). During the time the hospital switched to the safer PPT tubes, more than half of patients experienced false viral blips. This technical change resulted in repeat testing and clinic visits, as well as a medication change in at least one patient.

Viral load "blips" are followed by viral load measurements back below the level of detection without necessitating a decision about change in antiretroviral regimen (Greub et al. 2002). No new resistance mutations were detected during or immediately after a blip in a small study of 9 patients who were monitored intensively (Nettles et al. 2005), suggesting that low-level blips do not result from or trigger the evolution of resistant virus. Recurrent blips, however, or blips to increasingly higher levels of viremia, are more likely to lead to confirmed virologic failure (Greub et al. 2002). The clinician therefore may want to review patient adherence and tolerability issues upon the first such episode.

Additional studies that evaluate the clinical significance of both episodic and persistent low-level viremia may help to more precisely define the safety margin for continuing or the threshold for changing the regimen of a patient who experiences intermittent viremia from a base of optimally suppressed viremia (below 50 copies/mL).

References

Bangsberg DR, Guzman D, Riley ED, Clark R, Deeks SG. Nonnucleoside reverse transcriptase inhibitor (NNRTI) resistance occurs at lower levels of adherence than protease inhibitor (PI) resistance. In: Program and abstracts of the XV International AIDS Conference; July 11-16, **2004**; Bangkok, Thailand. Abstract 6061.

Deeks S, Barbour JD, Grant RM, Martin JN. Duration and predictors of CD4 T-cell gain in patients who continue combination therapy despite detectable plasma viremia. *AIDS*. **2002**;16:201-207.

DHHS. Panel on Clinical Practices for Treatment of HIV Infection. Guidelines for the Use of Antiretroviral Agents in HIV-1-Infected Adults and Adolescents. Washington, DC. October 29, **2004**; Available at: http://www.aidsinfo.nih.gov/guidelines/adult/AA_102904.pdf [accessed November 8, 2004].

Greub G, Cozzi-Lepri A, Ledergerber B, et al. Intermittent and sustained low-level HIV viral rebound in patients receiving potent antiretroviral therapy. *AIDS*. **2002**;16:1967-1969.

Havlir DV, Bassett R, Levitan D, et al. Prevalence and predictive value of intermittent viremia with combination HIV therapy. *JAMA*. **2001**;286:171-179.

Kieffer T, Finucane M, Nettles R, et al. Genotypic analysis of HIV-1 drug resistance at the limit of detection: virus production without evolution in treated adults with undetectable HIV loads. *J Infect Dis*. **2004**;189:1452-1465.

Lafeuillade, A, Hittinger G, Delbeke E, Poggi C. Resistance selection in patients with stable low levels of HIV-1 viremia. In: Program and abstracts of the XV International AIDS Conference; July 11-16, **2004**; Bangkok, Thailand. Abstract 5091.

Masquelier B, Peytavin G, Leport C, et al. Mechanisms of early virologic failure in antiretroviral naïve patients starting protease inhibitor-containing regimens: the APROVIR study. *J Infect Dis*. **2002**;186:1503-1507.

Mocroft A, Youle M, Moore A, et al. Reasons for modification and discontinuation of antiretrovirals: results from a single treatment centre. *AIDS*. **2001**;15:185-194.

Morse C, Maldarelli F, Dewar R, Rehm C, Kovacs J. Limited evolution of drug resistance in HIV-1-infected patients with persistent low-level viremia on stable antiretroviral regimen for longer than 1 year. In: Program and abstracts of the 12th Conference on Retroviruses and Opportunistic Infections; February 22-25, **2005**; Boston, Massachusetts. Poster 678

Murphy R, Berzins B, Leake A, et al. Effect of plasma preparation tubes vs standard EDTA tubes on viral "blips" in patients with optimally suppressed HIV-1 RNA. In: Program and abstracts of the 12th Conference on Retroviruses and Opportunistic Infections; February 22-25, **2005**; Boston, Massachusetts. Abstract 738.

Murri R, Cozzi-Lepri A, Phillips A, et al. Access to antiretroviral treatment, incidence of sustained therapy interruptions, and risk of clinical events according to sex. J Acquir Immune Defic Syndr. **2003**;34:184-190.

Nettles R, Kieffer T, Simmons R, et al. Genotypic resistance in HIV-1-infected patients with persistently detectable low-level viremia while receiving highly active antiretroviral therapy. *Clin Infect Dis*. **2004**;39:1030-1037.

Nettles RE, Kieffer T, Kwon P, et al. Intermittent HIV-1 viremia (blips) and drug resistance in patients receiving HAART. *JAMA*. **2005**; 293:817-829.

Parra-Ruiz J, Alvarez M, Munoz-Medina L, et al. Usefulness of drug resistance genotypic tests in HIV-infected patients with viral load lower than 1000 copies per mL. In: Program and abstracts of the XV International AIDS Conference; July 11-16, **2004**; Bangkok, Thailand. Abstract 5978.

Phillips AN, Staszewski S, Lampe F, et al. Human immunodeficiency virus rebound after suppression to below 400 copies/mL during initial highly active antiretroviral therapy regimens, and according to prior nucleoside experience and duration of suppression. *J Infect Dis*. **2002**;186:1086-1091.

Sklar PA, Ward DJ, Baker RK, et al. Prevalence and clinical correlates of HIV viremia ("blips") in patients with previous suppression below the limits of quantification. *AIDS*. **2002**;16:2035-2041.

van Valkengoed I, Gras L, Pogány K, et al. The effect of low level transient HIV viremia (blips) on the outcome of HAART. In: Program and abstracts of the 12th Conference on Retroviruses and Opportunistic Infections; February 22-25, **2005**; Boston, Massachusetts. Abstract 602.

(RLO-31)

IV.26. ANTIRETROVIRAL CROSS-RESISTANCE

LEARNING OBJECTIVE: Discuss antiretroviral cross-resistance resulting from prior therapy, including approach to agent selection based on resistance testing and treatment history.

Definition of Cross-Resistance and Factors Affecting Likelihood of Occurrence

When HIV is able to replicate in the presence of an inadequately suppressive antiretroviral regimen, the viral mutations that are selected by a specific agent may confer resistance not only to that agent but also possibly to other drugs in the same class. This has long been recognized for the protease inhibitor (PI) and nonnucleoside reverse transcriptase inhibitor (NNRTI) classes, but only relatively recently has the extent of cross-resistance among nucleoside reverse transcriptase inhibitors (NRTIs) become clear (Picard et al. 2001). This cross-resistance may or may not be apparent if resistance testing is performed. For example, stavudine resistance may confer cross-resistance to zidovudine despite little apparent change in genotypic or phenotypic stavudine resistance (Picard et al. 2001). The rate at which cross-resistance develops varies for the different classes of antiretroviral agents. Within the NNRTI class, there is almost complete cross-resistance. Among NRTIs, the potential for cross-resistance varies, although there is complete cross-resistance between lamivudine and emtricitabine. Among PIs, as more resistance mutations accumulate during virologic failure on any given drug, there is an increasing amount of resistance to the entire class (Hirsch et al. 2003).

Cross-Resistance Patterns in NRTIs

NRTI-associated mutations (NAMs)

NAMs (also referred to as "TAMs," or thymidine analog mutations) are a set of reverse transcriptase mutations that arise when HIV is exposed to the thymidine analogs zidovudine and stavudine. (See Objective IV.10 on Resistance Mutations in this Update.) The NAMs include M41L, E44D, D67N, K70R, V118I, L210W, T215Y/F, and K219Q/E. An accumulation of NAMs causes loss of susceptibility to the broad NRTI class independent of the specific mutations associated with resistance to other NRTIs (Whitcomb et al. 2003). This is even true for lamivudine, whose primary resistance mutation, M184V, counteracts the action of NAMs (Miller and Larder 2001). The resensitizing effect of M184V is itself overcome by additional NAMs, resulting in resistant virus (Whitcomb et al. 2003).

The NAMs function by increasing the rate at which reverse transcriptase reverses itself, uncoupling the last nucleoside in the new proviral DNA chain (Miller and Larder 2003). In this way, chain-terminating NRTIs are removed and reverse transcription of the complete proviral genome can resume. The extracted nucleoside most often ends up bound to ATP in a pharmacologically inactive complex. The effectiveness of this reaction is strongest for zidovudine but impacts other NRTIs to a considerable extent, hence the cross-resistance. A study of nearly 5000 clinical HIV isolates found that the cross-resistance correlation between zidovudine and a second drug was strongest for abacavir and stavudine (Harrigan and Larder 2002).

Multinucleoside resistance complexes

Two other resistance profiles also are associated with broad NRTI cross-resistance. One is the codon 69 insertion (Miller and Larder 2003). It is composed of a T69S mutation followed by the addition of two amino acids, serine plus, usually,

What's New

The development of the reverse transcriptase K65R mutation occurs during treatment with non-thymidine-analog HAART. The presence of thymidine analogs inhibits emergence of the K65R mutation because it counteracts the effect of mutations associated with thymidine resistance. The K65R and L74V mutations can lead to cross-resistance among non-thymidine NRTIs, reducing future treatment options.

Key Points

- Resistance to an individual drug within a class usually confers some degree of cross-resistance to other drugs within the same class.
- When switching therapy due to virologic failure, drugs in different classes will have retained antiviral activity because there is no cross-resistance between classes.
- Resistance testing can be helpful in assessing cross-resistance at the time of initial failure, although results are not always conclusive.

a second serine, alanine or glycine. It arises on a background of NAMs and a few other mutations to create resistance to all currently approved NRTIs including tenofovir. Fortunately, the codon 69 insertion is very rare.

Slightly less rare is the Q151M complex (Miller and Larder 2003). The Q151M mutation usually appears after HIV is exposed to didanosine plus either stavudine or zidovudine. Four other supporting mutations arise afterward (A62V, V75I, F77L and F116Y), with resulting loss of susceptibility to all NRTIs except tenofovir. Resistance occurs due to a selective loss of binding affinity between reverse transcriptase and the NRTIs (Deval et al. 2002).

The role of other mutations in cross-resistance

Most other drug-specific resistance mutations act, like the Q151M complex, by increasing reverse transciptase's ability to discriminate between NRTIs and the natural nucleosides. For these non-thymidine mutations, the implications of cross-resistance increase when drugs with similar resistance profiles are used together.

Recently, concern has arisen over the role of the K65R mutation in HIV reverse transcriptase. K65R is still comparatively rare but its frequency is increasing (Miller 2003). It confers broad resistance to drugs within the NRTI class, including abacavir, didanosine, emtricitabine, lamivudine, stavudine, tenofovir and zalcitabine. (See Objective IV.10 on Resistance Mutations in this Update.) Studies of tenofovir/lamivudine/abacavir versus efavirenz/lamivudine/abacavir have observed a high rate of virologic failure in subjects assigned to this triple-NRTI combination (Gallant et al. 2003). Over half of these patients had virus with the K65R mutation, which along with the M184V mutation diminishes susceptibility to all drugs in the regimen. In one study of this combination, 11 of 12 patients with virologic failure had HIV with both K65R and M184V mutations (Landman et al. 2004). The TONUS trial of abacavir/tenofovir/lamivudine found that initial treatment failure predominantly emerged with the appearance at 4 weeks of M184I/V reverse transcriptase mutations in viral isolates. By week 12, the majority of isolates contained both M184V or M184I and K65R (Delaunay et al. 2004).

Since pharmacokinetic studies of abacavir plus tenofovir have shown no negative drug-drug interactions in the plasma or within the cell (Kearney et al. 2003; Hawkins et al. 2004), the most likely explanation for the high rates of failure for this regimen—and the regimen of tenofovir, didanosine and lamivudine (Jemsek et al. 2004)—involves the simple evolution required to generate cross-resistance. The inferior potency of triple-NRTI regimens, which allows appreciable ongoing viral replication, makes it possible to climb over the low genetic barrier to resistance. The 2 together set the conditions for the rapid emergence of resistance and overt treatment failure. (For further discussion, see Objective IV.18 on Not-Recommended Antiretroviral Combinations in this Update.)

The use of thymidine analogs in a regimen appears to decrease the risk of this mutation emerging (Lanier et al. 2003) since K65R antagonizes the ability of NAMs to facilitate NRTI removal (Parikh et al. 2003). Data from quadruple-nucleoside studies evaluating once-daily zidovudine, abacavir, lamivudine and tenofovir exhibit high rates of virologic response with minimal evolution of K65R (Elion et al. 2004; Moyle et al. 2004). Good results were also obtained with a triple NRTI regimen of zidovudine/lamivudine/tenofovir (Rey et al. 2005). (When K65R is absent, tenofovir resistance can also arise from multiple NAMs [Maggiolo et al. 2005], which would affect on the drugs in these regimens.)

The influence of the L74V and M184V mutations is another area of uncertainty. L74V alone causes some decreased susceptibility to abacavir and didanosine (Underwood et al. 2005; Lanier et al. 2003). M184V promotes resistance mainly to lamivudine and emtricitabine. It reportedly *increases* susceptibility to tenofovir even in the presence of resistance mutations, but its contribution is modest in clinical isolates (Wolf et al. 2003). Data from Gilead Sciences' 902 and 907 tenofovir trials indicated that preexisting L74V mutations promote emergence of K65R-based tenofovir resistance unless thymidine analog resistance mutations are also present (Bae et al. 2004).

When either L74V or K65R occur combined with M184V, the result is loss of susceptibility to all NRTIs except the thymidine analogs (Underwood et al. 2005; Lanier et al. 2003). The L74V/M184V double mutation, however, is reportedly hypersusceptible to tenofovir in clinical samples (Underwood et al. 2005).

The L74V/K65R combination is not generally observed in clinical isolates, possibly because it impairs viral replication, but these mutations can be selected on different isolates within one person's blood (Wirden et al. 2005; Bae et al. 2004). Recent analysis of a Marseille database detected this double mutation in 12 of 3201 patients (Colson 2005). The patients had viral loads within the normal range, indicating that replication capacity was not compromised in these cases. Surprisingly, the study also found two patients with HIV isolates containing the K65R mutation along with the supposedly antagonistic thymidine analog resistance mutation T215Y. Compensatory mutations may be involved.

Distinct isolates containing K65R emerged while receiving tenofovir in 4 of 5 tenofovir recipients with L74V at baseline, compared with 10 of 106 without L74V. The implication is that NRTI-containing regimens need to include a thymidine analog—or else an especially potent agent from another drug class—to avoid a simple, 2-mutation evolution to general NRTI resistance (Wainberg and Turner 2004).

Cross-Resistance Patterns in NNRTIs and PIs

Mutations at reverse transcriptase positions 103 or 188 (K103N or Y188L) lead to high-level resistance to all current FDA-approved NNRTIs. (See Objective IV.10 on Resistance Mutations in this Update.) Mutations at position 181 lead to high-level resistance to nevirapine and subsequent rapid development of high-level resistance to the remainder of the approved NNRTIs. Prior NNRTI exposure in a nonsuppressive regimen is a key determinant of subsequent treatment responses to NNRTI-containing treatment, even when that exposure is single-dose nevirapine to prevent mother-to-child transmission (Jourdain et al. 2004). This incipient cross-resistance can still exist when resistance testing yields negative results (Lecossier et al. 2005).

Several protease mutations emerge during exposure to a variety of the PIs. The accumulation of 4 or more mutations at codons 10, 32, 46, 54, 82, 84 and 90 is associated with cross-resistance in this class. Some combinations containing fewer mutations may also confer cross-resistance. Unboosted PIs lose antiviral activity in the presence of fewer protease mutations than boosted PIs. (See Objective IV.10 on Resistance Mutations in this Update.)

Importance of Cross-Resistance for Designing Subsequent Regimens

In treatment-experienced patients experiencing virologic failure, cross-resistance is of great significance when designing effective subsequent regimens. For example, for a patient who is failing on zidovudine/lamivudine/nelfinavir, a clinician may consider switching to stavudine/lamivudine/indinavir. Such a regimen may work in some cases but has a relatively high risk of failure because of the likelihood of cross-resistance between the NRTI components. If there is complete cross-resistance (as can be conferred by the multinucleoside resistance mutations; see Objective IV.10 on Resistance Mutations in this

Update), the only effective drug in the proposed rescue regimen would be indinavir, and there may in some cases be a degree of cross-resistance between nelfinavir and indinavir.

Debate continues regarding the extent of cross-resistance between many antiretroviral agents. Cross-resistance may be affected by the agent that the patient was receiving at the time of virologic failure or the order in which drugs are taken. One study looked at heavily experienced, but atazanavir-naive pediatric patients (Aldrovandi et al. 2003). They harbored virus with multiple mutations associated with PI resistance. After failing on 1 or more PI regimens, their response to atazanavir was diminished. However, if a patient develops resistance while on atazanavir as the first PI (often with the I50L mutation), then phenotypic susceptibility to other PIs may be preserved (Colonno et al. 2003). In vitro, the I50L/A71V mutation pattern on the HIV protease increases the binding affinity to these other PIs (Yanchunas 2005). Convincing clinical documentation of the degree of susceptibility in that situation and for most other sequencing scenarios remains limited, unfortunately.

It is a good practice to add, if possible, a drug from a class that is new to the patient when switching therapy for virologic failure. This is usually possible for a second-line regimen, because most patients are treated with 2-class therapies at the outset. Studies among patients failing a first regimen of 2 NRTIs and a PI have shown that the proportion achieving a successful virologic response to a second-line regimen is much greater if an NNRTI is included in that subsequent regimen (Gulick et al. 2000; Deeks et al. 1999). In the example given above, for the patient failing zidovudine, lamivudine and nelfinavir, a switch to nevirapine, didanosine and a ritonavir-boosted PI such as lopinavir/ritonavir may be more likely to succeed. Then there is enfuvirtide. Belonging to a new class of antiretrovirals (entry inhibitors), it does not exhibit cross-resistance in cell culture to NRTIs, NNRTIs or PIs.

References

Aldrovandi G, Samson P, Fenton T, et al. Genotypic and phenotypic resistance to BMS232832 (atazanavir-ATV). In: Program and abstracts of the 9th Conference on Retroviruses and Opportunistic Infections; February 24-28, **2002**; Seattle, Washington. Abstract 811-W.

Bae AS, Waters JM, Margot NA, Borroto-Esoda K, Miller MD. Pre-existing L74V is a risk factor for virological non-response and development of K65R in patients taking tenofovir DF (TDF). *Antivir Ther.* **2004**;9:S174.

Colonno R, Rose R, Cianci C, Aldrovandi G, Parkin N, Friborg J. Emergence of atazanavir resistance and maintenance of susceptibility to other PIs is associated with an 150L substitution in HIV protease. In: Program and abstracts of the 10th Conference on Retroviruses and Opportunistic Infections; February 10-14, **2003**; Boston, Massachusetts. Abstract 597.

Colson P, Henry M, Tourres C, Ravaux I, Poizot-Martin I, Tamalet C. Evidence by cloning analysis of the rare coexistence of the K65R/L74V mutant in the same HIV genome. In: Program and abstracts of the 12th Conference on Retroviruses and Opportunistic Infections, **2005**; Boston, Massachusetts. Abstract 701.

Deeks SG, Hellmann N, Grant RM, et al. Novel four drug salvage treatment regimens after failure of a protease inhibitor-containing regimen: antiviral activity and correlation of baseline phenotypic drug susceptibility with virologic outcome. *J Infect Dis.* **1999**;179:1379-1381.

Delaunay C, Descamps D, Landman R, et al. Dynamic of selection of the K65R and M184V/I mutations in patients enrolled in TONUS trial. *Antivir Ther.* **2004**;9:S171.

Deval J, Selmi B, Boretto J, et al. The molecular mechanism of multidrug resistance by the Q151M human immunodeficiency virus type 1 reverse transcriptase and its suppression using alpha-boranophosphate nucleotide analogues. *J Biol Chem.* **2002**;277:42097-42104.

Elion R, Cohen C, DeJesus E, et al. COL40263: Resistance and efficacy of once-daily Trizivir and tenofovir DF in antiretroviral naïve subjects. In: Program and abstracts of the 11th Conference on Retroviruses and Opportunistic Infections; February 8-11, **2004**; San Francisco, California. Abstract 53.

Gallant JE, Rodriguez AE, Weinberg W, et al. Early non-response to tenofovir DF + abacavir (ABC) + lamivudine (3TC) in a randomized trial compared to efavirenz + ABC + 3TC: ESS30009. In: Program and abstracts of the 43rd Interscience Conference on Antimicrobial Agents and Chemotherapy; September 14-17, **2003**: Chicago, Illinois. Abstract H-1722a.

Gulick RM, Hu XJ, Fiscus SA, et al. Randomized study of saquinavir with ritonavir or nelfinavir together with delavirdine, adefovir or both in human immunodeficiency virus-infected adults with virologic failure on indinavir: AIDS Clinical Trials Group Study 359. *J Infect Dis.* **2000**;182:1375-1384.

Harrigan PR, Larder BA. Extent of cross-resistance between agents used to treat human immunodeficiency virus type 1 infection in clinically derived isolates. *Antimicrob Agents Chemother.* **2002**;46:909-912.

Hawkins T, Veikley W, St. Claire R, Hey A, Guyer B, Kearney BP. Intracellular pharmacokinetics of tenofovir-DF and carbovir-TP in patients receiving triple nucleoside regimens. In: Program and abstracts of the 5th International Workshop on Clinical Pharmacology of HIV Therapy; April 1-3, **2004**; Rome, Italy. Abstract 6.

Hirsch MS, Brun-Vezinet F, Clotet B, et al. Antiretroviral drug resistance testing in adults infected with HIV-1. Recommendations of an International AIDS Society-USA panel. *Clin Infect Dis.* **2003**;37:113-128.

Jemsek J, Hutcherson P, Harper E. Poor virologic responses and early emergence of resistance in treatment naive, HIV-infected patients receiving a once daily triple nucleoside regimen of didanosine, lamivudine, and tenofovir DF. In: Program and abstracts of the 11th Conference on Retroviruses and Opportunistic Infections; February 8-11, **2004**; San Francisco, California. Abstract 51.

Jourdain G, Ngo-Giang-Huong N, Le Coeur S, et al. Intrapartum exposure to nevirapine and subsequent maternal responses to nevirapine-based antiretroviral therapy. *N Engl J Med.* **2004**;351:229-240.

Kearney BP, Isaacson E, Sayre J, Ebrahimi R, Cheng AK. The pharmacokinetics of abacavir, a purine nucleoside analog, are not affected by tenofovir DF. In: Program and abstracts of the 43rd Interscience Conference on Antimicrobial Agents and Chemotherapy; September 14-17, **2003**: Chicago, Illinois. Abstract A-1615.

Landman R, Peytavin G, Descamps D, et al. Low genetic barrier to resistance is a possible cause of early virologic failures in once-daily regimen of abacavir, lamivudine, and tenofovir: the TONUS study. In: Program and abstracts of the 11th Conference on Retroviruses and Opportunistic Infections; February 8-11, **2004**; San Francisco, California. Abstract 52.

Lanier ER, Irlbeck D, Ross L, et al. Prediction of NRTI options by linking reverse transcriptase genotype to phenotypic breakpoints. In: Program and abstracts of the 10th Conference on Retroviruses and Opportunistic Infections; February 10-14, **2003**; Boston, Massachusetts. Abstract 586.

Lecossier D, Shulman NS, Morand-Joubert L, et al. Detection of minority populations of HIV-1 expressing the K103N resistance mutation in patients failing nevirapine. *J Acquir Immune Defic Syndr.* **2005**;38:37-42.

Maggiolo F, Callegaro A, Gregis G, et al. In vivo determination of tenofovir antiviral effect in the presence of TAMs. In: Program and abstracts of the 12th Conference on Retroviruses and Opportunistic Infections, **2005**; Boston, Massachusetts. Poster M124.

Miller MD, McColl DM, Whitle KL and Parkin N. Genotypic and phenotypic characterization of patient-derived HIV-1 isolates containing the K65R mutation in reverse transcriptase (RT). In: Program and abstracts of the 43rd Interscience Conference on Antimicrobial Agents and Chemotherapy; September 14-17, **2003**; Chicago, Illinois. Abstract H-904.

Miller V, Larder BA. Mutational patterns in the HIV genome and cross-resistance following nucleoside and nucleotide analogue drug exposure. *Antivir Ther.* **2001**;6(Suppl 3):25-44.

Moyle G, Nelson M, Higgs C, et al. A randomised open label comparative study of Combivir + efavirenz (2 class triple therapy) versus Trizivir + tenofovir (single class quadruple therapy) in initial therapy for HIV-1 infection. In: Program and abstracts of the 44th Interscience Conference on Antimicrobial Agents and Chemotherapy; October 30-November 2, **2004**; Washington, DC. Abstract H-1131.

Parikh U, Koontz D, Hammond J, et al. K65R: a multi-nucleoside resistance mutation of low but increasing frequency. *Antivir Ther.* **2003**;8:S152.

Picard V, Angelini E, Maillard A, et al. Comparison of genotypic and phenotypic resistance patterns of human immunodeficiency virus type 1 isolates from patients treated with stavudine and didanosine or zidovudine and lamivudine. *J Infect Dis.* **2001**;184:781-784.

Rey D, Krebs M, Partisani M, et al. Early virologic response at 1 month and 8 month median follow-up of a new triple NUCs combination (zidovudine, lamivudine, and tenofovir) in 42 antiretroviral-naive, HIV-1-infected patients. In: Program and abstracts of the 12th Conference on Retroviruses and Opportunistic Infections, **2005**; Boston, Massachusetts. Poster 599.

Underwood M, St Clair M, Ross L, Gerondelis P, Parkin N, Lanier R. Cross-resistance of clinical samples with K65R, L74V, and M184V mutations. In: Program and abstracts of the 12th Conference on Retroviruses and Opportunistic Infections, **2005**; Boston, Massachusetts. Abstract 714.

Wainberg M, Turner D. Resistance issues with new nucleoside/nucleotide backbone options. *J Acquir Immune Defic Syndr.* **2004**;37:S36-S43.

Whitcomb JM, Parkin NT, Chappey C, Hellmann NS, Petropoulos CJ. Broad nucleoside reverse-transcriptase inhibitor cross-resistance in human immunodeficiency virus type 1 clinical isolates. *J Infect Dis.* **2003**;188:992-1000.

Wirden M, Malet I, Derrache A, et al. Clonal analysis of HIV quasi-species in patients harboring plasma genotype with K65R mutation associated with thymidine analogue mutations or L74V substitution. In: Program and abstracts of the 12th Conference on Retroviruses and Opportunistic Infections, **2005**; Boston. Abstract 702.

Wolf K, Hauke W, Beerenwinkel N, et al. Tenofovir resistance and resensitization. *Antimicrobial Agents Chemother.* **2003**;47:3478-3484.

Yanchunas J, Langley D, Tao L, et al. Binding affinities of HIV-1 protease inhibitors are increased in the atazanavir-resistant I50L/A71V protease. In: Program and abstracts of the 12th Conference on Retroviruses and Opportunistic Infections, **2005**; Boston, Massachusetts. Abstract 695.

(RLO-32)

IV.28. VIRAL FITNESS AND REPLICATION CAPACITY

LEARNING OBJECTIVE: Discuss the distinction between viral fitness and replication capacity and the potential utility of reduced fitness on treatment-enhancing strategies.

Viral Fitness

Viral fitness refers to the ability of a virus to reproduce in a defined environment. HIV replication can be influenced by viral factors, such as efficiency of cell entry, reverse transcription and gene expression, as well as by innate and HIV-specific immune responses and antiretroviral drug pressure (Deeks et al. 2001; Nijhuis et al. 2001). The results of one study suggested that the envelope gene plays a role in the ability of HIV-1 to replicate and that early events in the life cycle (e.g., viral entry) may have a major impact on viral fitness (Rangel et al. 2003). Another study demonstrated that the *pol* gene may alter viral replication kinetics and possibly even virulence (Barbour et al. 2004).

A number of methods can be used to measure viral fitness, including growth kinetics, growth competition and recombinant virus-single cycle assays. Although growth competition is considered the gold standard for assessment of viral fitness in vitro, these assays are time-consuming and labor-intensive, making them impractical for clinical use (reviewed in Bates et al. 2003 and in Nijhuis et al. 2001). As described elsewhere (Prado et al. 2002; Deeks et al. 2001; Petropoulos et al. 2000), One company has developed an in vitro assay to measure RC by examining the HIV-1 *pol* gene. This assay has been shown to correlate with viral fitness measured by more traditional in vitro growth competition methods (Huang et al. 2003; Prado et al. 2002; Resch et al. 2002; Grant et al. 2001). The *pol* RC assay is currently reported as part of the resistance assay and phenotypic/genotypic resistance combination assay.

Replication Capacity

The above-cited ViroLogic *pol* RC assay is currently the only commercially available assay that measures in vitro viral fitness. This test uses a system whereby the HIV *pol* gene coding for reverse transcriptase and protease from plasma HIV-1 RNA is amplified and inserted into an HIV genomic vector that also carries a reporter gene that is used to measure the amount of replication. The amount of virus replication is compared with that of reference wild-type viruses during one round of replication. The RC of the reference wild-type isolate is set at 100%. Replication capacity values for the HIV isolate can thus range from 0% (unable to replicate) to greater than 100% (replicates better than wild-type HIV). The advantage of the ViroLogic *pol* RC assay is that it focuses on the HIV enzymes that are the current targets of most HIV therapy (reverse transcriptase and protease) and thus can assess the RC impact of mutations associated with therapeutic resistance (Campbell et al. 2003; Barbour et al. 2002; see also review by Nijhuis et al. 2001). A disadvantage is that other viral and host factors that contribute to the efficiency of virus replication in vivo are not measured (Trkola et al. 2003; Barbour et al. 2002; Deeks et al. 2001). For example, there frequently are mutations in the *gag* cleavage sites on which the protease enzyme acts. These can potentially influence the RC of HIV in the setting of drug-resistant mutations in protease (Koh et al. 2004). Because the RC assay is readily available, a substantial amount

What's New

New studies suggest that replication capacity may predict outcome independent of HIV RNA level and CD4 count.

Key Points

- Viral fitness indicates the ability of a given pathogen to replicate in vivo under a variety of forces, including the influence of drug therapy and immune responses.
- Replication capacity (RC) refers to the intrinsic ability of the pathogen to replicate in vitro relative to a specific reference isolate. An assay that measures the impact that a given individual's HIV reverse transcriptase and protease have on RC is commercially available.
- Certain HIV mutations that confer resistance also decrease RC, which may explain why some patients with highly resistant virus continue to benefit from antiretroviral therapy.
- The natural history of HIV-1 infection is heterogeneous, with wide variations in rates of disease progression. Research is under way to determine what influence, if any, viral fitness and RC may have on HIV disease (Hellman et al. 2002).

of the recent literature on the subject of viral fitness has employed this assay (including Campbell et al. 2003; Deeks et al. 2003, 2001; Huang et al. 2003; Sufka et al. 2003; Barbour et al. 2002; Maguire et al. 2002; Prado et al. 2002; Resch et al. 2002; White et al. 2002; and as reviewed in Bates et al. 2003).

Effect of antiretroviral drug resistance on *pol* RC

Although the initiation of combination antiretroviral therapy significantly suppresses HIV replication, resulting in extraordinary clinical benefits, genetic mutations associated with reduced drug susceptibility can be selected for in the setting of virologic rebound. Despite the presence of drug resistance, some patients maintain a viral load lower than levels measured prior to the initiation of antiretroviral therapy (reviewed in Barbour et al. 2002; Nijhuis et al. 2001). These observations suggest that antiretroviral therapy can exert some effect, even in the setting of drug resistance. Among the many possibilities is that the mutations that enable the virus to bypass the antiretroviral effect of the drugs may come at a cost to the virus. Their development may result in a decrease in the ability of HIV to replicate.

Investigators have demonstrated that certain mutations conferring resistance to reverse transcriptase inhibitors and protease inhibitors can decrease HIV RC (Barbour et al. 2004; Huang et al. 2003; Leigh Brown et al. 2003; Miller et al. 2003; Maguire et al. 2002; Prado et al. 2002; Resch et al. 2002; White et al. 2002; and as reviewed in Nijhuis et al. 2001). In addition, when individuals with high-level resistance and detectable plasma HIV-1 RNA levels interrupt their antiretroviral therapy, there is, in most cases, a shift in the predominant plasma virus population from drug-resistant to drug-sensitive virus. This coincides with a significant increase in plasma viremia and decrease in the CD4 count (Deeks et al. 2001). This suggests that the drug-sensitive HIV-1 is more replication-competent. Indeed, it was shown in these patients that the antiretroviral-sensitive virus has higher RC than the antiretroviral-resistant virus (Deeks et al. 2001). As seen in the studies discussed above, in cases where there is discordance between the CD4 counts and HIV-1 RNA levels, it appears that decreased *pol* RC may contribute to that phenomenon (Sufka et al. 2003; Deeks et al. 2001). This is not to say that drug resistance is good; in fact, additional mutations can eventually develop that would allow antiretroviral-resistant HIV-1 to become more replication-competent (reviewed in Nijhuis et al. 2001). Nevertheless, one study of 20 patients maintained on failing protease inhibitor-based regimens for a median of 26.2 months has shown that these compensatory mutations may evolve relatively slowly and may not readily compensate for impaired RC (Barbour et al. 2002). In these patients, RC remained stable and CD4 counts increased gradually while both viral load and phenotypic resistance to protease inhibitors gradually increased. It is also worth noting that a number of drug-resistance mutations do not appreciably impair RC, such as the K103N that confers resistance to NNRTIs (Koval et al. 2004). Additionally, in some settings, the mutations 41L/210W/215Y and 67N/70R/219Q have been associated with enhanced replication kinetics when compared with wild type (Hu et al. 2004).

Because of the effect that drug-resistant mutations can have on HIV-1 *pol* RC, highly treatment-experienced patients without alternative treatment options may derive continued benefit from remaining on drug therapy, despite evidence of resistance to most or all of the agents in the regimen. Nevertheless, such a strategy should not replace the goal of early detection of resistance with modification of therapy in order to achieve, whenever possible, complete viral suppression (Frenkel and Mullins 2001). One study found that for patients continuing a virologically failing regimen, any gain in CD4 count was lost by 3 years (Deeks et al. 2002) Another study found that patients with persistent low-level viremia while on therapy were also at considerable risk of treatment failure (Karlsson et al. 2004). Important to note is that resistance mutations will continue to accumulate with insufficient viral suppression, compromising future treatment options and perhaps taking away the chance to ever fully suppress the patient's virus.

Relationship between *pol* RC and the natural history of HIV-1 infection

A number of studies have now shown that RC is variable even in antiretroviral-naive individuals and that *pol* RC correlates with immunologic and clinical outcomes. In a study of 191 newly diagnosed drug-naive patients, it was shown that CD4 counts were significantly greater in those with decreased *pol* RC (Barbour et al. 2004). In addition, in a small study of patients not currently on therapy, RC was found to have a significant linear relationship with viral load (Campbell et al. 2003). There were similar findings in another study of patients receiving antiretroviral therapy who then underwent treatment interruption. In these subjects, both the viral load set point and the magnitude of viral rebound correlated with HIV-1 RC (Trkola et al. 2003). In addition, in those experiencing discordant responses to therapy (with stable or increasing CD4+ T cells despite increasing or persistently detectable HIV viral load), studies have shown a correlation between decreased RC and the degree of discordance (Deeks et al. 2001; Sufka et al. 2003). In a large prospective trial of phenotypic resistance testing in treated patients experiencing virologic failure, a correlation was further found between lower RC at baseline and greater increases in CD4+ T cells at months 6 and 12 (Haubrich et al. 2002). Finally, a recent study measured RC from baseline samples obtained from a cohort of minimally antiretroviral-treated HIV-infected hemophiliacs. In this case it was shown that RC was correlated with plasma HIV-1 RNA levels and CD4 counts and was predictive of clinical progression, even after controlling for HIV-1 RNA level and CD4 count (Daar et al. 2003).

The rapidly growing body of data related to the clinical relevance of viral fitness may help us to understand why those with antiretroviral-resistant virus continue to derive benefit from therapy to which they are resistant. Although additional research will be needed to definitively show how RC measurements might best be used to make more informed therapeutic decisions, the studies discussed here do provide evidence that RC may be an important factor in HIV-1 pathogenesis.

References

Barbour JD, Win T, Grant RM, et al. Evolution of phenotypic drug susceptibility and viral replication capacity during long-term virologic failure of protease inhibitor therapy in human immunodeficiency virus-infected adults. *J Virol.* **2002**;76:11104-11112.

Barbour JD, Hecht FM, Wrin T, et al. Higher CD4+ T cell counts associated with low viral *pol* replication capacity among treatment-naive adults in early HIV-1 infection. *J Infect Dis.* **2004**;190:251-256.

Bates M, Wrin T, Huang W, Petropoulos C, Hellmann N. Practical applications of viral fitness in clinical practice. *Curr Opin Infect Dis.* **2003**;16:11-18.

Campbell TB, Schneider K, Wrin T, Petropoulos CJ, Connick E. Relationship between in vitro human immunodeficiency virus type 1 replication rate and plasma virus load. *J Virol.* **2003**;77:12105-12112.

Daar E, Kesler K, Donfield S, et al. HIV replication capacity predicts HIV clinical progression. [Abstract 273]. *Antiviral Ther.* **2003**;8(suppl 1):251.

Deeks SG, Wrin T, Liegler T, et al. Virologic and immunologic consequences of discontinuing combination antiretroviral-drug therapy in HIV-infected patients with detectable viremia. *N Engl J Med.* **2001**;344:472-480.

Deeks SG, Barbour JD, Grant RM, Martin JN. Duration and predictors of CD4+ T cell gains in patients who continue combination therapy despite detectable plasma viremia. *AIDS.* **2002**;16:201-207.

Deeks SG, Grant RM, Wrin T, et al. Persistence of drug-resistant HIV-1 after a structured treatment interruption and its impact on treatment response. *AIDS.* **2003**;17:361-370.

Frenkel LM, Mullins JI. Should patients with drug-resistant HIV-1 continue to receive antiretroviral therapy? *N Engl J Med.* **2001**;344:520-521.

Grant RM, Liegler T, Elkin C, et al. Protease inhibitor resistant HIV-1 has marked decreased fitness in vivo. In: Program and abstracts of 8th Conference on Retroviruses and Opportunistic Infections; February 4-8, **2001**; Chicago, Illinois. Abstract LB4.

Haubrich R, Wrin T, Hellmann N, et al. Replication capacity as a predictor of immunological and virological benefit despite virological failure of an antiretroviral regimen [Abstract 121]. *Antiviral Ther.* **2002**;7:S101.

Hellmann N, Wrin T, Bates M, et al. Modeling the effect of HIV replication capacity on treatment outcomes [abstract 63]. *Antiviral Ther.* **2002**;7:S53.

Hu ZX, Reid P, Lu J, Kuritzkes DR. Fitness of T215Y vs T215F mutants in HIV-1 RT: comparison of specific thymidine analogue-resistance mutation patterns. In: Program and abstracts of the 11th Conference on Retroviruses and Opportunistic Infections; February 8-11, **2004**; San Francisco, California. Abstract 638.

Huang W, Gamarnik A, Limoli K, Petropoulos CJ, Whitcomb JM. Amino acid substitutions at position 190 of human immunodeficiency virus type 1 reverse transcriptase increase susceptibility to delavirdine and impair virus replication. *J Virol.* **2003**;7:1512-1523.

Karlsson AC, Younger SR, Martin JN, et al. Immunologic and virologic evolution during periods of intermittent and persistent low-level viremia. *AIDS.* **2004**;18:981-989.

Koh Y, Aoki M, Ogata H, Yoshimura K, Mitsuya H. Role of *gag* mutations in HIV in its replication fitness and acquisition of resistance to protease inhibitors. In: Program and abstracts of the 11th Conference on Retroviruses and Opportunistic Infections; February 8-11, **2004**; San Francisco, California. Abstract 634.

Koval C, Dykes C, Demeter L. Ex vivo replication fitness of efavirenz-resistant HIV mutants. In: Program and abstracts of the 11th Conference on Retroviruses and Opportunistic Infections; February 8-11, **2004**; San Francisco, California. Abstract 640.

Leigh Brown AJ, Frost SDW, Good B, et al. Genotypic basis of variation in protease susceptibility in primary HIV infection analyzed with machine learning. In: Program and abstracts of the 10th Conference on Retroviruses and Opportunistic Infections; February 10-14, **2003**; Boston, Massachusetts. Abstract 594.

Maguire MF, Guinea R, Griffin P, et al. Changes in human immunodeficiency virus type 1 Gag at positions L449 and P453 are linked to I50V protease mutants in vivo and cause reduction of sensitivity to amprenavir and improved viral fitness in vitro. *J Virol.* **2002**;76:7398-7406.

Miller MD, White KL, Petropoulos CJ, Parkin NT. Decreased replication capacity of HIV-1 clinical isolates containing K65R or M184V RT mutations. In: Program and abstracts of the 10th Conference on Retroviruses and Opportunistic Infections; February 10-14, **2003**; Boston, Massachusetts. Abstract 616.

Nijhuis M, Deeks S, Boucher C. Implications of antiretroviral resistance on viral fitness. *Curr Opin Infect Dis.* **2001**;14:23-28.

Petropoulos CJ, Parkin NT, Limoli KL, et al. A novel phenotypic drug susceptibility assay for human immunodeficiency virus type 1. *Antimicrob Agents Chemother.* **2000**;44:920-928.

Prado, J, Wrin T, Beauchaine J, et al. Amprenavir-resistant HIV-1 exhibits lopinavir cross-resistance and reduced replication capacity. *AIDS.* **2002**;16:1009-1017.

Rangel H, Weber J, Chakraborty B, et al. Role of the human immunodeficiency virus type 1 envelope gene in viral fitness. *J Virol.* **2003**;77:9069-9073.

Resch W, Ziermann R, Parkin N, Gamarnik A, Swanstrom R. Nelfinavir-resistant, amprenavir-hypersusceptible strains of human immunodeficiency virus type 1 carrying an N88S mutation in protease have reduced infectivity, reduced replication capacity, and reduced fitness and process the Gag polyprotein precursor aberrantly. *J Virol.* **2002**;76:8659-8666.

Sufka SA, Ferrari G, Gryszowka VE, et al. Prolonged CD4+ cell/virus load discordance during treatment with protease-inhibitor based highly active antiretroviral therapy: immune response and viral control. *J Infect Dis.* **2003**; 187:1027-1037.

Trkola A, Kuster H, Leemann C, et al. Human immunodeficiency virus type 1 fitness is a determining factor in viral rebound and set point in chronic infection. *J Virol.* **2003**;77:13146-13155.

White KL, Margot NA, Wrin T, Petropoulos CJ, Miller MD, Naeger LK. Molecular mechanisms of resistance to human immunodeficiency virus type 1 with reverse transcriptase mutations K65R and K65R+M184V and their effects on enzyme function and viral replication capacity. *Antimicrob Agents Chemother.* **2002**;46:3437-3446.

(RLO-33)

IV.29. TREATMENT INTERRUPTIONS

LEARNING OBJECTIVE: Discuss various approaches to, the rationale for, and the risks and benefits of treatment interruption in: (a) HIV-infected patients who are on successful antiretroviral therapy; (b) HIV-infected patients for whom antiretroviral therapy is failing.

Introduction

Treatment interruption as discussed in this Objective is defined as any discontinuation of antiretroviral therapy in a patient for a reason other than drug toxicity or an immediate change to another antiretroviral regimen. This idea seems to go against every basic tenet of antiretroviral therapy in that we have always assumed that suppressing viral load as much and for as long as possible was the main goal of therapy. However, the alternative strategy of not having patients on continuous antiretroviral therapy may have some advantages. These include the following possibilities: (1) the same efficacy with less drug use; (2) fewer chronic medication side effects; (3) increased medication compliance; (4) improved restoration of immune function; and (5) reduced costs.

However, there are significant concerns about treatment interruptions. The biggest fear is the emergence of resistance to antiretrovirals and the consequent life-long loss of medications to treat HIV in that particular patient. Other worries include increased HIV transmission, the conversion of HIV to more virulent phenotypes, severe illnesses associated with rapid HIV rebound and the increased risk of central nervous system disease or malignancies. Another consideration is whether the impetus for treatment interruption is currently as strong now that easier and less toxic antiretrovirals are available. Clearly, if treatment interruptions were shown to be a safe and effective strategy, then this strategy would be a tremendous benefit for patients. However, treatment interruptions have not yet been shown to be beneficial in patients with HIV infection, and the current bottom line is that treatment interruptions should not be generally recommended outside the closely observed confines of a clinical study (DHHS 2004).

Types of Treatment Interruptions

Treatment interruptions can be broken down into 4 general types: (1) interruptions in patients started on antiretroviral therapy during acute infection; (2) regularly scheduled therapy hiatuses in stable, virologically suppressed patients; (3) interruptions in therapy in stable patients having an excellent response to therapy that are not regularly scheduled but are based on CD4 and/or viral load measurements ("CD4-driven" or "viral load-driven" interruptions); and (4) interruptions in patients who are failing their current antiretroviral regimen, with the hypothesis that the rebound of "wild-type" virus will improve the effectiveness of subsequent antiretroviral treatment.

Treatment interruptions in patients started on antiretroviral therapy during acute infection

Patients who are treated with antiretrovirals during or very shortly after seroconversion have preservation of HIV-specific immune responses as compared with patients with chronic infection (Malhotra et al. 2000; Oxenius et al. 2000;

What's New

The role of antiretroviral treatment interruption as a therapeutic strategy remains uncertain. Conflicting results have been reported for structured intermittent therapy and for the viral load- and CD4-driven interruptions. Results of studies of treatment interruption to restore HIV-specific immune responses or to improve response to salvage therapy do not support recommending treatment interruptions for these purposes.

Key Points

- HIV-specific immune response can control viral replication but is lost soon after primary infection.
- Antiretroviral treatment during acute infection, if commenced in time, might preserve HIV-specific immunity in selected cases, but the long-term effects on viral load set point, rate of CD4 count decline or clinical benefit remain unknown.
- Results from treatment interruption studies in patients with established, chronic HIV infection that attempt to restore HIV-specific immunity have not been encouraging.
- Results from short-cycle structured intermittent therapy studies designed to reduce toxicity have been mixed and may depend on the regimen chosen.
- CD4-driven treatment interruption studies are still under study.

Rosenberg et al. 2000, 1997). One strategy to maintain this immunity during acute infection involves initial treatment shortly after infection followed by structured treatment interruptions. In one small study of 8 patients with acute HIV infection, therapy was discontinued in a protocol that required restarting therapy for viral rebound before the set point was achieved (Rosenberg et al. 2000). Although the short-term findings showed functional improvements in HIV-specific CD4 and CD8 responses, recent updates on an increased cohort of 14 patients have noted that nearly all of the study subjects have experienced viral rebound when therapy was withdrawn for a prolonged period (Kaufmann et al. 2004). The long-term clinical implications of these immune benefits are unknown. Although treatment interruptions in patients treated during acute HIV infection appear to confer some improvement in laboratory-measured immune responses, these treatment strategies cannot be considered standard of care at this time. (See also Objective IV.1 on Treatment of Acute HIV in this Update.)

Treatment interruptions in clinically stable patients with virologic suppression

In contrast to patients diagnosed during acute infection, most patients who begin therapy during chronic infection have already lost whatever HIV-specific immunity they may have developed in the early stages of infection. It has been theorized that repeat exposure to viremia might serve as a form of "autoimmunization" that can reinvigorate the HIV-specific immune response. The rationale for treatment interruptions in such patients is to try to restore, rather than to preserve, HIV-specific immunity (reviewed in Abbas et al. 2002; Havlir 2002; Hogg et al. 2002). This is clearly a more challenging goal, and results from clinical trials testing this approach have not been encouraging (Hirschel et al. 2002). The other rationales for treatment interruption — less exposure to drug, fewer side effects, economic benefits — appear to be more compelling than boosting the immune response.

There are several varieties of treatment interruption strategies for patients with chronic infection who have had a good response to therapy, but they can generally be divided into 2 categories: (1) scheduled interruptions in treatment; and (2) CD4- or viral load-driven treatment interruptions. In the scheduled-interruption strategy, patients with undetectable viral loads and preserved CD4 counts have therapy stopped and restarted according to a defined schedule (e.g., cycles of 1 week on therapy and 1 week off therapy). In the CD4-driven strategies, patients with undetectable viral loads and preserved CD4 counts have their therapies stopped, and are followed closely. Therapy is restarted when the CD4 count drops below and/or viral load rises above some threshold value. The CD4 threshold is always above the 250- to 300-cell/mm^3 level so as to avoid exposing patients to opportunistic complications.

Scheduled interruptions

In the scheduled-interruption strategy, patients with undetectable viral loads and preserved CD4 counts have their antiretroviral medications stopped and restarted according to a defined schedule. A variety of antiretroviral regimens and interruption times have been studied. In general, the trials using relatively short periods of interruption (1 week or less) have been associated with better preservation of CD4 counts and less development of virologic resistance as compared with trials using longer periods of interruption (weeks to months). It is thought that the longer interruption times allow for greater viral rebound in the face of subtherapeutic drug levels and thus an increased risk of resistance. Also, some patients have shown dramatic decreases in CD4 counts during long treatment interruptions, especially if their baseline viral loads were elevated (Ruiz et al. 2004). In addition, no trial has convincingly demonstrated the combination of CD4 preservation, lack of virologic resistance and reduction of long-term side effects. Preliminary data from trials employing very short periods of interruption (5 days on, 2 days off) are provocative, but further, long-term data are needed to confirm that "taking the weekend off your medications" is safe and effective.

- A week on/week off regimen using a once-daily regimen containing efavirenz in 7 patients maintained viral suppression for at least 60 weeks. There were no significant changes in the CD4 counts or lipid levels of the patients in this trial (Dybul et al. 2004). The development of antiretroviral resistance during treatment interruptions is a particular concern when using drugs that have both a low genetic barrier to resistance and very long half-lives (such as efavirenz and lamivudine, both of which were used in this trial). No resistance was detected in 2 patients who had viral load increases (1 due to going off the regimen temporarily and the other due to elective permanent discontinuation of therapy). Efavirenz drug concentrations did stay at subtherapeutic levels for lengthy periods during the treatment interruptions, and this provides an opportunity for drug resistance to emerge. Drug levels of efavirenz measured on the seventh day of treatment interruption in 7 patients varied from 70 to 720 ng/mL, well below the assumed the optimal level of over 1000 ng/mL. Six of 7 patients had levels over 1000 ng/mL within 36 hours of resuming therapy, with 4 reaching this threshold within 12 hours.

- The 1-week on/1-week off arm of the STACCATO trial included ritonavir-boosted saquinavir once daily in some patients , but it recorded a virologic failure rate of 53% (i.e., 19 of 36 evaluable patients had 2 consecutive viral load measurements of over 500 HIV RNA copies/mL) (Ananworanich et al. 2003). This led to the termination of that arm of the study. It is unclear why this trial had so much more frequent virologic failure than the study mentioned above.

- A trial using longer-cycle treatment interruptions (8 weeks on/4 weeks off) was prematurely terminated after 5 of the 26 patients in the treatment-interruption arm developed resistance mutations during the trial (Dybul et al. 2003). In this trial, 8 patients in the treatment-interruption arm were treated with efavirenz, and 3 of these patients developed nonnucleoside reverse transcriptase inhibitor (NNRTI) and/or nucleoside reverse transcriptase inhibitor (NRTI) resistance-associated mutations (2 had K103N and M184V, 1 had only M184V). Also, 2 patients on interruption from a protease inhibitor-based regimen developed either an M184V or T215Y NRTI resistance-associated mutation. Trial participants exhibited no benefit from treatment interruption in terms of toxicity and immunologic parameters. The data from this trial suggest that scheduled interruptions using long cycles should be avoided, with the risk of developing resistance greatest for drugs with a long half-life and low genetic barrier to resistance.

- An 8-week on/2-week off study found a fairly large proportion of patients developing resistance in subpopulations of virus during treatment interruptions (Metzner et al. 2003). Using reverse transcriptase PCR and allele-discriminating oligonucleotides to identify small subpopulations of virus harboring resistance mutations, these authors found that 56% and 12% of the subjects had evidence for the M184V and L90M mutations, respectively.

CD4-guided interruptions

CD4-guided treatment interruptions are still under extensive study. The bulk of studies suggest that the leading predictor for requiring resumption of therapy is a lower nadir CD4 count before starting suppressive treatment. It is important to emphasize that all of these studies enrolled or will enroll clinically stable patients with relatively high CD4 counts and suppressed viral loads.

- The STACCATO trial is an open-label, randomized trial of 600 treatment-experienced patients in Thailand, Switzerland, Australia, Argentina and Canada, comparing 3 arms: continuous therapy, 1-week on/1-week off therapy and CD4-guided therapy with therapy restarted when CD4 counts fall below 350 cells/mm^3 (Ananworanich et al. 2003; Ananworanich et al. 2004). All 74 Thai patients were treated with 2 NRTIs and ritonavir-boosted saquinavir dosed once daily. As mentioned above, the treatment-interruption arm was discontinued due to virologic failure, especially in the Thai participants. At the end of 96 weeks, all patients were placed on continuous HAART for 12 weeks, and then laboratory values were assessed (Ananworanich et al. 2004). At week 108, 96% (24/25) of patients and 100% (23/23) of patients in the continuous and CD4-driven arms, respectively, had CD4 counts over 350 cells/mm^3, and 100% and 91% had viral loads under 400 copies/mL, respectively. There were no differences between the 2 arms in adverse events, lipid levels or quality-of-life outcomes.

- The Tibet Study is another open-label study, enrolling 201 patients with CD4 counts above 500 cells/mm^3 for over 6 months and undetectable viral loads for over 1 year (Ruiz et al. 2004). It randomized trial participants into continuous therapy or CD4- and viral load-guided therapy. Therapy was restarted in the guided-therapy group for CD4 counts under 350 cells/mm^3 or viral loads above 100,000 copies/mL. Treatment continued until CD4 count rose above 500 or viral load fell below 80 copies/mL (Ruiz et al. 2003). Preliminary data show that only 9 of 101 patients in the continuous-therapy group had a viral load over 50 copies/mL at 96 weeks. Sixty-eight of the 100 patients in the intermittent therapy had to reinitiate therapy. The median time off of antiretrovirals during the first treatment interruption was 44 weeks. Acute retroviral syndrome was noted in 6% of the patients who stopped therapy. In a report assessing drug resistance development during the treatment interruption, 31 of the 87 (36%) patients tested had resistant virus (Ruiz et al. 2005). Owing to the new NNRTI mutations detected, the researchers cautioned that treatment interruption should not be used for patients on NNRTI-containing regimens.

- The BASTA study is a reasonably large, prospective, controlled trial of a CD4-driven treatment-interruption strategy (Maggiolo et al. 2004). Sixty-nine patients with CD4 counts above 800 cells/mm^3 were randomized in a 1:2 ratio to continue their therapy or stop. Therapy was restarted for patients in the treatment-interruption arm when the CD4 count fell below 400 cells/mm^3 (Maggiolo et al. 2004). All patients who restarted therapy experienced rapid increases in CD4 counts. The length of time that therapy could be safely discontinued was tied to nadir CD4 counts: The mean duration of time off therapy for those with a nadir below 200 cells/mm^3 was only 5.4 months; for those with a nadir of 200-350 cells/mm^3, it was 11.7 months; and for those with a nadir of 351-500 cells/mm^3, it was 15.1 months. No patient with a nadir CD4 count over 500 cells/mm^3 was required to resume therapy during the study's 64 weeks of follow-up.

- The SMART study (CPCRA 065) is an ambitious, long-term trial that will attempt to definitively test a CD4-driven treatment-interruption strategy (SMART Study 2003). Patients with CD4 counts above 350 cells/mm^3 are randomly assigned to the virologic-suppression group or the drug-conservation group. The virologic-suppression group will use antiretroviral therapy in a conventional manner to maintain viral load as low as possible without regard to CD4 counts. The drug-conservation group will defer therapy until CD4 counts drop below 250 cells/mm^3. These patients will resume therapy for as long as it takes to get their CD4 counts to rise above 350 cells/mm^3, and then they will stop again. The primary endpoint is clinical disease progression or death, and the duration of follow-up required for the study is estimated to be 6 to 9 years. (More information about this ongoing trial is available at the study's Web site: http://www.smart-trial.org.)

Treatment interruptions in patients failing therapy before initiation of a rescue regimen

It is well established that continued treatment with a failing antiretroviral regimen serves to maintain the persistence of drug-resistant virus. Once therapy is discontinued, wild-type virus — which in most cases has greater "fitness" or ability to replicate than does drug-resistant virus (Nijhuis et al. 2001) — reemerges as the predominant viral strain. For this reason, it has been suggested that failing combination antiretroviral regimens be discontinued before initiation of a rescue regimen, on the premise that the rescue regimen may then be more active against the predominant wild-type virus than it would be against drug-resistant virus.

Work by Miller and colleagues (2000) showed both the risks with and a possible short-term benefit of such an approach. Despite extensive resistance in the heavily pretreated patients in this study, therapy interruption resulted in increases in viral load and decreases in CD4 counts, illustrating the clinical risk of discontinuing treatment in this group. A possible benefit was seen in some patients who experienced a shift toward wild-type virus during treatment interruption — a shift that was associated with short-term improved virologic response when therapy was restarted. However, this retrospective study was not able to show whether there was a possibility of long-term benefit. Similarly, a 68-person randomized French study preceded a 7- to 8-drug salvage regimen with an 8-week structured treatment interruption (STI) (Katlama et al. 2004). It reported significant virologic benefit compared with immediately switching therapy, but that was after just 12 weeks on the new regimen.

Other studies indicate that drug-resistant virus remains permanently archived, even when overgrown by wild-type virus (Deeks et al. 2001; Siliciano 2001). Once combination antiretroviral therapy is reinitiated and selective pressure resumes, resistant virus rapidly reemerges and predominates. Furthermore, because wild-type virus often replaces protease inhibitor-resistant virus in an average of 8 weeks, a fairly lengthy "drug holiday" is required. Moreover, the outgrowth of wild-type virus is associated with an increase in the rate of CD4 count decline in patients who stop therapy, presumably because the wild-type virus is more fit (Deeks et al. 2001). This CD4 count decline is of particular concern among those patients with low CD4 cell counts. The published results of the larger CPCRA 064 trial found that subjects who had a 16-week STI before restarting a new combination had an increased risk for AIDS-defining clinical events compared with subjects who switched therapy without an STI (Lawrence et al. 2003). In addition, the subjects who interrupted therapy experienced a decline in CD4 count that persisted, while those subjects who switched therapy without an STI maintained stable CD4 counts (Lawrence et al. 2003). The final results of this study with a median 36 months of follow-up found that STI had no benefit — no matter what study parameter was evaluated (Lawrence et al. 2005). Two other notable studies of STI prior to salvage therapy that failed to observe benefit are the 48-week AIDS Clinical Trials Group study A5086 using a 16-week STI (Benson et al. 2004) and a 60-week Canadian Trials Network study 164 trying a 12-week STI (Walmsley et al. 2005).

Based on the above studies, treatment interruption strategies to improve the response to salvage regimens are not recommended. They may be particularly dangerous in patients who have advanced HIV disease, as outgrowth of a fitter wild type virus will lead to further CD4 declines.

Adjunctive Therapies During Treatment Interruptions

It is possible that the use of some adjunctive therapies can extend the length of time before antiretroviral therapy has to ultimately be restarted. One report on the use of granulocyte-macrophage colony-stimulating factor (GM-CSF) given during the first 4 weeks of a 12-week interruption suggested that this cytokine may blunt the viral rebound and CD4 decline when antiretrovirals are withdrawn (Fagard et al. 2003). A second study administered three cycles of interleukin (IL)-2 for 5 days every 8 weeks prior to treatment interruption. It found that the CD4 increase resulting from IL-2 treatment prolonged the period of time before the CD4 count fell below the threshold value for restarting therapy (Katzenstein et al. 2004).

The M184V mutation confers lamivudine resistance and also reduces viral replicative capacity (see Objective IV.10 on Resistance Mutations in this Update). Maintaining M184V by continuing lamivudine monotherapy during a treatment interruption could hypothetically reduce viral fitness and slow CD4 count decay. A 50-person trial randomized patients with breakthrough M184V-containing HIV to either stop all antiretrovirals or continue with lamivudine alone (Castagna et al. 2004). Patients discontinued the study and resumed therapy if their CD4 counts fell below 350 cells/mm^3. Results at 24 weeks were available for 40 study participants. Ten of 24 (42%) on complete treatment interruption maintained that interruption through week 24. By contrast, 12 of 21 (57%) on lamivudine monotherapy maintained that course. HIV rebounds and CD4+ T cell losses were attenuated in the lamivudine arm, but no statistical analysis was reported for these modest results.

Conclusions

CD4-driven treatment interruptions in patients with relatively high CD4 cell counts and suppressed viral loads are still under study. Short-term data do not demonstrate an elevated risk of resistance or disease progression. Scheduled interruptions involving long periods of time (weeks to months) have been associated with viral resistance, and are inadvisable. Shorter scheduled interruptions (days) are still under study. Risk factors for rapid viral rebound and CD4 decline during a treatment interruption include: high viral set point, low CD4 nadir prior to initial treatment and shorter duration of viral suppression prior to stopping treatment. Treatment interruptions in chronically infected patients may result in increases in laboratory-measured immune responses, but these have not correlated with any clinical or virologic benefit. Treatment interruptions in patients failing therapy with low CD4 counts are associated with significant disease progression, and should not be undertaken. The use of adjunctive therapy to maintain resistant virus during the treatment interruption may have some promise, but data from larger trials are necessary before any conclusions can be drawn.

References

Abbas UL, Mellors JW. Interruption of antiretroviral therapy to augment immune control of chronic HIV-1 infection: risk without reward. *Proc Natl Acad Sci U S A*. **2002**;99:13377-13378.

Ananworanich J, Nuesch R, Le Braz M, et al. Failures of 1 week on, 1 week off antiretroviral therapies in a randomized trial. *AIDS*. **2003**;17:F33-F37.

Ananworanich J, Siangphoe U, Cardiello, et al. A randomized trial of continuous, CD4-guided and one week on – one week off HAART in 74 patients with chronic HIV infection: week 108 results. In: Program and abstracts of the XV International AIDS Conference; July 11-16, **2004**; Bangkok, Thailand. Abstract WeOrB1283.

Benson C, Downey G, Havlir DV, et al. A 16-week treatment interruption does not improve the virologic response to multidrug salvage therapy in treatment-experienced patients: 48-week results from ACTG A5086. In: Program and abstracts of the 11th Conference on Retroviruses and Opportunistic Infections; February 8-11, **2004**; San Francisco, California. Abstract 58.

Castagna A, Danise A, Carini E, et al. E-184V. Pilot study to evaluate immunological response to lamivudine monotherapy vs treatment interruption in failing HIV-1 infected subjects, harbouring the M184V mutation. In: Program and abstracts of the XV International Conference on AIDS; July 11-16, **2004**; Bangkok, Thailand. Abstract WeOrB1286.

Deeks SG, Wrin T, Liegler T, et al. Virologic and immunologic consequences of discontinuing combination antiretroviral-drug therapy in HIV-infected patients with detectable viremia. *N Engl J Med*. **2001**;344:472-480.

Department of Health and Human Services (DHHS). Guidelines for the use of antiretroviral agents in HIV-1-infected adults and adolescents. October 29, **2004**. Available at: http://www.aidsinfo.nih.gov/guidelines [accessed February 25, 2005].

Dybul M, Nies-Kraske E, Daucher M, et al. Long-cycle structured intermittent versus continuous highly active antiretroviral therapy for the treatment of chronic infection with human immunodeficiency virus: effects on drug toxicity and on immunologic and virologic parameters. *J Infect Dis*. **2003**;188:388-396.

Dybul M, Nies-Kraske E, Dewar R, et al. A proof-of-concept study of short-cycle intermittent antiretroviral therapy with a once-daily regimen of didanosine, lamivudine, and efavirenz for the treatment of HIV infection. *J Infect Dis*. **2004**;189:1974-1982.

Fagard C, Le Braz M, Gunthard H, et al. A controlled trial of granulocyte macrophage-colony stimulating factor during interruption of HAART. *AIDS*. **2003**;17:1487-1492.

Havlir DV. Structured intermittent treatment for HIV disease: necessary concession or premature compromise? [commentary]. *Proc Natl Acad Sci U S A*. **2002**;99:4-6.

Hirschel B, Fagard C, Oxenius A, et al. SSITT: a prospective trial of treatment interruption in HIV infection. In: Program and abstracts of the 9th Conference on Retroviruses and Opportunistic Infections; February 24-28, **2002**; Seattle, Washington. Abstract 528.

Hogg RS, Havlir DV, Miller V. To stop or not to stop: that is the question, but what is the answer? *AIDS*. **2002**;16:787-789.

Katlama C, Dominguez S, Gourlain K, et al. Benefit of treatment interruption in HIV-infected patients with multiple therapeutic failures: a randomized controlled trial (ANRS 097). *AIDS*. **2004**;18:217-226.

Katzenstein DA, Henry K, Tebas P, et al. Interrupting antiretroviral therapy (ART) using CD4+ T cell counts <350/mm^3 to restart ART (ACTG A5102). In: Program and abstracts of the XV International AIDS Conference; July 11-16, **2004**; Bangkok, Thailand. Abstract TuPeB4585.

Kaufmann DE, Lichterfeld M, Altfeld M, et al. Limited durability of viral control following treated acute HIV infection. *PLoS Med*. **2004**;1:e36.

Lawrence J, Huppler Hullsiek K, Thackeray L, et al. Final results of CPCRA 064: a randomized trial examining structured treatment interruption for patients failing therapy with multi-drug resistant HIV. In: Program and abstracts of the 12th Conference on Retroviruses and Opportunistic Infections, February 22-25, **2005**; Boston, Massachusetts. Abstract 579.

Lawrence J, Mayers DL, Hullsiek KH, et al. Structured treatment interruptions in patients with multidrug-resistant human immunodeficiency virus. *N Engl J Med*. **2003**;349:837-846.

Maggiolo F, Ripamonti D, Gregis G, Quinzan G, Callegaro A, Suter F. Effect of prolonged discontinuation of successful antiretroviral therapy on CD4 T cell: a controlled, prospective trial. *AIDS*. **2004**;18:439-446.

Malhotra U, Berrey MM, Huang Y, et al. Effect of combination antiretroviral therapy on T-cell immunity in acute human immunodeficiency virus type 1 infection. *J Infect Dis*. **2000**;181:121-131.

Metzner KJ, Bonhoeffer S, Fischer M, et al. Emergence of minor populations of human immunodeficiency virus type 1 carrying the M184V and L90M mutations in subjects undergoing structured treatment interruptions. *J Infect Dis*. **2003**;188:1433-1443.

Miller V, Sabin C, Hertogs K, et al. Virological and immunological effects of treatment interruptions in HIV-1 infected patients with treatment failure. *AIDS*. **2000**;14:2857-2867.

Nijhuis M, Deeks S, Boucher C. Implications of antiretroviral resistance on viral fitness. *Curr Opin Infect Dis*. **2001**;14:23-28.

Oxenius A, Price DA, Easterbrook PJ, et al. Early highly active antiretroviral therapy for acute HIV-1 infection preserves immune function of CD8+ and CD4+ T lymphocytes. *Proc Natl Acad Sci U S A*. **2000**;97:3382-3387.

Rosenberg ES, Altfeld M, Poon SH, et al. Immune control of HIV-1 after early treatment of acute infection [Letter]. *Nature*. **2000**;407:523-526.

Rosenberg ES, Billingsley JM, Caliendo AM, et al. Vigorous HIV-1-specific CD4+ T cell responses associated with control of viremia. *Science*. **1997**;278:1447-1450.

Ruiz L, Gómez G, Domingo P, et al. A multicenter, randomized controlled clinical trial of continuous vs. intermittent HAART guided by CD4+ T cell counts and plasma HIV-1 RNA levels. In: Program and abstracts of the 10th Conference on Retroviruses and Opportunistic Infections; February 10 -February 14, **2003**; Boston, Massachusetts. Abstract 65.

Ruiz L, Gómez G, Domingo P, et al. A multicenter, randomized controlled clinical trial of continuous vs. intermittent HAART guided by CD4+ T cell counts and plasma HIV-1 RNA levels: two-year follow-up. In: Program and abstracts of the XV International Conference on AIDS; July 11-16, **2004**; Bangkok, Thailand. Abstract TuPeB4567.

Ruiz L, Romeu J, Martínez-Picado J, et al. Selection of drug-resistance mutations in chronic HIV-infected patients during therapy interruptions guided by CD4+ T cell counts and viral load levels: the Tibet study. In: Program and abstracts of the 12th Conference on Retroviruses and Opportunistic Infections, February 22-25, **2005**; Boston, Massachusetts. Abstract 679.

Siliciano R. Viral reservoirs and ongoing virus replication in patients on HAART: implications for clinical management. In: Program and abstracts of the 8th Conference on Retroviruses and Opportunistic Infections; February 4-8, **2001**; Chicago, Illinois. Abstract L5.

SMART Study (CPCRA 065). Protocol Synopsis Version 2.0, August 18, **2003**. Available at: www.smart-trial.org [accessed February 14, 2005].

Walmsley S, LaPierre N, Loutfy M, et al. CTN 164: a prospective randomized trial of structured treatment interruption vs immediate switching in HIV-infected patients experiencing virologic failure on HAART. In: Program and abstracts of the 12th Conference on Retroviruses and Opportunistic Infections, February 22-25, **2005**; Boston, Massachusetts. Abstract 580.

(RLO-34)

IV.30. TREATMENT CESSATION

LEARNING OBJECTIVE: Discuss the pharmacokinetic and resistance considerations and approaches to stopping antiretroviral regimens containing drugs with different half-lives.

At some point in the course of antiretroviral therapy, physicians may find the need to stop therapy. This need may arise because of severe side effects, or in other cases patients may request participation in supervised (or unsupervised) treatment interruption. Until recently, a general principle has been that patients who stop therapy should stop taking all of their antiretroviral medications simultaneously. However, advances in the understanding of the pharmacokinetics of highly active antiretroviral therapy (HAART) suggest that some drugs, particularly drugs of the nonnucleoside reverse transcriptase inhibitor (NNRTI) class, have substantially longer plasma half-lives than other antiretroviral agents (Cressey et al. 2004; Muro et al. 2004; Taylor et al. 2004). Because of the prolonged plasma levels associated with NNRTIs, cessation of all components of an NNRTI-containing regimen may lead to a situation analogous to NNRTI monotherapy. Because licensed drugs of the NNRTI class have a low genetic barrier to resistance (Bangsberg 2004), treatment cessation with this class increases the risk of developing resistance to NNRTIs.

On the basis of available, but limited, pharmacokinetic and resistance data, strategies for minimizing the development of antiretroviral drug resistance during treatment cessation have been suggested. However, it is important to bear in mind that these strategies have not been tested in randomized controlled trials.

NNRTIs Have Prolonged Plasma Levels

Taylor and colleagues (2004) conducted pharmacokinetic monitoring of 8 HIV-infected patients who were taking efavirenz (Sustiva) prior to undergoing an interruption in treatment. Plasma levels of this drug were monitored for up to 3 weeks after treatment cessation. The team found that low but detectable levels of efavirenz persisted after patients stopped taking the drug and were still present at 3 weeks. On the basis of these findings, the study team recommended stopping efavirenz 2 weeks prior to ceasing the rest of the regimen. The theory underpinning this concept is that the other drugs in the regimen would provide continued antiviral activity and reduce the subsequent development of NNRTI-resistant mutations.

Muro and colleagues (2004) conducted a similar study using a single dose of the NNRTI nevirapine in 44 HIV-negative, healthy females. In 40 subjects (91%), nevirapine was still detectable after 2 weeks, and in 7 subjects (16%), nevirapine plasma levels remained low but detectable 3 weeks after the drug was first taken.

Temporary, continued use of antiretroviral therapy for 1 week after cessation of the NNRTI component had seemed to be a reasonable course of action, as determined by an expert review panel—the British HIV Association (BHIVA 2003); however, although evidence from randomized controlled trials to support the approach suggested by Taylor has not been

What's New

This learning objective is new to the AAHIVM Core Curriculum. See Key Points below for information highlights.

Key Points

- Currently available antiretroviral drugs differ in their relative plasma elimination half-lives. Drugs with longer half-lives, particularly nonnucleoside reverse transcriptase inhibitors (NNRTIs), may be stopped prior to those with shorter half-lives in order to minimize the potential for selecting NNRTI resistance, although this strategy has not been tested formally.
- Current recommendations include continuing nucleoside reverse transcriptase inhibitors (NRTIs) 7 days after stopping NNRTIs or switching to a "boosted" protease inhibitor for 1 to 2 weeks before stopping treatment to cover residual NNRTI levels. However, these options are based on limited data.
- Longer half-lives of NNRTIs may explain increased risk of drug resistance found in studies of treatment interruption.
- Structured treatment interruption continues to be explored in clinical trials but is not currently recommended as treatment.
- Drug resistance mutations that arise following single-dose nevirapine exposure have an effect on the efficacy of subsequent NNRTI-based therapies.

published, pharmacologic data suggest that continuing treatment for 2 weeks might be better. Additional possible scenarios include switching from an NNRTI to a ritonavir-boosted protease inhibitor (PI) for 1 to 2 weeks before stopping the entire regimen (BHIVA 2003). This approach can be justified by the observation that few resistance mutations to the PI class have thus far been reported in those with incomplete suppression while on effective boosted-PI regimens.

Race and Ethnicity May Have a Role

Analyses of plasma samples from two studies, ACTG A5095 and A5097, conducted over 24 weeks suggest that African American and Hispanic subjects have decreased clearance of efavirenz compared with white subjects (Ribaudo et al. 2004). Supporting this finding, another study made the association between the presence of a mutation of the hepatic enzyme cytochrome P450 2B6 in African Americans and the presence of increased side effects (Haas et al. 2004). Researchers studied this mutation because efavirenz is cleared through the activity of CYP2B6 (Sustiva 2004). (CYP3A4 is also involved in efavirenz metabolism.) All in all, these results underscore the need for caution when implementing treatment cessation in African American and Hispanic patients, particularly when NNRTIs are used. (These findings also suggest a potential role for therapeutic drug monitoring when NNRTIs are prescribed for these patients.)

Drug Resistance and Structured Treatment Interruption

Evidence from clinical trials of structured treatment interruption (8 weeks on, 2 weeks off) indicates that 14 of 25 subjects developed mutations associated with resistance to nucleoside analogues. Also, 3 of 25 subjects had a mutation associated with resistance to PIs, L90M. (Metzner et al. 2003); however, this was associated with treatment failure in only in 1 patient. The L90M mutation can confer primary resistance to nelfinavir and, in combination with other mutations, also to other PIs.

The other mutation that commonly developed was M184V (Metzner et al. 2003); this confers resistance to lamivudine and emtricitabine—both of the nucleoside reverse transcriptase inhibitor (NRTI) class. Lamivudine has a prolonged intracellular half-life (Yuen et al. 2004) and a relatively low genetic barrier to the development of resistance (Rodriguez-French et al. 2004; Yuen et al. 2004; Rousseau et al. 2003). In summary, the results from studies support the use of caution when undertaking structured treatment interruption (Martinez-Picado et al. 2002).

The above issues are focused on interruptions of sufficient length to lead to viral rebound. A different approach involves "short-cycle" interruptions designed to minimize the risk of viral rebound while still providing some time off of daily medication. The FOTO study reported on 20 HIV-infected, virally suppressed patients on continuous HAART who were treated for 5 consecutive days and interrupted on 2 consecutive days, to mimic a 5-day workweek and 2-day weekend (Cohen et al. 2004). In this open-label study, 10 participants were receiving efavirenz-based regimens and the other 10 were receiving PI-based regimens (with lopinavir/ritonavir in 8 and nelfinavir in 2). After approximately 1 year, the only two cases of virologic failure were reported in the PI arm, both in lopinavir/ritonavir users. The underlying factors for this are under study. Quality-of-life assessments indicate that participants preferred the FOTO regimen to standard schedules; in fact, all 19 patients who took the survey indicated a "very strong preference" for the 5-days-on/2-days-off schedule. The preliminary results from FOTO suggest that use of NNRTI-based regimens in very short but repeated treatment interruptions may not be associated with the development of viral resistance. It should be kept in mind that this was a small study that lasted only 1 year, and a more detailed report is required before further conclusions about the efficacy of this approach can be made.

All in all, the benefits of treatment interruption over the long term are not clear. Treatment interruption continues to be the subject of investigation and is not a preferred therapeutic strategy at this point (DHHS 2004). (See also Objective IV.29 on Treatment Interruptions in this Update.)

NNRTI Mutations Develop in Vertical Transmission Studies

NNRTI resistance has also been found in low-income countries, where HAART is not yet widely available, and is being used in vertical transmission studies at different stages of pregnancy. Brief exposure to a nevirapine was associated with subsequent development of clinically relevant resistance (for details, please see Objective IV.35 on Antiretroviral Agent Toxicity and Contraindication in Pregnancy, in this Update).

References

Bangsberg DR, Moss AR, Deeks SG. Paradoxes of adherence and drug resistance to HIV antiretroviral therapy. *J Antimicrob Chemother.* **2004**;53:696-699.

British HIV Association Treatment Guidelines, **2003**. Available at: http://www.bhiva.org/guidelines/2003/hiv/index.html [accessed February 22, 2005].

Cohen CJ, Morris A, Bazner S, et al. The FOTO Study: A pilot study of short-cycle treatment interruption, taking antiretroviral medications for five days on, two days off (FOTO) for those with viral load suppression on either PI or EFV-based regimens. In: Program and abstracts of the XV International Conference on AIDS; July 11-16, **2004**; Bangkok, Thailand. Abstract TuPeB4575.

Cressey TR, Kunkeaw S, Ruttana-Aroongorn PN, et al. Duration of nevirapine (NVP) postpartum exposure in women who received single dose NVP during labor in addition to standard zidovudine (ZDV) prophylaxis for the prevention of mother-to-child transmission of HIV-1 in Thailand. In: Program and abstracts of the 15th International Conference on AIDS; July 11-16, **2004**; Bangkok, Thailand. Abstract ThOrB1352.

Department of Health and Human Services (DHHS). guidelines for the use of antiretroviral agents in HIV-1-infected adults and adolescents. October 29, **2004**. Available at: http://aidsinfo.nih.gov/guidelines [accessed February 22, 2005].

Fagard C, Oxenius A, Günthard H, et al. A prospective trial of structured treatment interruptions in human immunodeficiency virus infection. *Arch Intern Med.* **2003**;163:1220-1226.

Haas D, Ribaudo H, Kim R, et al. A common *CYP2B6* variant is associated with efavirenz pharmacokinetics and central nervous system side effects: AACTG Study NWCS214. In: Program and abstracts of the 11th Conference on Retroviruses and Opportunistic Infections; February 8-11, **2004**; San Francisco, California. Abstract 133.

Martinez-Picado J, Morales-Lopetegi K, Wrin T, et al. Selection of drug-resistant HIV-1 mutants in response to repeated structured treatment interruptions. *AIDS.* **2002**;16:895-899.

Metzner KJ, Bonhoeffer S, Fischer M, et al. Emergence of minor populations of human immunodeficiency virus type 1 carrying the M184V and L90M mutations in subjects undergoing structured treatment interruptions. *J Infect Dis.* **2003**;188:1433-1443.

Muro E, Droste J, ter Hofstede H, Bosch M, Dolmans W, Burger D. Nevirapine plasma concentrations are still detectable after more than 2 weeks in the majority of women receiving single-dose NVP: implications for intervention studies. In: Program and abstracts of the 11th Conference on Retroviruses and Opportunistic Infections; February 8-11, **2004**; San Francisco, California. Abstract 891.

Ribaudo H, Clifford D, Gulick R, et al. Relationships between efavirenz pharmacokinetics, side effects, drug discontinuation, virologic response, and race: results from ACTG A5095/A5097s. In: Program and abstracts of the 11th Conference on Retroviruses and Opportunistic Infections; February 8-11, **2004**; San Francisco, California. Abstract 132.

Rodriguez-French A, Boghossian J, Gray GE, et al. The NEAT study: a 48-week open-label study to compare the antiviral efficacy and safety of GW433908 versus nelfinavir in antiretroviral therapy–naive HIV-1-infected patients. *J Acquir Immune Defic Syndr.* **2004**;35:22-32.

Rousseau FS, Wakeford C, Mommeja-Marin H, et al. Prospective randomized trial of emtricitabine versus lamivudine short-term monotherapy in human immunodeficiency virus–infected patients. *J Infect Dis.* **2003**;188;1652-1658.

Sustiva (efavirenz) [prescribing information]. Princeton, NJ: Bristol-Myers Squibb; December **2004**.

Taylor S, Allen S, Fidler S, et al. Stop Study: after discontinuation of efavirenz, plasma concentrations may persist for 2 weeks or longer. In: Program and abstracts of the 11th Conference on Retroviruses and Opportunistic Infections; February 8-11, **2004**; San Francisco, California. Abstract 131.

Yuen GJ, Lou Y, Bumgarner NF, et al. Equivalent steady-state pharmacokinetics of lamivudine in plasma and lamivudine triphosphate within cells following administration of lamivudine at 300 milligrams once daily and 150 milligrams twice daily. *Antimicrob Agents Chemother.* **2004**;48:176-182.

(RLO-35)

IV.32. INVESTIGATIONAL ANTIRETROVIRAL AGENTS

LEARNING OBJECTIVE: Describe the antiretroviral agents currently in advanced-phase clinical trials and expanded/early-access programs in terms of their class, resistance profile, toxicities, and the means by which to access them prior to pharmacy availability.

What's New

As of March 2005, tipranavir is the only antiretroviral available through an expanded-access program and the only new antiretroviral under FDA licensing review. Compounds in advanced phase III clinical trials as of March are the NRTI reverset, the NNRTI capravirine, the PI TMC114, and the CCR5 antagonist maraviroc (UK-427,857). Several promising compounds have entered phase II trials.

Key Points

- A limited expanded-access program for tipranavir began at the end of November 2004.
- As of December 2004, 6 nucleoside reverse transcriptase inhibitors (NRTIs) were in advanced (phase II or III) human development: alovudine, elvucitabine, SPD754, D-d4FC (reverset), RCV-201 (racivir), and amdoxovir (DAPD); all of which target viruses that are currently resistant to the current NRTIs.
- Four nonnucleoside reverse transcriptase inhibitors (NNRTIs) were also in advanced development, the most advanced being capravirine (phase III) and etravirine (TMC125), Calanolide A, and TMC278 (all Phase II). These compounds target several mutant viruses resistant to currently approved NNRTIs.
- The protease inhibitor (PI) tipranavir is under review at the FDA for approval, and another, TMC114 is in phase III. Both require boosting by ritonavir and demonstrate activity against drug-resistant isolates. Preliminary phase III clinical trial data suggest that tipranavir/ritonavir is superior to standard therapy in treatment-experienced patients, including those with highly PI-resistant virus.

Expanded/Early Access

Expanded-access programs are often created to make a drug available to patients in particular need before the drug is licensed (see also Objective V.4 on Access to Clinical Trials in the AAHIVM 2003 Study Guide). Tipranavir, for which a new drug application (NDA) has been filed, began a limited expanded-access program in late fall 2004 (Boehringer Ingelheim 2004). (Physicians can register by calling 888-524-8675 or via the Internet at http://www.tpv-eap.com.) As of this Update's publication date, the FDA approval hearing for tipranavir was imminent.

Investigational Agents: NRTIs, NNRTIs and PIs

Nucleoside reverse transcriptase inhibitors (NRTIs)

Alovudine (MIV-310) is a fluorinated thymidine analog nucleoside reverse transcriptase inhibitor (NRTI). In vitro, the agent has demonstrated activity against virus with multiple thymidine analog mutations (TAMs). In a small 4-week phase II pilot study (Katlama et al. 2004), the median viral load decrease was 1.13 $\log_{10}$ copies/mL, but an attenuated virologic response was observed in regimens that combined alovudine with stavudine and may indicate an antagonism between the 2 drugs.

Amdoxovir (DAPD) is active against various NRTI-associated mutations (Thompson et al. 2003, abstract). Clinical research was canceled in January 2004 for strategic reasons by the manufacturer, who returned its license along with toxicity, efficacy, and other data to Emory University and the University of Georgia (Gilead Sciences 2004). The AIDS Clinical Trials Group of the National Institutes of Health (NIH) is continuing phase II trials (DHHS 2004).

Elvucitabine (ACH-126,443 or beta-L-Fd4C) is an L-cytidine analog with in vitro activity against HIV that is resistant to NRTIs, nonnucleoside reverse transcriptase inhibitors (NNRTIs), and protease inhibitors (PIs). An initial comparative trial enrolled 59 adults with lamivudine-resistant virus who were still receiving a triple antiretroviral lamivudine-containing regimen (Dunkle et al. 2003). Mean baseline viral load was 10,300 copies/mL. Participants continued lamivudine 300 mg/day or replaced it with a daily dose of either 50 mg or 100 mg elvucitabine. Forty-six of the volunteers completed the 28-day observation period. Those on elvucitabine experienced a viral load decline of 0.67 and 0.78 $\log_{10}$ copies/mL in the 50 mg and 100 mg arms, respectively, whereas the lamivudine group had an increase of 0.01 $\log_{10}$ copies/mL ($P < .0001$ for all). More myelosuppression was observed in the higher-dose elvucitabine arm. Pharmacokinetic modeling data suggest that with an estimated elimination half-life of approximately 200 hours, elvucitabine might be effectively given once weekly (Stypinski et al. 2004).

Racivir is a cytidine analog NRTI that is being investigated for use in patients with drug resistance. A 14-day dose-finding study of Racivir given once daily with stavudine and efavirenz as initial treatment showed mean viral load reductions ranging from 2.02 to 2.43 $\log_{10}$ copies/mL across the dose groups; these reduc-

Key Points (cont.)

- One HIV entry inhibitor maraviroc (UK-427,857) has entered phase III testing, and several have also entered phase II testing: BMS-488043, PRO-542, TNX-355, SCH D, and GW873140 .
- Other novel HIV drug targets in development include integrase inhibitors and maturation inhibitors; all are only in preclinical or phase I development, except for the maturation inhibitor PA-457 (phase II).

tions were maintained for at least 2 weeks following the end of treatment (Otto et al. 2003). A phase II study is under way to investigate the efficacy and safety of Racivir as a replacement for lamivudine in treatment-experienced patients who have lamivudine drug resistance (Pharmasset 2004).

Reverset (D-d4FC) is another cytidine analog NRTI that is active in vitro against HIV resistant to other NRTIs. In a phase II study, 30 treatment-naive participants with viral loads above 5000 copies/mL received 10 once-daily doses of D-d4FC monotherapy or placebo. Preliminary results showed mean viral load declines of 1.67 $\log_{10}$ copies/mL for the 50 mg dose, 1.74 $\log_{10}$ copies/mL for 100 mg and 1.77 $\log_{10}$ copies/mL for 200 mg. Maximum reductions ranged from 1.2 to 2.3 $\log_{10}$ copies/mL (Murphy et al. 2004a). In a phase II study of 10 heavily NRTI-experienced patients failing their current therapy with a mean HIV RNA level of 4.53 $\log_{10}$ copies/mL, Reverset 200 mg once daily was added to the failing regimens of 8 patients for 10 days. At day 11, the Reverset regimen achieved a mean viral load decrease of 0.8 $\log_{10}$ copies/mL, with 4 of the 8 patients achieving viral loads below 400 copies/mL. Prior to receiving Reverset, 5 of the 8 patients had the M184V mutation and 4 had 3 or more thymidine analog resistance mutations (Murphy et al. 2004b).

SPD754 is also a cytidine analog NRTI in phase II testing. Like, D-d4FC, it shows in vitro activity against thymidine analog- and lamivudine-resistant isolates (Bethell et al. 2003). A 10-day randomized, placebo-controlled monotherapy study in 63 treatment-naive patients observed reductions of 1.16 to 1.65 $\log_{10}$ copies/mL in viral load using a range of doses (Cahn et al. 2003). Adverse events were mild to moderate and similar in both treatment groups. No new NRTI mutations were identified during 24 days of follow-up. A recent in vitro study showed that lamivudine antagonized the antiviral activity of SPD754 through an intracellular drug-drug interaction (Bethell et al. 2004).

Nonnucleoside reverse transcriptase inhibitors (NNRTIs)

Capravirine (AG1549) is an NNRTI with potent activity against HIV, including strains with the K103 mutation. Preliminary phase II data from an ongoing study showed that 50% of those receiving capravirine had viral loads below 400 copies/mL at 12 weeks. Moderate nausea, vomiting, and diarrhea were reported (Wolfe et al. 2001). Clinical research was put on partial hold by the FDA in January 2001 when toxicology studies revealed vasculitis in dogs that had received high doses of capravirine. In November 2001, FDA allowed research to resume after clinical monitoring showed no increase in vasculitis compared with subjects receiving placebo (Hawley et al. 2002). Thirty-six of the participants who achieved viral loads below 400 copies/mL in the phase II capravirine study continued in an open-label extension phase (Hammond et al. 2003). Sixteen of those still had viral loads below 400 copies/mL after 28 to 34 months of capravirine. Six of the 20 discontinuations were due to virologic failure, and 5 were due to adverse events. Several phase II and III trials are ongoing.

TMC125 (etravirine), a diaminopyrimidine (DAPY) derivative, is a new NNRTI with potent in vitro activity against both wild-type and resistant HIV by virtue of its flexible binding site. In a phase II study of patients with phenotypic resistance to NNRTIs, the median viral load decrease from baseline was 0.9 $\log_{10}$ copies/mL after 7 days of replacing patients' current NNRTI with TMC125 (Gazzard et al. 2002). Mild diarrhea and headache were the most common adverse events. A second study involved 1 week of TMC125 monotherapy (900 mg twice daily) or placebo in 19 treatment-naive patients. In the 12 patients receiving TMC125, a sharp median decline of 1.99 $\log_{10}$ copies/mL in viral load compared with a mean 0.06-$\log_{10}$ copies/mL decline in the placebo group ($P < .001$) (Gruzdev et al. 2003). Initial problems with the cumbersome formulation have been overcome, and the drug is undergoing larger clinical trials.

Another DAPY derivative, TMC278, is also being developed as a once-daily oral NNRTI. In vitro data show TMC278 to be highly active against wild-type and resistant HIV-1. In healthy volunteers, this investigational NNRTI was well tolerated and displayed a pharmacokinetic profile indicative of once-daily dosing (de Béthune et al. 2005). In a dose-finding phase II study of TMC278 given as monotherapy twice daily to treatment-naive HIV-infected patients, all doses produced a greater than 1 log_{10} drop in HIV RNA level by day 8 (Goebel et al. 2005). The lowest dose tested, 25 mg, was as potent as higher doses. Given the low dose required for potent antiviral activity, this agent has the potential to be used as part of a fixed-dose combination. TMC278 is also being evaluated in treatment-experienced patients.

Protease inhibitors (PIs)

Tipranavir is active in vitro against a variety of strains resistant to all of the current PIs (Cooper et al. 2003; Gathe et al. 2003; Yeni et al. 2003; Back et al. 2000; Larder et al. 2000; Rusconi et al. 2000). Phase I/II testing demonstrated efficacy and tolerability of a range of doses of tipranavir coadministered with ritonavir (Gathe et al. 2003). It must be boosted with ritonavir to reduce its pill burden and achieve adequate plasma levels. Although it does have significant gastrointestinal toxicity, little laboratory toxicity was seen in a clinical trial (McCallister et al. 2004). In a study (BI 1182.51) of patients with multiple PI resistance mutations, short-term (2-week) response to tipranavir/ritonavir alone was better than with comparator boosted-PI regimens (Mayers et al. 2004). However, in another study, when tipranavir was added to other PIs as part of a dual-PI-boosted regimen, substantial decreases occurred in the other PI concentrations (Walmsley et al. 2004).

Tipranavir is currently under accelerated approval review at the FDA. The basis for the safety and efficacy of tipranavir are the results from the RESIST-1 and -2 phase III studies. In the RESIST-1 study, a total of 620 heavily treatment-experienced patients were randomized to receive either tipranavir/ritonavir or an optimized comparator PI boosted with ritonavir. A planned 24-week analysis demonstrated that tipranavir/ritonavir was superior to the comparator PI in terms of the proportion of patients achieving undetectable viral loads (34.7% vs. 16.5%) and in median increases in CD4 counts (36 vs. 6 cells/mm^3) (Hicks et al. 2004). The RESIST-2 study is of similar study design but was conducted in Europe and Latin America. The planned interim 24-week results were similar to those of the RESIST-1 study: An intent-to-treat analysis showed that 41.0% in the boosted tipranavir arm and 14.9% in the comparator arm had achieved viral load decreases of more than 1 log_{10} copies/mL, with both arms having a similar incidence of serious adverse events (13.8% vs. 12.1%) (Cahn 2004). Of note, patients in both studies had to have at least 1 primary PI mutation but no more than 2 mutations associated with tipranavir resistance (i.e., mutations at codons 33, 82, 84 and 90). In a further analysis of the 24-week data from over 1100 patients in the RESIST trials, the treatment response of tipranavir/ritonavir was compared with that of lopinavir/ritonavir. The results showed that the tipranavir regimen was superior for all efficacy variables tested, even when controlling for the number of other active agents in the regimen and enfuvirtide use (Cooper et al. 2005). However, there were no statistically significant differences in the proportions of subjects achieving a decline in viral load of 1 log_{10} copies/mL or more when comparing tipranavir/ritonavir and lopinavir/ritonavir in subjects who were not on lopinavir/ritonavir at study entry or in subjects with virus susceptible to lopinavir. This report also demonstrated superior outcomes in subjects who received enfuvirtide as part of their background combination, whether or not they were enfuvirtide naive at study entry.

TMC114 is a PI with activity against PI-resistant HIV. It is now being studied in phase III trials. In a 14-day open-label randomized study, TMC114 with low-dose ritonavir (TMC114/r) replaced 50 patients' PI in their previously failing regimen. The TMC114/r replacement effected a median viral load reduction of 1.35 log_{10} copies/mL. The most common adverse events were gastrointestinal. Interim analysis of 24 week data from two 96-week dose-finding trials of TMC114 showed that all doses produced significantly better virologic responses compared with patients who received an investigator-determined optimized PI-based regimen (Katlama et al. 2005). The highest dose studied, 600 mg twice daily plus ritonavir 100 mg twice daily, produced the greatest reduction in viral load, more than 1.8 $\log_{10}$ copies/mL below baseline levels, and 67% of enfuvirtide-naive subjects who received enfuvirtide plus TMC114 600 mg twice daily achieved a viral load below 50 copies/mL after 24 weeks of therapy.

Investigational Agents: New Antiretroviral Classes

Entry inhibitors

Entry inhibitors are an attractive area for drug development due to the multiple steps involved in entry, including viral attachment, coreceptor binding, and fusion (Doms 2004). HIV entry into cells begins with attachment of HIVgp120 to the cellular CD4 receptor. This leads to conformational changes in gp120 which, in turn, lead to exposure of areas on the molecule that attach to one of the chemokine coreceptors (CXCR4 for lymphotropic viruses or CCR5 for macrophage-tropic viruses). The interaction results in gp120 exposure and viral gp41 release, leading to fusion with the cell membranes and viral entry into the cell. The entry inhibitors can be broken down into subgroups: attachment inhibitors, coreceptor CXCR4 and CCR5 inhibitors, and fusion inhibitors. The fusion inhibitor enfuvirtide (Fuzeon or T-20) is the first drug of this class approved by the FDA. By simultaneously targeting multiple entry steps, synergistic drug activity may emerge (Doms 2004).

The lead follow-on compound to enfuvirtide was T-1249, which was effective in patients with virus resistant to other antiretrovirals, including enfuvirtide (Lalezari et al. 2003). In January 2004, the manufacturer indefinitely suspended study of this fusion inhibitor, "due to challenges in achieving the technical profile of the current formulation" (Roche 2004).

Attachment by HIV to a CD4 cell can be inhibited by blocking host cell receptors, e.g., by using humanized monoclonal anti-CD4 antibodies (TNX-355) or by blocking viral antigens, e.g., with compounds that bind to gp120 (BMS-488043 and PRO-542).

A phase IIa trial investigating the attachment inhibitor BMS-488043 enrolled 30 untreated HIV-infected individuals (Bristol-Myers Squibb 2004; Hanna et al. 2004). Twelve received 800 mg BMS-488043 twice daily, 12 received 1800 mg twice daily, and 6 received placebo. After 8 days, the 800 mg arm had a mean drop in viral load of 0.72 $\log_{10}$ copies/mL. The majority of participants in both treatment arms experienced viral load decreases greater than 1 $\log_{10}$ copies/mL.

PRO 542 is a recombinant immunoglobulin that targets the gp120 envelope protein. The drug must be given parenterally, and phase I/II testing demonstrated viral load reductions greater than 0.7 $\log_{10}$ copies/mL in pediatric patients (PACTG 351) (Shearer et al. 2000). In a single-dose study of PRO 542 in infected adults with advanced HIV disease, significant mean viral load reductions of approximately 0.5 $\log_{10}$ copies/mL were seen for 4 to 6 weeks in all patients (Jacobson et al. 2004).

Entry of HIV into the host cell can also be blocked by inhibition of the chemokine coreceptors CCR5 and CXCR4. SCH C and SCH D are both orally available small molecules that are highly active antagonists of the CCR5 receptor. A dose-escalation study of SCH C monotherapy observed 10-day viral load declines of 0.68, 1.23 and 1.50 $\log_{10}$ copies/mL at twice-daily doses of 25, 50 and 100 mg, respectively (Schurmann et al. 2004). Cardiac arrhythmia (QTc prolongation) has been seen with SCH C, and research on this drug has been discontinued. SCH D is 10 times more potent in vitro than SCH C. A 14-day dose-ranging trial for SCH D monotherapy enrolled 48 HIV-infected volunteers (Schurmann et al. 2004). Participants, who were not currently receiving treatment, took placebo or twice-daily doses of SCH D 10 mg, 25 mg or 50 mg. Mean viral load reductions were

1.08, 1.56 and 1.62 log_{10} copies/mL, respectively. No significant QTc prolongation has been observed with this compound to date. A phase II study of SCH-D is currently under way within the ACTG.

Another oral CCR5 antagonist with potent in vitro activity is maraviroc (UK-427,857). Twenty-five asymptomatic HIV-infected patients received 25 mg once daily, 100 mg twice daily or placebo for 10 days in a dose-ranging study (Pozniak et al. 2003). Trial participants were prescreened for the presence of only R5 HIV strains. Those receiving 100 mg twice daily had a mean viral load reduction of 1.42 log_{10} copies/mL by day 11, whereas those receiving 25 mg once daily experienced a mean viral load drop of 0.42 log_{10} copies/mL. Phase III studies of maraviroc in treatment-naive and treatment-experienced patients are in progress.

GW873140 is a CCR5 antagonist in phase II trials. It has been shown to have a prolonged duration (over 100 hours) of binding to the CCR5 coreceptor (Demarest 2004). A 10-day monotherapy study showed mean viral load reductions of up to 1.66 log_{10} copies/mL in treatment-naive and -experienced patients (Lalezari at al. 2004).

A concern with CCR5 coreceptor inhibitors is whether blocking this coreceptor will induce HIV to switch to using the CXCR4 coreceptor for entry. CXCR4 tropism has correlated with disease progression. So far, no definitive conclusions can be drawn, but all CCR5 coreceptor inhibitors tested clinically so far appear safe (Kuritzkes 2005). A retrospective analysis of a coreceptor study in which CXCR4-using HIV emerged in 2 patients during treatment concluded that these HIV variants most likely came from a pretreatment viral reservoir (Lewis et al. 2004). CCR5 and CXCR4 coreceptor inhibitors will likely need to be combined in the treatment of patients with mixed HIV populations of this sort as well as those with dual tropic viruses.

Integrase inhibitors

Integration of viral DNA into the host's genomic DNA is required for both viral transcription and latent infection. Integrase is the viral enzyme responsible for this action. The 2 lead compounds developed as integrase inhibitors were S-1360 and L-870,810, but the development of both of these compounds has been discontinued (Merck 2004; Glaxo 2003). However, a 10-day dosing study of L-870,810 documented a greater than 1.7 log_{10} copies/mL mean reduction in viral load in subjects receiving either of two doses of L-870,810 (Little et al. 2005), demonstrating that in vivo activity of an integrase inhibitor can be achieved. One follow-up compound, C-2507, is in phase I trials (Merck 2004), but no data are available.

Maturation inhibitors

PA-457 is the first in the class of maturation inhibitors (Li et al. 2003). This drug prevents conversion of capsid precursor proteins to mature capsid proteins (p24), resulting in release of virus that is noninfectious. PA-457 has demonstrated in vitro activity against wild-type and resistant viruses. PA-457 appears to have a suitable half-life, is orally bioavailable, and does not interact with the cytochrome P450 system. It is now in phase II testing.

Table IV.32-1. Status of investigational agents: NRTIs, NNRTIs, and PIs as of March 2005.

Drug code/Generic name	Development phase I	II	III	FDA review	Comment
NRTIs					
Reverset (D-d4FC)			X		
Alovudine (MIV-310)		X			
Amdoxovir (DAPD)		X			
Elvucitabine (beta-L-Fd4C)		X			
Racivir (RCV-201)		X			
SPD 754 (DOTC)		X			
GS 7340 (Gilead)		X			Discontinued
D-FDOC	X				
SN1212	Preclin				
NNRTIs					
Capravirine			X		
Calanolide A		X			
Etravirine (TMC125)		X			
TMC278		X			
GW678248X (prodrug = GW695634)	X				
CSIC	Preclin				
DAPY/DATA	Preclin				
UC781	Preclin				
PIs					
Tipranavir (BI)				X	
TMC114			X		
AG 1859		X			
640385 (GSK)	X				
Ro-033-4649	X				
P-1946	Preclin				
GS 9005 (Gilead)	Preclin				Discontinued

Table IV.32-2. Investigational agents: new antiretroviral classes.

Drug code/Generic name	Development phase I	II	III	FDA review	Comment
		Entry inhibitors			
CCR5 coreceptor antagonists					
Maraviroc (UK-427,857)			X		
GW873140		X			
SCH 417690 (SCH-D)		X			
PRO 140	X				
AK602	Preclin				
RANTES analogs	Preclin				
TAK-220	Preclin				
Attachment inhibitors					
BMS-488043		X			Binds gp120
PRO 542		X			Anti-gp120 antibody
TNX-355		X			Anti-CD4 antibody
Fusion inhibitors					
NB-2, NB-64	Preclin				
T-649	Preclin				
CXCR4 coreceptor antagonists					
AMD070	X				
AL40-YV	Preclin				
KRH-2731-5HCL	Preclin				
T-22	Preclin				
TAK-779	Preclin				
		Maturation inhibitors			
PA-457		X			
		Integrase inhibitors			
C-2507	X				
L-870,810	X				On hold
S-1360	X				On hold
Styrylquinolones	Preclin				
V-165	Preclin				
		Others			
D-amino acid peptides	Preclin				
RNAse H inhibitors	Preclin				
Zinc finger inhibitors	Preclin				

Note: Additional agents may have entered advanced-phase clinical trials after the time of this publication (early 2005). More current information about clinical trial eligibility and locations may be available from AIDSinfo, sponsored by the U.S. Department of Health and Human Services, at http://www.aidsinfo.nih.gov.

References

Arasteh K, Clumeck N, Pozniak A, et al. Antiretroviral activity, safety and pharmacokinetics of TMC114, a next-generation protease inhibitor (PI) in multiple PI-experienced patients. In: Program and abstracts of the 2nd International AIDS Society Conference on Pathogenesis and Treatment; July 13-16, **2003**; Paris, France. Abstract LB16.

Back NK, van Wijk A, Remmerswaal D, et al. In-vitro tipranavir susceptibility of HIV-1 isolates with reduced susceptibility to other protease inhibitors. *AIDS*. **2000**;14:101-102.

Bethell R, Adams J, De Muys J, et al. Pharmacological evaluation of a dual deoxycytidine analogue combination: 3TC and SPD754. In: Program and abstracts of the 11th Conference on Retroviruses and Opportunistic Infections; February 8-11, **2004**; San Francisco, California. Abstract 138.

Bethell RC, Parkin N, Lie Y. Antiviral activity of SPD754 against clinical isolates of HIV-1 resistant to other nucleoside reverse transcriptase inhibitors. *Antivir Ther.* **2003**;8:S6.

Boehringer Ingelheim. Boehringer Ingelheim Announces U.S. Expanded Access In: Program for Anti-HIV Drug Tipranavir [PR Newswire]. November 20, **2004**. Available at: http://www.prnewswire.com/cgi-bin/stories.pl?ACCT=109&STORY=/www/story/11-30-2004/0002555041&EDATE [accessed January 5, 2005].

Bristol-Myers Squibb. Bristol-Myers Squibb presents data providing proof-of-concept for novel experimental oral attachment inhibitor, a potential new class of antiretroviral therapy [press release]. February 11, **2004**. Available at: http://www.bms.com/news/press/data/pf_press_release_4337.html [accessed March 7, 2004].

Cahn P. 24-week data from RESIST-2: phase 3 study of the efficacy and safety of either tipranavir/ritonavir (TPV/r) or an optimized ritonavir-boosted standard-of-care (SOC) comparator PI (CPI) in a large randomized multicenter trial in treatment-experienced HIV+ patients. In: Program and abstracts of the 7th International Congress on Drug Therapy and HIV Infection; November 14-18, **2004**; Glasgow, United Kingdom. Abstract PL14.3.

Cahn P, Lange J, Cassetti I, et al. Anti HIV-1 activity of SPD754 a new NRTI: results of a 10 day monotherapy study in treatment naïve patients. In: Program and abstracts of the 2nd International AIDS Society Conference on Pathogenesis and Treatment, July 13-16, **2003**; Paris, France. Abstract LB15.

Cooper D, Hall D, Jayaweera D, et al. Baseline phenotypic susceptibility to tipranavir/ritonavir is retained in isolates from patients with multiple protease inhibitor experience (BI 1182.52). In: Program and abstracts of the 10th Conference on Retroviruses and Opportunistic Infections: February 10-14, **2003**; Boston, Massachusetts. Abstract 596.

Cooper D, Hicks C, Cahn P, et al. 24-Week RESIST study analyses: the efficacy of tipranavir/ritonavir is superior to lopinavir/ritonavir, and the TPV/r treatment response is enhanced by inclusion of genotypically active antiretrovirals in the optimized background regimen. In: Program and abstracts of the 12th Conference on Retroviruses and Opportunistic Infections, February 22-25, **2005**; Boston, Massachusetts. Abstract 560.

de Béthune MP, Andries K, Azijn H, et al. TMC278, a new potent NNRTI, with an increased barrier to resistance and good pharmacokinetic profile. In: Program and abstracts of the 12th Conference on Retroviruses and Opportunistic Infections, February 22-25, **2005**; Boston, Massachusetts. Abstract 556.

Demarest J, Sparks S, Watson C, McDanal C, Kenakin TP, Shibayama S. Prolonged and unique binding of a novel CCR5 antagonist, 873140. In: Program and abstracts of the 44th Interscience Conference on Antimicrobial Agents and Chemotherapy; October 30-November 2, **2004**; Washington, DC. Abstract H-211.

Department of Health and Human Services (DHHS). Amdoxovir: Technical Version. AIDSinfo Drug Database. May 20, **2004**. Available at: http://aidsinfo.nih.gov/drugs/htmldrug_tech.asp?int_id=0359 [accessed January 6, 2005.]

Doms RW. Unwelcome guests with master keys: how HIV enters cells and how it can be stopped. *Top HIV Med.* **2004**;12:100-103.

Dunkle LM, Gathe JC, Pedevillano DE, et al. Elvucitabine: Potent antiviral activity demonstrated in multidrug resistant HIV infection. *Antivir Ther.* **2003**;8:S5.

Gathe J, Kohlbrenner VM, Pierone G, et al. Tipranavir/ritonavir demonstrates potent efficacy in multiple protease inhibitor experienced patients: BI 1182-52. In: Program and abstracts of the 10th Conference on Retroviruses and Opportunistic Infections; February 10-14, **2003**; Boston, Massachusetts. Abstract 179.

Gazzard B, Pozniak A, Arasteh A, et al. TMC125, a next-generation NNRTI, demonstrates high potency after 7 days therapy in treatment-experienced HIV-1-infected individuals with phenotypic NNRTI resistance. In: Program and abstracts of the 9th Conference on Retroviruses and Opportunistic Infections; February 24-28, **2002**; Seattle, Washington. Abstract 4.

Gilead Sciences. Gilead, Emory University and the University of Georgia Research Foundation end licensing agreement for amdoxovir, investigational agent for HIV [press release]. Foster City, California. January 28, **2004**. Available at: http://www.gilead.com/wt/sec/pr_1075260536 [accessed March 7, 2004].

GlaxoSmithKline. Results announcement for the second quarter 2003. London, United Kingdom. July 23, **2003**. Available at http://213.219.8.102/pdfs/gsk/q2_2003/gsk_q22003_results.pdf [accessed February 8, 2005].

Goebel F, Yakovlev A, Pozniak A, et al. TMC278: Potent anti-HIV activity in antiretroviral therapy-naïve patients. In: Program and abstracts of the 12th Conference on Retroviruses and Opportunistic Infections, February 22-25, **2005**; Boston, Massachusetts. Abstract 160.

Gruzdev B, Rakhmanova A, Doubovskaya E, et al. A randomized, double-blind, placebo-controlled trial of TMC125 as 7-day monotherapy in antiretroviral naïve, HIV-1 infected subjects. *AIDS.* **2003**;17:2487-2494.

Hammond JL, Amantea M, Raber S, et al. Long-term virologic response to capravirine in HIV-infected, NNRTI-experienced patients. In: Program and abstracts of the 43rd Interscience Conference on Antimicrobial Agents and Chemotherapy; September 14-17, **2003**; Chicago, Illinois. Abstract H-871.

Hanna G, Lalezari J, Hellinger J, et al. Antiviral activity, safety, and tolerability of a novel, oral small-molecule HIV-1 attachment inhibitor, BMS-488043, in HIV-1-infected subjects. In: Program and abstracts of the 11th Conference on Retroviruses and Opportunistic Infections; February 8-11, **2004**; San Francisco, California. Abstract 141.

Hawley P, Diniz-Piraino W, Paxton W, et al. Absence of risk of vasculitis in a HIV population taking capravirine-results of an active monitoring plan. In: Program and abstracts of the 14th International AIDS Conference, July 7-12, **2002**; Barcelona, Spain. Abstract TuPeB4549.

Hicks C. RESIST-1: a phase 3, randomized, controlled, open-label, multicenter trial comparing tipranavir/ritonavir (TPV/r) to an optimized comparator protease inhibitor/r (CPI/r) regimen in antiretroviral (ARV) experienced patients: 24-week data. In: Program and abstracts of the 44th Interscience Conference on Antimicrobial Agents and Chemotherapy; October 30-November 2, **2004**; Washington, DC. Abstract H-1137a.

Jacobson JM, Israel RJ, Lowy I, et al. Treatment of advanced human immunodeficiency virus type 1 disease with the viral entry inhibitor PRO 542. *Antimicrob Agents Chemother.* **2004**;48:423-429.

Katlama C, Ghosn J, Tubiana R, et al. MIV-310 reduces HIV viral load in patients failing multiple antiretroviral therapy: results from a 4-week phase II study. *AIDS.* **2004**;18:1299-1304.

Katlama C, Berger D, Bellos N, et al. Efficacy of TMC114/r in 3-class experienced patients with limited treatment options: 24-week planned interim analysis of 2 96-week multinational dose-finding trials. In: Program and abstracts of the 12th Conference on Retroviruses and Opportunistic Infections, February 22-25, **2005**; Boston, Massachusetts. Abstract 164LB.

Kuritzkes D. Clinical activity and efficacy trials of chemokine receptor inhibitors. In: Program and abstracts of the 12th Conference on Retroviruses and Opportunistic Infections, February 22-25, **2005**; Boston, Massachusetts. Abstract 57.

Lalezari JP, Bellos N, Richmond G, et al. Final analysis of T1249-102: T-1249 retains potent short term antiviral activity in patients who have failed a regimen containing enfuvirtide (ENF). In: Program and abstracts of the 43rd Interscience Conference on Antimicrobial Agents and Chemotherapy; September 14-17, **2003**. Chicago, Illinois. Abstract H-444.

Lalezari J, Thompson M, Kumar P, et al. 873140, a novel CCR5 antagonist: antiviral activity and safety during short-term monotherapy in HIV-infected adults. In: Program and abstracts of the 44th Interscience Conference on Antimicrobial Agents and Chemotherapy; October 30-November 2, **2004**; Washington, DC. Abstract H-1137b.

Larder BA, Hertogs K, Bloor S, et al. Tipranavir inhibits broadly protease inhibitor-resistant HIV-1 clinical samples. *AIDS.* **2000**;14:1942-1948.

Lewis ME, Van der Ryst E, Youle M, et al. Phylogenetic analysis and co-receptor tropism of HIV-1 envelope sequences from two patients with emergence of CXCR4 using virus following treatment with the CCR5 antagonist UK-427,857. In: Program and abstracts of the 44th Interscience Conference on Antimicrobial Agents and Chemotherapy; October 30-November 2, **2004**; Washington, DC. Abstract H-584b.

Li F, Goila-Gaur R, Salzwedel K, et al. PA-457: a potent HIV inhibitor that disrupts core condensation by targeting a late step in Gag processing. *Proc Natl Acad Sci U S A.* **2003**;100:13555-13560.

Little S, Drusano G, Schooley R, et al. Antiretroviral effect of L-000870810, a novel HIV-1 integrase inhibitor, in HIV-1-infected patients. In: Program and abstracts of the 12th Conference on Retroviruses and Opportunistic Infections, February 22-25, **2005**; Boston, Massachusetts. Abstract 161.

McCallister S, Valdez H, Curry K, et al. A 14-day dose-response study of the efficacy, safety, and pharmacokinetics of the nonpeptidic protease inhibitor tipranavir in treatment-naive HIV-1-infected patients. *J Acquir Immune Defic Syndr.* **2004**;35:376-382.

Mayers D, Leith J, Valdez H, et al. Impact of three or four protease mutations at codons 33, 82, 84 and 90 on 2 week virological responses to tipranavir, lopinavir, amprenavir and saquinavir all boosted by ritonavir in Phase 2B trial BI 1182.51. [Abstract 147]. *Antivir Ther.* **2004**;9:S163

Merck & Co. Annual Report 2003. Whitehouse Station, NJ. March 1, **2004**. Available at: http://www.merck.com/finance/annualreport/ar2003/home/index.html [accessed February 8, 2005].

Murphy RL, Schürmann D, Beard A, Cartee L, Schinazi RF, Otto MJ. Tolerance and potent anti-HIV-1 activity of Reverset following 10 days of monotherapy in treatment-naive individuals. In: Program and abstracts of the 11th Conference on Retroviruses and Opportunistic Infections; February 8-11, **2004a**; San Francisco, California. Abstract 137.

Murphy RL, Schurmann D, Levy R, et al. Tolerance and anti-HIV activity of Reverset following 10 days as add-on therapy to current regimens in treatment-experienced HIV-infected individuals. In: Program and abstracts of the 44th Interscience Conference on Antimicrobial Agents and Chemotherapy; October 30-November 2, **2004b**; Washington, DC. Abstract H-1130.

Otto MJ, Arasteh K, Kreckel P, et al. Sustained anti-HIV-1 effect of Racivir combined with d4T and Sustiva following a 14-day treatment of infected volunteers. In: Program and abstracts of the 10th Conference on Retroviruses and Opportunistic Infections; February 10-14, **2003**; Boston, Massachusetts. Abstract 552.

Pharmasset. Pharmasset Initiates Racivir Phase II HIV Study [Press Release]. Atlanta, Georgia: November 10, **2004**. Available at: http://www.pharmasset.com [accessed January 6, 2005].

Pozniak AL, Fätkenheuer G, Johnson M, et al. Effect of short-term monotherapy with UK-427,857 on viral load in HIV-infected patients. In: Program and abstracts of the 43rd Interscience Conference on Antimicrobial Agents and Chemotherapy; September 14-17, **2003**; Chicago, Illinois. Abstract H-443.

Roche. Following the successful development of Fuzeon, Roche and Trimeris sign new research agreement to develop next generation HIV fusion inhibitors [press release]. Basel, Switzerland. January 6, **2004**. Available at: http://www.roche.com/med-corp-detail-2004?id=1107&media-language=e [accessed March 7, 2004].

Rusconi S, La Seta Catamancio S, Citterio P, et al. Susceptibility to PNU-140690 (tipranavir) of human immunodeficiency virus type 1 isolates derived from patients with multidrug resistance to other protease inhibitors. *Antimicrob Agents Chemother.* **2000**;44:1328-1332.

Schurmann D, Rouzier R, Nougarede R, et al. SCH D: antiviral activity of a CCR5 receptor antagonist. In: Program and abstracts of the 11th Conference on Retroviruses and Opportunistic Infections; February 8-11, **2004**; San Francisco, California. Abstract 140LB.

Shearer WT, Israel RJ, Starr S, et al. Recombinant CD4-IgG2 in human immunodeficiency virus type 1-infected children: phase 1/2 study. *J Infect Dis.* **2000**;182:1774-1779.

Stypinski D, Pottage JC Jr, Gustavson LM, Gorski HA, Lavigne J, Ducharme MP. Optimization of the therapeutic index of elvucitabine through PK/PD modeling. In: Program and abstracts of the 5th International Workshop on Clinical Pharmacology of HIV Therapy; April 1-3, **2004**; Rome, Italy. Abstract 38.

Thompson M, Richmond G, Kessler H, et al. Preliminary results of dosing of amdoxovir in treatment-experienced patients. In: Program and abstracts of the 10th Conference on Retroviruses and Opportunistic Infections; February 10-14, **2003**; Boston, Illinois. Abstract 554.

Walmsley S, Leith J, Katlama C, et al. Pharmacokinetics and safety of tipranavir/ritonavir (TPV/r) alone or in combination with saquinavir (SQV), amprenavir (APV), or lopinavir (LPV): interim analysis of BI1182.51. In: Program and abstracts of the XV International AIDS Conference; July 11-16, **2004**; Bangkok, Thailand. Abstract WeOrB1236.

Wolfe P, Hawley P, Boccia G, et al. Safety and efficacy of capravirine versus placebo in HIV-infected patients failing a nonnucleoside-reverse-transcriptase-inhibitor-containing regimen: results of a phase II, double-blind, placebo-controlled study. In: Program and abstracts of the 8th Conference on Retroviruses and Opportunistic Infections; February 4-8, **2001**; Chicago, Illinois. Abstract 323.

Yeni P, MacGregor T, Gathe J, et al. Correlation of viral load reduction and plasma levels in multiple protease inhibitor experienced patients taking tipranavir/ritonavir in a phase IIB trial: BI 1182.52. In: Program and abstracts of the 10th Conference on Retroviruses and Opportunistic Infections: February 10-14, **2003**; Boston, Massachusetts. Abstract 528.

(RLO-36)

IV.33. INVESTIGATIONAL STRATEGIES UTILIZING APPROVED ANTIRETROVIRALS

LEARNING OBJECTIVE: Discuss current data on investigational strategies utilizing FDA-approved antiretroviral agents.

Initial Therapy

Current treatment guidelines for treatment-naive patients recommend pairing a dual nucleoside reverse transcriptase inhibitor (NRTI) backbone with either a protease inhibitor (PI) or nonnucleoside reverse transcriptase inhibitor (NNRTI). Recent studies have challenged this treatment paradigm by proposing novel combinations of available drugs. The rationale for such research includes attempts at reducing side effects, preserving treatment options and minimizing treatment costs. The following update describes various studies looking into novel antiretroviral combinations and strategies for treatment-naive patients.

NRTI-sparing regimens

NRTIs may cause a wide variety of toxicities, such as lactic acidosis, hepatic steatosis, pancreatitis, myopathy, peripheral neuropathy and lipoatrophy (see Objectives IV.8 on Common Antiretroviral Toxicities, and IV.49 on Metabolic Complications in this Update). One plausible way to avoid these adverse effects is to avoid NRTIs altogether by using so-called "NRTI-sparing" regimens. NRTI-sparing regimens would also prevent HIV from developing resistance to this class of drugs, permitting their full impact in salvage therapy. Non-NRTI regimens employ either an NNRTI-PI combination or a boosted PI as monotherapy.

NNRTI-PI combinations. DMP 006, the pivotal trial for efavirenz, incorporated an efavirenz/indinavir arm in the study design. The efavirenz/indinavir arm was found to be inferior compared with the zidovudine/lamivudine/efavirenz arm but better than zidovudine/lamivudine/indinavir. Indinavir was dosed three times daily while efavirenz was given once daily. Also, combining efavirenz with indinavir accelerated the metabolism of indinavir, leading to suboptimal serum levels even though the indinavir dose was increased from 800 mg three times daily to 1000 mg three times daily (Sustiva 2004).

The concurrent use of ritonavir improves the pharmacokinetics of most PIs (see Objective IV.17 on Boosted Protease Inhibitors in this Update). By achieving increased interdose plasma levels (C_{min}) and overall drug exposure (AUC), ritonavir boosting leads to better viral suppression. Improved pharmacokinetics permits simplified dosing schedules. Various studies have looked at boosted PIs as part of an NRTI-sparing regimen. Stek and colleagues (2003) randomized patients to receive indinavir (800 mg) and ritonavir (100 mg), both twice daily, along with once daily efavirenz (600 mg), with or without stavudine. (Patients on stavudine received either 30 or 40 mg twice daily depending on weight.) After 48 weeks, 53% of patients on the NRTI-sparing arm had viral loads below 50 copies/mL compared with 61% of patients on the stavudine-containing arm (using an intent-to-treat analysis with noncompleters considered failures). Adverse event-related discontinuations were 23% and 17%, respectively. (See also the study by Boyd and colleagues below in treatment-experienced patients.)

The BIKS study (Ferré et al. 2003) tested a combination of efavirenz and lopinavir/ritonavir (Kaletra). BIKS enrolled 86 participants, 65 of whom were treatment-naive. The remaining 21 were NNRTI-naive and had HIV with less than five lopinavir-associated resistance mutations. All participants received an increased dose

What's New

This learning objective is new to the AAHIVM Core Curriculum. See Key Points below for highlights.

Key Points

- Any off-label use of drugs, especially when there is little literature supporting it, should be undertaken with extreme caution and preferably within the context of a controlled trial. The poor outcomes with triple-nucleoside reverse transcriptase inhibitor (NRTI) combinations, such as tenofovir/abacavir/lamivudine, serve as a warning about untested combinations.
- Initial trials have found that NRTI-sparing regimens can have acceptable efficacy, especially with the inclusion of ritonavir-boosted protease inhibitors (PIs).
- Pilot studies have reported indications that ritonavir-boosted lopinavir (Kaletra) might be effective as single-agent therapy.
- Investigations are continuing into induction/maintenance treatment strategies with the aim of inducing prolonged virologic suppression while improving treatment tolerability.
- Maintenance with coformulated zidovudine/lamivudine/abacavir (Trizivir) was effective after four-drug induction therapy, although the latter resulted in a high discontinuation rate. Due to lack of a standard therapy comparator arm, no assumption can be made about the relative efficacy of this induction/maintenance approach.
- Use of double-PI combinations boosted with low-dose ritonavir is a an approach that is under evaluation in deep salvage therapy, but there is as yet no evidence that a double boosted PI offers superior efficacy to single boosted PIs. Pharmacokinetic studies will be critical in determining the drug-drug interactions between the three agents if this strategy is to be useful in the future.

of lopinavir/ritonavir (533.3/133.3 mg twice daily) plus efavirenz (600 mg once daily). After 24 weeks, 76% of patients on treatment had viral loads below 50 copies/mL. The mean CD4+ T cell increase was 162 cells/mm^3. Week-48 response data have yet to be released. Grade 3/4 clinical adverse events occurred in 34 patients, and mostly consisted of central nervous system symptoms and diarrhea. Twenty-nine patients experienced grade 3/4 blood lipid elevations. The median increase in LDL/HDL ratio was 27% at week 24.

Lopinavir/ritonavir single-agent therapy. The absence of lopinavir mutations in treatment-naive studies of lopinavir/ritonavir as well as the high AUC and C_{min} of the drug relative to the inhibitory levels for wild-type HIV have led some investigators to try lopinavir/ritonavir in novel ways. They have tested it either as a single agent, as a component of an induction-maintenance approach or as a once-daily PI.

Gathe and colleagues (2004a) studied 30 treatment-naive volunteers who received lopinavir/ritonavir monotherapy at doses of either 400/100 mg twice daily or 533/133 mg twice daily, depending on body weight (above or below 70 kg). At the end of 48 weeks, 16 (54%) patients still on lopinavir/ritonavir monotherapy had viral loads below 50 copies/mL. Another 3 patients had viral loads below 400 copies/mL. Lopinavir resistance was not detected. There were 11 (37%) discontinuations in this study, including 3 for virologic failures. (See also the study by Arribas and colleagues using induction/maintenance therapy below.)

Once-daily PIs

Once-daily therapy promises to markedly improve patient adherence by simplifying the dosing schedule. Once-daily NRTIs and NNRTIs have become common, supported by plasma and intracellular half-life studies. To date, atazanavir is the only PI approved by the FDA for once-daily dosing without ritonavir boosting. Ritonavir-boosted fosamprenavir is approved for once-daily dosing in treatment-naive patients. (See also Objective IV.11 on Once-Daily Regimens in this Update.)

There are a number of studies investigating the use of other boosted PIs as part of once-daily regimens. One such trial, the SPRINT study, compared once-daily saquinavir/ritonavir (1600/100 mg) with twice-daily indinavir/ritonavir (800/100 mg), both given as components of standard regimens (Montaner et al. 2004). Study participants included 147 patients with viral loads over 5000 copies/mL; patients were PI-naive (90%) or had discontinued PI therapy without viral rebound. Background NRTIs were individually determined. At the end of 24 weeks of therapy, 51% of the saquinavir/ritonavir recipients had viral loads below 50 copies/mL versus 42% of the indinavir/ritonavir recipients. This difference was not statistically significant. Adverse event-related discontinuations were higher in the indinavir/ritonavir arm: seven participants (10%) on saquinavir/ritonavir and 20 (26%) on indinavir/ritonavir discontinued study drugs.

Abbott study 418 compared once- versus twice-daily lopinavir/ritonavir (Kaletra) at doses of 800/200 mg once daily or 400/100 mg twice daily (Gathe et al. 2004b). Trial participants also received once-daily tenofovir (300 mg) and emtricitabine (200 mg) as the NRTI backbone. The study enrolled 190 treatment-naive participants. Virologic results were essentially the same for both arms: An intent-to-treat analysis found that 64% of the twice daily arm and 70% of the once daily arm had viral loads below 50 copies/mL at the end of 48 weeks of therapy. Discontinuations due to grade 3/4 diarrhea were markedly higher among those on once-daily lopinavir/ritonavir: 16% of those in the once daily arm compared with 5% in the twice daily arm. A separately conducted pharmacokinetics study demonstrated lower lopinavir C_{min} when lopinavir/ritonavir was administered once daily as compared with twice daily (Burger et al. 2004).

Induction/maintenance therapy

The induction/maintenance approach, patterned after chemotherapeutic strategies, hypothesizes that an antiretroviral regimen can be simplified by cutting the number of antiretrovirals after achieving virologic suppression. Earlier studies started patients on triple therapy and then maintained them on a reduced regimen of either two NRTIs or one unboosted PI. Patients who continued their initial triple-drug regimen had considerably better virologic outcomes (Flandre et al. 2002; Havlir et al. 1998).

One renewed attempt at maintenance therapy used lopinavir/ritonavir single agent therapy due to its enhanced pharmacokinetics. The Only Kaletra (OK) study enrolled 42 volunteers who were taking lopinavir/ritonavir plus two NRTIs, and had viral loads below 50 copies/mL for at least 6 months (Arribas et al. 2004). Study participants were randomized to either continue their current regimen or to take lopinavir/ritonavir alone. Treatment failure was defined as two viral load measurements above 400 copies/mL or a change in therapy. At the end of 24 weeks, 3 of the 21 patients in the lopinavir/ritonavir single agent therapy arm met the criteria for treatment failure. There were no treatment failures among patients who continued on triple therapy. Investigators found no new PI mutations among the three single-agent failures.

Another variation on the induction-maintenance strategy involves starting with a four-drug regimen in the hopes of rapidly driving down viral loads and subsequently maintaining patients on a more conventional three-drug regimen after viral suppression is achieved. A 2004 meta-analysis of nine trials comparing initial three- and four-drug regimens suggested no difference in outcome (Hill and Moyle 2004). Using either an intent-to-treat or on-treatment analysis, one clinical trial (ACTG 388) found that maintaining a triple-class regimen of zidovudine/lamivudine/indinavir/efavirenz was superior to combinations that either replaced efavirenz with nelfinavir (resulting in a dual PI-containing regimen) or omitted it altogether (resulting in three-drug therapy).

Further information on the benefits of initial quadruple therapy will be available in 2005 from the ACTG A5095 study, a direct comparison of fixed-dose zidovudine/lamivudine/abacavir (Trizivir) plus efavirenz versus fixed-dose zidovudine/lamivudine (Combivir) plus efavirenz in approximately 1000 treatment-naive patients. Interim results led to early termination of a third trial arm, Trizivir alone, due to a nearly two-fold higher failure rate than the other two arms combined (Gulick et al. 2004).

The TIME study administered Trizivir as maintenance therapy after viral load suppression with a four-drug combination (Markowitz et al. 2004). Participants received Trizivir plus efavirenz for one year. At the end of 48 weeks on quadruple therapy, the trial randomized those participants with viral loads below 50 copies/mL to either discontinue efavirenz or continue on quadruple therapy. Only 282 of the initial 448 participants (63%) were available for randomization. At week 96, 79% of those remaining on the four-drug regimen had viral loads below 50 copies/mL compared with 77% of those switched to the triple-NRTI maintenance regimen. The proportions of patients completing the second phase of the trial were 85% for the four-drug arm and 89% for the triple-NRTI maintenance arm. Drug toxicities were reduced and adherence increased on the triple-NRTI combination compared with the four-drug arm. A major limitation of the TIME data is that this study did not include a comparator arm receiving a standard three-drug, two-class combination from the beginning.

The FORTE induction/maintenance trial did include such a comparator arm (Williams et al. 2004). The trial's 122 participants started on a triple-class, four-drug regimen (2 NRTIs/NNRTI/PI) or a three-drug, PI-sparing treatment. Those in the four-drug arm entered maintenance therapy by discontinuing the PI if their viral loads declined to below 50 copies/mL after 24 to 32 weeks. At week 48, 81% of trial participants on induction/maintenance and 65% on standard therapy had viral loads below 50 copies/mL. This difference approached statistical significance (P = .07).

In ACTG A5116, the trend went the other way (Fischl et al. 2005). This trial included 236 patients who had achieved undetectable viral loads on their initial HAART regimen. Subjects were randomized to switch to lopinavir/ritonavir plus efavirenz (an NRTI-sparing combination) or 2 NRTIs plus efavirenz (a PI-sparing combination). At randomization, subjects' median baseline CD4 count was 475 cells/mm^3. During a median 110 weeks follow-up, there were more regimen changes due to toxicity in the lopinavir/ritonavir/efavirenz arm than in the 2 NRTI/efavirenz arm (17% vs. 5%). This difference arose mainly because of triglyceride elevations with the NRTI-sparing regimen. Recipients of this regimen also exhibited higher cholesterol levels. The total virologic failure rate in the two arms was 7%, with a trend favoring the 2 NRTI/efavirenz (P = .088). Finally, in the metabolic sub-study (ACTG A51125S), investigators found that those in the NRTI-sparing group gained limb fat whereas those on the other group lost it (P = .002) (Tebas et al. 2005).

Treatment-Experienced Patients

NRTI-sparing regimens may have a particular niche as salvage therapy. Many patients have experienced treatment failure with multiple standard pre-HAART and HAART therapies. They may either exhibit severe NRTI-related intolerance or develop HIV with broad resistance against NRTIs.

For example, a Thai trial enrolled 61 volunteers who had failed single-class NRTI regimens (Boyd et al. 2004). They had a median viral load of 12,300 copies/mL. All received 800 mg indinavir twice daily/100 mg ritonavir twice daily plus 600 mg efavirenz once daily At week 96, 42 patients (69%) had viral loads below 50 copies/mL. Unfortunately, blood lipids and glucose rose significantly in approximately half of the remaining patients.

Boosted double-PI therapy in PI failures

The use of ritonavir as a PI booster has proven beneficial in overcoming low-level protease resistance, prompting some investigators to investigate boosted double-PI combinations in PI-experienced populations.

The rationale for boosted double-PI combinations comes from the potential synergy between PIs, especially in the setting of mixed viral populations. An isolate resistant to one of the PIs may be susceptible to the other. Because some PIs have the capacity to induce P450 enzymes, the use of PIs in combination can increase the clearance of the other PI and ritonavir, attenuating the boosting effect. The end result may be that neither PI is present at as high a concentration as would be the case if it were the only PI being used with ritonavir. Fosamprenavir taken with lopinavir/ritonavir, for example, results in reduced levels of both lopinavir and amprenavir (Kashuba et al. 2005). Adding on PIs also has its drawbacks in terms of cumulative toxicity. (For additional information on these combinations, see Objective IV.17 on Boosted Protease Inhibitors in this Update.)

Boosted PIs have a very high mutational barrier to resistance and whether boosting two PIs together will necessarily elevate this mutational barrier any further, and increase efficacy in salvage, is an unanswered question. It may turn out that protease inhibitors with demonstrated ability to treat protease resistant strains, such as boosted tipranavir and the experimental compound TMC-114, will prove superior for treating protease resistant virus than boosted double-PI regimens – with less pill burden and toxicity. Additional active agents, including enfuvirtide, may be helpful, too, especially in patients with high PI resistance (as reviewed in Staszewski 2004).

Several small studies indicate that boosted double-PI regimens are at least feasible:

- In the LOPSAQ trial (Staszewski et al. 2004), volunteers from the Frankfort cohort received no NRTIs, just saquinavir-sgc/lopinavir/ritonavir at doses of 1000/400/100 mg twice daily Participants had extensive exposure to antiretrovirals and prior to enrollment had been on failing regimens due to drug resistance or systemic toxicity. Nearly 70% had treatment interruptions before entering the trial. At week 48, only 67 of 126 patients (53%) were still receiving the study drugs. Thirty-seven patients (29%) discontinued due to intolerance. Seventy-seven patients (61%) responded to therapy at some point in the trial, with 50 (40%) achieving viral loads below 50 copies/mL. Nonresponders tended to be those with CD4 counts below 200 cells/mm^3 and extensive PI resistance at the end of their last therapy.
- A related Frankfort cohort study, CRIXILOP (Dauer et al. 2003), evaluated the non-NRTI combination of indinavir/lopinavir/ritonavir at doses of 800/400/100 mg twice daily The trial cohort consisted of 32 highly treatment-experienced patients. Of the 28 evaluable patients at week 24, 10 had discontinued the study regimen: 7 due to indinavir intolerance and 3 because of virologic failure. Among the remaining patients, viral loads decreased to a median of 80 copies/mL from a baseline median of 158,000 copies/mL.
- Another study took place in patients who had no choice – they were either resistant or intolerant to all NRTIs and NNRTIs (Duvivier et al. 2005). Forty-one patients were in each category. In the intolerant group, 71% had baseline viral loads below 400 copies/mL. Active regimens, consisting solely of boosted double-PI combinations, were chosen on the basis of genotypic resistance tests. The most frequent combinations were saquinavir 800 mg/lopinavir 400 mg/ritonavir 100 mg twice daily; indinavir 400 mg/lopinavir 400 mg/ritonavir 100 mg twice daily; and indinavir 400 mg/amprenavir 600 mg/ritonavir 100 mg twice daily. Five cases of virologic failure occurred by week 24. At that point, 82% of the trial participants had viral loads below 400 copies/mL by intent-to-treat analysis. There was considerable gastrointestinal intolerance in the group as a whole, the main reason why 20 persons switched dual PI regimen in the course of the trial.

These results suggest that a boosted double PI alone can be an effective salvage option in situations in which NRTIs are not viable. There remains insufficient information to determine when boosted double PIs are appropriate. Toxicities appear to be great, and there are no data comparing them to boosted single PI regimens, either in terms of toxicity or efficacy.

Note: *All of the strategies described in this Objective remain investigational. The absence of controlled trials in many cases makes it impossible to know how the investigational strategy compares to more conventional therapeutic combinations. The rapid virologic failure in patients treated with triple-nucleoside combinations such as tenofovir, abacavir, and lamivudine, serve as warning that untested or poorly tested combinations may be ineffective due to unanticipated factors such as cross-resistance or drug-drug interactions (see Objective IV.18 on Not-Recommended Antiretroviral Combinations in this Update).*

References

Arribas JR, Pulido F, Lorenzo A, et al. Simplification to lopinavir/r single-drug HAART: 24 weeks results of a randomized controlled, open label, pilot clinical trial (OK study). In: Program and abstracts of the XV International AIDS Conference; July 11-16, **2004**; Bangkok, Thailand. Abstract TuBe4486.

Boyd MA, Siangphoe U, Duncombe CJ, et al. Indinavir/ritonavir 800/100mg bid and efavirenz 600mg qd in patients with combination nucleoside failure: 96 week outcomes of HIV-NAT 009. In: Program and abstracts of the XV International AIDS Conference; July 11-16, **2004**; Bangkok, Thailand. Abstract MoOrB1084.

Burger DM, La Porte CJL, Schippers EF, et al. Pharmacokinetics of once-daily (QD) lopinavir/ritonavir (LPV/r) as part of a regimen also containing two nucleosides administered QD: the influence of dose modifications. In: Program and abstracts of the XV International AIDS Conference; July 11-16, **2004**; Bangkok, Thailand. Abstract TuPeB4607.

Dauer B, Von Hentig N, Müller A, et al. The CRIXILOP cohort study: preliminary results from a salvage study of the boosted double protease inhibitor (PI) regimen containing indinavir (IDV) plus lopinavir/ritonavir (LPV/r) without the addition of reverse transcriptase inhibitors (RTI) in heavily therapy-experienced HIV+ patients. In: Program and abstracts of the 9th European AIDS Conference; October 25-29, **2003**; Warsaw, Poland. Abstract 7.4/4.

Duvivier C, Ghosn J, Wirden M, et al. Efficacy and safety of dual boosted PI regimen without RT inhibitors in HIV-1-infected patients. In: Program and abstracts of the 12th Conference on Retroviruses and Opportunistic Infections; February 22-25, **2005**; Boston, Massachusetts. Abstract 578.

Ferré V, Allavena C, Poizot-Martin I, et al. BIKS study (lopinavir/ritonavir-efavirenz combination): complete 24-week results. *Antivir Ther.* **2003**;8(suppl 1):S193. Abstract 36.

Fischl M, Bassett R, Collier A, et al. Randomized, controlled trial of lopinavir/ritonavir + efavirenz vs efavirenz + 2 nucleoside reverse transcriptase inhibitors following a first suppressive 3- or 4-drug regimen in advanced HIV disease. In: Program and abstracts of the 12th Conference on Retroviruses and Opportunistic Infections; February 22-25, **2005**; Boston, Massachusetts. Abstract 162.

Flandre P, Raffi F, Descamps D, et al. Final analysis of the Trilège induction-maintenance trial: results at 18 months. *AIDS.* **2002**;16:561-568.

Gathe JC, Washington MY, Mayberry C, Piot D, Nemecek J. IMANI-1 TC3WP single drug HAART – proof of concept study. Pilot study of the safety and efficacy of Kaletra (LPV/r) as single drug HAART in HIV+ ARV-naive patients – interim analysis of subjects completing final 48 week data. In: Program and abstracts of the XV International AIDS Conference; July 11-16, **2004a**; Bangkok, Thailand. Abstract MoOrB1057.

Gathe J, Podzamczer D, Johnson M, et al. Once-daily vs. twice-daily lopinavir/ritonavir in antiretroviral-naïve patients: 48-week results. In: Program and abstracts of the 11th Conference on Retroviruses and Opportunistic Infections; February 8-11, **2004b**; San Francisco, California. Poster 570.

Girard PM, Cabie A, Michelet C, et al. EFV/TDF vs EFV/3TC/TDF as maintenance regimen in virologically controlled patients under HAART: a 6-month analysis of the COOL Trial. In: Program and abstracts of the XV International Conference on AIDS; July 11-16, **2004**; Bangkok, Thailand. Abstract TuPeB4493.

Gulick RM, Ribaudo HJ, Shikuma CM, et al. Triple-nucleoside regimens versus efavirenz-containing regimens for the initial treatment of HIV-1 infection. *N Engl J Med.* **2004**;350:1850-1861.

Havlir DV, Marschner IC, Hirsch MS, et al. Maintenance antiretroviral therapies in HIV infected subjects with undetectable plasma HIV RNA after triple-drug therapy. *N Engl J Med.* **1998**;339:1261-1268.

Hill A, Moyle G. A meta-analysis of the virological efficacy of regimens containing four versus three active antiretroviral agents as initial therapy for HIV-1 infection. In: Program and abstracts of the 13th International HIV Drug Resistance Workshop; June 8-12, **2004**; Tenerife, Canary Islands. Poster 164. Available at: http://www.informedhorizons.com/resistance2004 [accessed February 16, 2005].

Kashuba ADM, Tierney C, Downey GF, et al. Combining fosamprenavir with lopinavir/ritonavir substantially reduces amprenavir and lopinavir exposure: ACTG protocol A5143 results. *AIDS.* **2005**;19:145-152.

Markowitz M, Hill-Zabala C, Lang J, et al. Maintenance with Trizivir (TZV) or TZV + efavirenz (EFV) for 48 weeks following a 48-week induction with TZV + EFV in antiretroviral-naive HIV-1 infected subjects (ESS40013). In: Program and abstracts of the XV International AIDS Conference; July 11-16, **2004**; Bangkok, Thailand. Abstract LbOrB14.

Montaner JSG, Press N, Harris M, et al. Simplified Protease Inhibitor Trial (SPRINT): Antiviral effect of once daily saquinavir SGC plus ritonavir (SQV/r) vs twice daily indinavir plus ritonavir (IDV/r). In: Program and abstracts of the XV International AIDS Conference; July 11-16, **2004**; Bangkok, Thailand. Abstract TuPeB4488.

Staszewski S. Potential therapeutic strategies using double-boosted protease inhibitor regimens [iMedOptions, LLC]. June 11, **2004b**. Available at: http://clinicaloptions.com/hiv/manage/doubleboost/# staszewski [accessed February 16, 2005].

Staszewski S, Dauer B, Carlebach A, et al. The LOPSAQ salvage study: 48 week analysis of the full cohort treated with lopinavir (LPV/r) plus saquinavir (SQV) without any additional antiretroviral (ART) therapy. In: Program and abstracts of the XV International AIDS Conference; July 11-16, **2004a**; Bangkok, Thailand. Abstract B10840.

Stek M, Hirschel B, Benetucci J, et al. Comparison of PI-boosted indinavir with efavirenz plus stavudine regimens in EASIER (European and South American study of indinavir, efavirenz, and ritonavir). [Abstract 39.] *Antiviral Ther.* **2003**;8(suppl.1):S194.

Sustiva (efavirenz) [prescribing information]. Princeton, NJ: Bristol-Myers Squibb; December **2004**.

Tebas P, J Zhang J, K Yarasheski K, et al. Switch to a protease inhibitor-containing/nucleoside reverse transcriptase inhibitor-sparing regimen increases appendicular fat and serum lipid levels without affecting glucose metabolism or bone mineral density. The results of a prospective randomized trial, ACTG 5125s. In: Program and abstracts of the 12th Conference on Retroviruses and Opportunistic Infections; February 22-25, **2005**; Boston, Massachusetts. Abstract 40.

Williams I, Asboe D, Babiker A, et al. A virological benefit from an induction/maintenance strategy compared with a standard 3-drug regimen in antiretroviral naïve patients: the FORTE trial. In: Program and abstracts of the 11th Conference on Retroviruses and Opportunistic Infections; February 8-11, **2004**; San Francisco, California. Abstract 564.

(RLO-37)

IV.35. ANTIRETROVIRAL AGENT TOXICITY AND CONTRAINDICATION IN PREGNANCY

LEARING OBJECTIVE: Identify the toxicity of antiretroviral agents in pregnancy and those that are contraindicated in pregnancy and in reproductive-age women not actively avoiding pregnancy.

Many experts would initiate antiretroviral therapy in pregnant HIV-infected women regardless of gestational age of the fetus. Others would not commence treatment during the first trimester unless it is urgently indicated, because of concern about possible teratogenicity during this critical period of organogenesis (Connor et al. 1994). This objective describes specific antiretroviral drugs to avoid or use cautiously during pregnancy. (For further information on considerations and antiretroviral regimens for HIV-infected women during pregnancy and labor, see the other Objectives in Chapter 43 on Pregnancy in the AAHIVM 2003 Study Guide, and Objective IV.38 on Pharmacokinetics of Antiretrovirals in Pregnancy in this Update.)

Pregnancy Categories of Antiretrovirals

The U.S. Food and Drug Administration (FDA) has placed over half of the currently FDA-approved antiretroviral agents in pregnancy category C (USPHS 2004), indicating that "safety in human pregnancy has not been determined, animal studies are either positive for fetal risk or have not been conducted, and the drug should not be used unless the potential benefit outweighs the potential risk to the fetus." The exceptions are atazanavir, didanosine, emtricitabine, enfuvirtide, nelfinavir, ritonavir, saquinavir, and tenofovir, which are in category B, indicating that "animal reproduction studies fail to demonstrate a risk to the fetus but adequate and well-controlled studies of pregnant women have not been conducted." Among these category B drugs, however, the Department of Health and Human Services Guidelines note "insufficient data to recommend use" of atazanavir, enfuvirtide and tenofovir in pregnant women.

As of a labeling change in December 2004, efavirenz, which was previously in pregnancy category C (risk of fetal harm cannot be ruled out), has now been placed in pregnancy category D (positive evidence of fetal risk) (Sustiva 2004). Drugs in this category may cause fetal harm when administered during the first trimester to a pregnant woman. This label change followed four reports of neural tube defects in infants: three newborns with meningomyelocele and one with Dandy Walker syndrome, an abnormality of the cerebellum and fourth ventricle (BMS 2005). The women who gave birth to these children were exposed to efavirenz during the first trimester of their pregnancies. These cases follow the report of myelomeningocele in an infant exposed to efavirenz early in gestation (Fundarò et al. 2002). These abnormalities are consistent with malformations observed in fetuses born to efavirenz-treated animals (USPHS 2004). Therefore, efavirenz should not be used in pregnancy.

Adverse Events With Implications for Pregnancy

A recent search of the Adverse Event Reporting System database of the FDA for hepatic adverse events in HIV-infected women of childbearing age found that hepatic events were

What's New

Pregnancy-related data on atazanavir, fosamprenavir, emtricitabine, and enfuvirtide are limited. Antiretroviral therapy and especially HAART before pregnancy may be associated with pre-eclampsia and fetal death.

Key Points

- Most antiretroviral agents are in pregnancy category C, indicating that safety in pregnancy has not been determined; these drugs should be used only when the potential benefit outweighs the potential risk to the fetus.
- Efavirenz is now classified in pregnancy category D. Efavirenz should not be used during the first trimester because of concerns about fetal abnormalities.
- Antiretroviral agents that are in pregnancy category B are atazanavir, didanosine, emtricitabine, enfuvirtide, nelfinavir, ritonavir, saquinavir and tenofovir.
- The combination of stavudine and didanosine is contraindicated in pregnancy because fatal maternal lactic acidosis has been associated with prolonged use.
- Hepatic adverse events have been reported more frequently with the use of nevirapine and stavudine/didanosine regimens.
- Antiretroviral therapy in general may increase the risk of pre-eclampsia and fetal death.
- Despite concerns about the use of medications during pregnancy, the benefits of antiretroviral therapy clearly outweigh the risks. An axiom of care in pregnant women is to "maximize maternal health."

more frequently associated with the use of nucleoside reverse transcriptase inhibitors and/or nevirapine than with protease inhibitors (Baylor et al. 2004). No events were reported for tenofovir, emtricitabine, atazanavir, or enfuvirtide. Severe hepatotoxicity in this patient population was associated with the use of nevirapine, and with regimens containing stavudine/didanosine. Based on postmarketing surveillance data and the manufacturer's clinical trial database for nevirapine, the product labeling for nevirapine has been amended to include updated information about hepatotoxicity associated with nevirapine (Boehringer Ingelheim 2004). Women with CD4 counts over 250 cells/mm^3, including pregnant women receiving chronic treatment for HIV infection, are at considerably higher risk (12-fold) of serious hepatotoxicity. Atazanavir administration is associated with a significant incidence of hyperbilirubinemia in adults (Reyataz 2004). Thus, a concern for the use of atazanavir in pregnancy is that the drug might cause hyperbilirubinemia in the mothers (USPHS 2004) and subsequently lead to kernicterus in the neonates (Reyataz 2004). No data are available, but this issue makes many prescribers reluctant to use atazanavir during pregnancy. The manufacturer recommends considering additional monitoring for this effect during the prepartum period as well as the use of an alternative antiretroviral (Reyataz 2004).

Some in vitro studies of tenofovir have been associated with reduced fetal growth and bone porosity (USPHS 2004), leading to a concern among some clinicians when prescribing tenofovir during pregnancy. Preclinical studies have shown reduced survival, developmental delays, and low body weight due to endocrine deficiencies in fetuses exposed to tenofovir. However, no human studies of pregnant women have been conducted (USPHS 2004).

The combination of stavudine and didanosine with other antiretroviral agents is contraindicated in pregnancy because there have been instances of fatal maternal lactic acidosis associated with prolonged use of this combination in pregnant women (Bristol-Myers Squibb 2001).

Pharmacokinetics of Antiretrovirals During Pregnancy

Pregnancy can affect the pharmacokinetics of some antiretrovirals, particularly the protease inhibitors. For details, please see Objective IV.38 on Pharmacokinetics in Pregnancy, in this Update.

Nevirapine Resistance in Vertical Transmission Prevention Studies

The use of HAART during pregnancy in HIV-infected women has greatly reduced the risk of vertical transmission. However, in low-income countries, HAART is not yet widely available, and experiments using single or dual antiretroviral agents during different stages of pregnancy are under way to assess their efficacy (Jourdain et al. 2004). These studies have found high rates of NNRTI resistance. In one placebo-controlled study, a single intrapartum dose of nevirapine was given to 1390 of 1844 HIV-infected pregnant women, all of whom were also receiving zidovudine (Jourdain et al. 2004). Follow-up data are available from 221 women who received intrapartum nevirapine and 48 women who received placebo HAART postpartum. Of these, 209 nevirapine users and 48 placebo recipients had blood samples available for genotyping. Analysis of these blood samples 10 days postpartum found that 32% of 209 women who received nevirapine intrapartum developed mutations conferring resistance to nevirapine. Thus, a relatively high degree of resistance can occur after limited exposure to an NNRTI in a viremic patient.

Also in this study, 269 of the women mentioned above received postpartum antiretroviral therapy in a regimen that included nevirapine. However, 6 months after initiation of HAART, only 49% of the women who received intrapartum nevirapine were able to sustain viral suppression below 50 copies/mL. In contrast, 68% of the women who received placebo instead of nevirapine during delivery were able to suppress their viral load below the 50-copy mark (Jourdain et al. 2004). This study shows a relationship between brief exposure to a drug and the subsequent development of clinically relevant resistance. These data are also relevant to the concerns about treatment cessation of a suppressive regimen that contains an NNRTI (see objective IV.30 on Treatment Cessation in this Update).

Another study involving 623 HIV-infected mothers in South Africa also found that when nevirapine was given to mothers during labor and to infants within 72 hours of birth, relatively high rates of resistance to this drug were detected in both mothers and infants (Martinson et al. 2004). Moreover, these mutations persisted in 35% of women and 65% of children 6 months after the initial exposure (Morris et al. 2004), and it is likely that these mutations are archived in latent HIV within long-lived memory cells. Clearly, more potent antiretroviral therapy during and after delivery would minimize the risks of developing resistance if treatment cannot be sustained (Cressey et al. 2004).

HAART and Pregnancy Complications

Recently, a group of Spanish investigators reported a significantly higher incidence of pre-eclampsia and fetal death in HIV-infected mothers compared with all other mothers delivering at their institution (Suy et al. 2004). In total, 11% of 82 HIV-infected mothers suffered pre-eclampsia, vs. 2.8% of 242 non-HIV-infected mothers; sudden fetal death was reported in 6.1% of infants of HIV-infected mothers vs. 0.5% of infants of non-HIV-infected mothers. They compared these complications in women during three time periods: pre-antiretroviral period (1985-1994), mono/double therapy period (1994-1998), and HAART period (1998-2003). They found a higher incidence of complications associated with antiretroviral therapy and HAART; furthermore, HAART before pregnancy as well as tobacco use were independently associated with a higher risk for these outcomes. This finding should prompt caution in the management of HIV-infected pregnant women but should not dissuade physicians from using antiretroviral therapy in this population.

References

Acosta EP, Bardeguez A, Zorrilla CD, et al. Pharmacokinetics of saquinavir plus low-dose ritonavir in human immunodeficiency virus-infected pregnant women. *Antimicrob Agents Chemother.* **2004**;48:430-436.

Baylor M, Truffa M, Gibbs N. Hepatic toxicity of antiretrovirals in HIV-infected pregnant women: a review of the FDA's Adverse Event Reporting System. In: Program and abstracts of the 11th Conference on Retroviruses and Opportunistic Infections; February 8-11, **2004**; San Francisco, California. Abstract 944.

Boehringer Ingelheim. Important new safety information [letter]. February **2004**. Available at: http://www.fda.gov/medwatch/SAFETY/2004/viramune_deardoc_Feb04.pdf [accessed February 14, 2005].

Bristol-Myers Squibb. Healthcare provider important drug warning letter. Princeton, NJ; January 5, **2001**. Available at: http://www.thebody.com/fda/zerit-videx_letter.html [accessed February 14, 2005].

Bristol-Myers Squibb. Important change in Sustiva (efavirenz) package insert—change from pregnancy category C to D. Dear health care provider letter, March **2005**. Bristol-Myers Squibb, Princeton, NJ.

Connor EM, Sperling RS, Gelber R, et al. Reduction of maternal-infant transmission of human immunodeficiency virus type 1 with zidovudine treatment. *N Engl J Med.* **1994**;331:1173-1180.

Cressey TR, Kunkeaw S, Ruttana-Aroongorn PN, et al. Duration of nevirapine (NVP) postpartum exposure in women who received single dose NVP during labor in addition to standard zidovudine (ZDV) prophylaxis for the prevention of mother-to-child transmission of HIV-1 in Thailand. In: Program and abstracts of the 15th International Conference on AIDS; July 11-16, **2004**; Bangkok, Thailand. Abstract ThOrB1352.

Fundarò C, Genovese O, Rendeli C, Tamburrini E, Salvaggio E. Myelomeningocele in a child with intrauterine exposure to efavirenz. *AIDS*. **2002**;16:299-300.

Jourdain G, Ngo-Giang-Huong N, Le Coeur S, et al. Intrapartum exposure to nevirapine and subsequent maternal responses to nevirapine-based antiretroviral therapy. *N Engl J Med*. **2004**;351:229-240.

Martinson N, Morris L, Gray G, et al. HIV resistance and transmission following single-dose nevirapine in a PMTCT cohort. In: Program and abstracts of the 11th Conference on Retroviruses and Opportunistic Infections; February 8-11, **2004**; San Francisco, California. Abstract 38.

McIntyre J, Martinson N, Investigators for Trial 1413, et al. Addition of short course Combivir (CBV) to single dose Viramune (sdNVP) for prevention of mother to child transmission (MTCT) of HIV-1 can significantly decrease the subsequent development of maternal NNRTI-resistant virus. In: Program and abstracts of the XV International AIDS Conference; July 11-16, **2004**; Bangkok, Thailand. Abstract LbOrB09.

Morris L, Martinson N, Pillay C, et al. Persistence of nevirapine resistance mutations 6 months following single dose nevirapine. In: Program and abstracts of the 15th International Conference on AIDS; July 11-16, **2004**; Bangkok, Thailand. Abstract ThOrB1353.

Reyataz (atazanavir [prescribing information]. Princeton, NJ: Bristol-Myers Squibb; October **2004**.

Sustiva (efavirenz) [prescribing information]. Princeton, NJ: Bristol-Myers Squibb; December 2004.

Suy A, Coll O, Martinez E, et al. Increased risk of pre-eclampsia and fetal death in HIV-infected pregnant women receiving highly active antiretroviral therapy. In: Program and abstracts of the XV International AIDS Conference; July 11-16, **2004**; Bangkok, Thailand. Abstract ThOrB1359.

United States Public Health Service USPHS. Public Health Service Task Force recommendations for the use of antiretroviral drugs in pregnant HIV-1-infected women for maternal health and interventions to reduce perinatal HIV-1 transmission in the United States. June 23, **2004**. Available at: http://aidsinfo.nih.gov/guidelines [accessed February 14, 2005].

(RLO-38)

IV.38. PHARMACOKINETICS IN PREGNANCY

LEARNING OBJECTIVE: Discuss the variations in antiretroviral pharmacokinetics (PK) that may occur during pregnancy, as well as potential strategies to avoid the development of viral resistance or toxicity as a consequence.

Many HIV-infected pregnant women are taking antiretroviral regimens for their own health as well as to prevent mother-to-child transmission (MTCT) of HIV. Protecting the mother's and baby's health are convergent goals: Studies indicate that use of highly active antiretroviral therapy (HAART) and viral suppression are independent factors associated with reduced MTCT to less than 2% with viral loads under 30,000 copies/mL (Cooper et al. 2002). HAART drugs may specifically protect the fetus and neonate by crossing the placenta and acting prophylactically. They may also reduce HIV in genital secretions to a greater extent than they do plasma viral load.

This optimistic picture is not without its complications. Studies with a limited number of antiretroviral drugs indicate that many have different pharmacokinetics in pregnant women than in the rest of the population. The mechanisms behind such variations have not been determined. Prior research has reported changes in the hepatic drug metabolism, gastrointestinal activity, placental drug transport and increases in body water and fat (Rakhmanina et al. 2004). Other complications include placental and fetal compartmentalization of the drugs and their resulting biotransformation.

These factors can change over the course of a pregnancy, with concomitant alterations in drug levels. Adjusting for these changes poses hazards in the clinic. Too-low levels will allow for viral breakthrough, with the possibility of MTCT or the emergence of drug resistance. High drug levels increase the likelihood of such adverse effects as mitochondrial dysfunction, end-organ toxicity, and poor pregnancy outcome, including birth defects (Perinatal HIV Guidelines Working Group 2005; Rakhmanina et al. 2004).

A U.S. Public Health Service task force has issued guidelines for the use of antiretroviral therapies in pregnant women (Perinatal HIV Guidelines Working Group 2005). The recommended drugs are the nucleoside reverse transcriptase inhibitors (NRTIs) zidovudine and lamivudine, the nonnucleoside reverse transcriptase inhibitor (NNRTI) nevirapine, and the protease inhibitors nelfinavir and ritonavir-boosted saquinavir.

The panel based its advice on what was known about pharmacokinetics and adverse effects during pregnancy (see also Objective IV.35 on Antiretroviral Agent Toxicity and Contraindication in Pregnancy in this Update). Pharmacokinetic studies are slowly accumulating, and the more recent significant findings are listed below. (All patients were on HAART regimens that included the study drug.)

Stavudine

The perinatal HIV guidelines qualify zidovudine and lamivudine as the preferred NRTIs for pregnancy due to the long experience and extensive research with this combination.

What's New

This learning objective is new to the AAHIVM Core Curriculum. See Key Points below for highlights.

Key Points

- Pregnancy alters drug processing in the body and, consequently, drug levels frequently become suboptimal.
- The passage of medications through the placenta, which can also lower drug levels, is both advantageous and risky.
- The United States Public Health Service has issued guidelines on antiretroviral treatment during pregnancy. Its recommendations attempt to take pregnancy pharmacokinetics into account.
- Recent research has focused on stavudine (no change in PK), nevirapine (mixed results), nelfinavir (reduced drug levels), saquinavir (compromised drug levels unless boosted with ritonavir) and lopinavir/ritonavir (suboptimal drug levels).
- Even when drug levels declined, loss of viral control and HIV transmission to the baby occurred rarely.

Stavudine is an alternative to zidovudine in cases of intolerance or treatment failure. A recent study of stavudine plus lamivudine found no decline in stavudine pharmacokinetics during pregnancy or labor, compared with historical nonpregnant adult controls (Wade et al. 2003). Cord blood concentrations at delivery were similar to those in maternal blood.

Nevirapine

The Perinatal HIV Guidelines Working Group favored nevirapine over efavirenz because of the latter's teratogenicity. (Because of the risk of life-threatening hepatotoxicity, the guidelines recommend nevirapine only if "benefit clearly outweighs risk." Women who enter pregnancy already on nevirapine may continue if they are tolerating it well.) The panel noted that one study, presented in 2004, reported no change in nevirapine pharmacokinetic during pregnancy. That study (Aweeka et al. 2004) found no significant difference in nevirapine levels between 12 pregnant women and a historic control cohort of 35 men and 8 women. Second-trimester levels tended to be lower than third-trimester or postpartum levels. Another study at the XV International AIDS Conference (Haberl et al. 2004) involving 13 men and 10 nonpregnant and 16 pregnant women reported no significant difference between the men and nonpregnant women in maximum or trough levels or in weight-adjusted AUC (area under the concentration time curve). Pregnant women, however, exhibited a significant, though moderate, decrease in peak nevirapine levels and AUC compared with nonpregnant women. There was no observed effect on viral suppression. Another study at the International AIDS Conference noted suboptimal nevirapine levels in 21 women undergoing cesarean sections (Gingelmaier et al. 2004). The researchers noted that nevirapine's free passage through the placenta was the source of these apparent reductions.

In one study of 9 patients (postpartum women as well as men and other women), nevirapine persisted for an average of 7 days as its levels gradually declined (Mackie et al. 2004). Prolonged suboptimal exposure can lead to the emergence of nevirapine-resistant HIV, so it may help to continue background NRTIs for at least 5 days longer than nevirapine if discontinuing therapy after birth.

Nelfinavir

Although nelfinavir has had a lower rate of virologic response in some comparative clinical trials, it was 1 of 2 protease inhibitors recommended by the Perinatal Guidelines Working Group. This recommendation stems from extensive experience with the drug in pregnancy without the appearance of serious toxicity or other issues. PACTG trial 353 found that nelfinavir AUCs were lower compared with postpartum levels (Bryson et al. 2002). Nonetheless, 82% of the women had antepartum viral loads below 400 copies/mL, compared with 77% postpartum. Little nelfinavir passed through the placenta; it was undetectable in 7 of 16 cord blood samples. A more recent study found that nelfinavir levels were reduced by about one-quarter in pregnant women compared with nonpregnant ones (Nellen et al. 2004). Here, too, pregnant women with suboptimal nelfinavir levels largely maintained viral suppression.

Note that "ritonavir boosting" is generally not used with nelfinavir. Concurrent ritonavir has only a relatively small effect on nelfinavir levels compared with the effect on other protease inhibitors (Zelkin and Petruschke 2004), such as saquinavir and lopinavir.

Saquinavir

The second recommended protease inhibitor regimen is saquinavir plus low-dose ritonavir. Unboosted saquinavir (soft gel capsules [sgc], 1200 mg three times daily) was rejected after a phase I study found that it yielded compromised drug levels—well below those attained by nonpregnant adults—in the first 4 trial participants evaluated (Acosta et al. 2001). This trial resumed in 13 women using saquinavir sgc plus ritonavir (800/100 mg twice daily) (Acosta et al. 2004). The exposure to both drugs tended to decrease during pregnancy and birth, and despite a high degree in variability, all trial participants achieved sufficient saquinavir concentrations. Six-week postpartum saquinavir levels did not differ significantly from those observed during pregnancy and delivery. However, ritonavir levels, which were also highly variable, were significantly different when compared with higher postpartum levels.

Lopinavir

Lopinavir/ritonavir (Kaletra) was listed as an alternative protease inhibitor in the Perinatal Guidelines. A study presented at the XV International AIDS Conference warned that drug levels for this agent are often suboptimal (Stek et al. 2004). The mean third-trimester lopinavir AUC was 67% of that achieved by trial participants postpartum and 55% of that in nonpregnant historical controls. Cord blood levels at delivery were only about a quarter of those in maternal blood.

Conclusions

It is remarkable that these studies have observed little virologic failure in the mother or HIV transmission to her baby. It may be that a few months of suboptimal drug exposure is not enough to select for viral resistance, at least as continuation of a previously suppressive HAART regimen. Still, there is a risk of virologic failure, and the risk is highest in treatment-naive women with substantial viral burdens that they must quickly reduce. Investigators frequently suggest the need for the use of therapeutic drug monitoring and possibly increasing medication doses (Nellen et al. 2004). Ritonavir boosting is another option. This method was successful with saquinavir, but, otherwise, the needed dose changes have not been confirmed by clinical study. The paucity of data is worrisome since excessive drug levels pose a risk to the mother and developing fetus. Until there are more data, therapy choices need to be made in discussion with the mother and take into account her drug tolerances and adherence abilities (Rakhmanina et al. 2004). Physicians should perform frequent monitoring during treatment to check for emerging signs of drug resistance and toxicity (Perinatal HIV Guidelines Working Group 2005).

References

Acosta EP, Bardeguez A, Zorrilla CD, et al. Pharmacokinetics of saquinavir plus low-dose ritonavir in human immunodeficiency virus-infected pregnant women. *Antimicrob Agents Chemother.* **2004**; 48:430-436.

Acosta EP, Zorrilla C, Van Dyke R, et al. Pharmacokinetics of saquinavir-SGC in HIV-infected pregnant women. *HIV Clin Trials*. **2001**;2:460-465.

Aweeka F, Lizak P, Frenkel L, et al. Steady state nevirapine pharmacokinetics during second and third trimester pregnancy and postpartum: PACTG 1022. In: Program and abstracts of the11th Conference on Retroviruses and Opportunistic Infections; February 8-11, **2004**; San Francisco, California. Abstract 932.

Bryson Y, Stek A, Mirochnick M, et al. for the PACTG 353 Team. Pharmacokinetics, antiviral activity and safety of nelfinavir (NFV) in combination with ZDV/3TC in pregnant HIV-infected women and their infants: PACTG 353 Cohort 2. In: Program and abstracts of the 9th Conference on Retroviruses and Opportunistic Infections; Seattle, Washington; February 24-28, **2002**. Abstract 795-W.

Cooper ER, Charurat M, Mofenson L, et al. Combination antiretroviral strategies for the treatment of pregnant HIV-1-infected women and prevention of perinatal HIV-1 transmission. *J Acquir Immune Defic Syndr.* **2002**;29:484-494.

Gingelmaier A, Grubert TA, Kurowski M, Kaestner R, Kriegel S, Friese K. Nevirapine and different protease inhibitors - pharmacokinetics and placental transfer at the delivery of HIV-positive women. In: Program and abstracts of the XV International Conference on AIDS; July 11-16, **2004**; Bangkok, Thailand. Abstract ThPeB7100.

Haberl A, Hentig N, Carlebach A, Kurowski M, Harder S, Staszewski S. Nevirapine plasma exposure is decreased in pregnant women. In: Program and abstracts of the XV International Conference on AIDS; July 11-16, **2004**; Bangkok, Thailand. Abstract TuPeB4644.

Mackie NE, Fidler S, Tamm N, et al. Clinical implications of stopping nevirapine-based antiretroviral therapy: relative pharmacokinetics and avoidance of drug resistance. *HIV Med.* **2004**;5:180-184.

Nellen JF, Schillevoort I, Wit FW, et al. Nelfinavir plasma concentrations are low during pregnancy. *Clin Infect Dis.* **2004**;39:736-740.

Perinatal HIV Guidelines Working Group. Recommendations for use of antiretroviral drugs in pregnant HIV-1-infected women for maternal health and interventions to reduce perinatal HIV-1 transmission in the United States. United States Public Health Service. Washington, DC. February 25, **2005**. Available at: http://AIDSinfo.nih.gov [accessed April 26, 2005].

Rakhmanina NY, van den Anker JN, Soldin SJ. Safety and pharmacokinetics of antiretroviral therapy during pregnancy. *Ther Drug Monit.* **2004**;26:110-115.

Stek A, Mirochnick M, Capparelli E, et al. Reduced lopinavir exposure during pregnancy: preliminary pharmacokinetic results from PACTG 1026. In: Program and abstracts of the XV International Conference on AIDS; July 11-16, **2004**; Bangkok, Thailand. Abstract LBOrB08.

Wade N, Unadkat J, Huang S, et al. Pharmacokinetics and safety of d4T and 3TC in HIV-infected pregnant women and their infants (PACTG 332). In: Program and abstracts of the 10th Conference on Retroviruses and Opportunistic Infections; February 10-14, **2003**; Boston, Massachusetts. Abstract 886.

Zeldin RK, Petruschke RA. Pharmacological and therapeutic properties of ritonavir-boosted protease inhibitor therapy in HIV-infected patients. *J Antimicrob Chemother.* **2004**;53:4-9.

(RLO-39)

IV.39. ADHERENCE PRINCIPLES

LEARNING OBJECTIVE: Identify the degree of adherence necessary for successful antiretroviral therapy and discuss how various levels of adherence affect the probability of developing antiretroviral resistance.

Adherence Requirements for Treatment Success

The success of all currently approved antiretroviral therapies lies in their ability to reduce viral replication to below the level of detection. The 2004 guidelines from the U.S. Public Health Service define optimal therapy as that which reduces plasma HIV RNA to below 50 copies/mL (using PCR assay; below 75 copies/mL using bDNA assay; and below 80 copies/mL using QT-assay), and state that such reductions are associated with more complete and durable viral suppression (DHHS 2004). Studies have found that near-perfect adherence, greater than 95%, is necessary to optimally suppress viral replication (Low-Beer et al. 2000; Paterson et al. 2000). Even a minor drop in average adherence from higher than 95% to 90% resulted in a marked reduction in rates of viral suppression: 84% of patients with adherence of higher than 95% achieved HIV RNA below 500 copies/mL on at least two occasions, compared with only 64% of patients whose adherence rates ranged from 90% to 95% (Low-Beer et al. 2000).

At first, the adherence demands of HIV/AIDS treatment may seem especially challenging, particularly for long-term care. But bear in mind that many patients and their doctors can successfully collaborate in identifying barriers to adherence and ultimately maintaining the benefits of therapy. Strategies for improving adherence that have proved useful in other chronic disease states are often relevant in the case of HIV/AIDS (Chesney 2003).

Improving Adherence

Given the chaotic and often unstructured lives of some patients with HIV/AIDS, particularly those with mental health, substance use and housing issues, it is not surprising that rates of adherence in this population are perceived to be less than optimal. Just as public health programs attempt to teach the uptake of healthier lifestyles (better food choices, exercise, avoiding and quitting tobacco smoking), it seems logical that improved adherence can also be taught.

Adherence can be improved by counseling when patients begin antiretroviral therapy. Such counseling should include discussion of proper antiretroviral therapy administration, food restrictions, and side-effect management while monitoring patient progress over a number of weeks. Persons receiving such counseling in one 28-week study achieved greater adherence and viral suppression compared with those who did not receive this counseling (Rathbun et al. 2004).

The association between adherence and successful viral suppression is not as straightforward as it first seemed. A recent study from San Francisco among patients who remained on a stable regimen for the 6-month observation period found, once again, that suppression of viral loads to below 50 copies/mL correlated with better adherence

What's New

Patients with suboptimal adherence may be at risk for development of drug resistance. Individualized adherence support was more successful than medication alarms in ensuring and maintaining adherence.

Key Points

- Antiretroviral adherence rates of greater than 95% are necessary for optimal suppression of HIV.
- Repeated counseling sessions can improve adherence and increase the frequency of successful viral suppression.
- Lowest adherence has been correlated with significantly higher levels of NNRTI resistance compared with PI resistance mutations.
- Each antiretroviral class may have a unique adherence-resistance relationship, and different patient populations may require different interventions to improve adherence.
- Maintaining high adherence to a nonsuppressive therapy carries the risk for evolution of further drug resistance but may be necessary if no viable follow-up therapy is available.

(Bangsberg et al. 2003). However, in patients who failed to achieve complete virologic suppression, higher levels of adherence were associated with a greater risk of selection of resistant virus than was seen in patients with poor adherence levels. Overall, 23% of the drug-resistance mutations occurred in study participants with 92% to 100% adherence, and half of the new resistance mutations appeared in patients with at least 79% adherence. A similar finding was described in a trial comparing either a lopinavir/ritonavir (Kaletra)-based regimen with a nelfinavir-based regimen. King and colleagues (2003) found that 80% to 95% adherence resulted in the greatest risk of having detectable resistance. In this study, higher levels of adherence were associated with less resistance because of greater virologic suppression, and lower levels of adherence were associated with a decreased risk of resistance, perhaps because of less selective pressure.

Strengthening the doctor-patient bond

Studies have found that physicians often misjudge their patients' adherence to medication (reviewed in Murri et al. 2002); yet physicians play a critical role in helping their patients understand the importance of adherence. To avoid misjudgments, Murri and colleagues suggest that several objective ways of assessing adherence are available that enable physicians to understand their patients' barriers to adherence. A good first step involves maintaining and improving the quality of communication between patients and doctors. Clear and concise explanations about the risks and benefits of antiretroviral therapy, as well as continuing discussions with active patient participation about therapy, are essential to the success of the therapeutic relationship. Further discussion between the multidisciplinary team and the patient can only enhance avenues for raising the topic of adherence and reinforcing physician-framed instructions.

These conversations between the care team and patient should continue beyond the initiation of therapy. At least one study has found that adherence begins to wane after the first month of therapy in patients with HIV/AIDS (Gross et al. 2001). This finding may serve as an additional time frame in which to monitor adherence and intervene if necessary.

Overcoming other barriers to adherence

An important barrier to adherence is depressive illness. Early diagnosis (and treatment) of this condition has the potential to lay the groundwork for improved patient quality of life, social functioning, and adherence (Starace et al. 2002).

Different patients and subpopulations may require different interventions to improve adherence. The interventions may take the form of simplified treatment regimens; management of comorbid conditions, such as anxiety, depression, and substance use; reduction of drug side effects; suggestions about lifestyle changes; and maintaining and enhancing the patient-provider relationship (Chesney 2003). All in all, one or more of these interventions (as necessary) has the potential to improve adherence and the patient's willingness to remain on long-term therapy.

Adherence and Class of Therapy

Bangsberg and colleagues (2004) explored the relationship between different degrees of adherence and the development of resistance to the nonnucleoside reverse transcriptase inhibitor (NNRTI) and PI classes of therapies. They recruited subjects who were homeless or marginally housed. Adherence was assessed by means of unannounced visits or pill counts over a period of 1 year. Forty-three subjects were on an NNRTI-based regimen and 59 were taking PI-based regimens. Data analysis of the lowest adherence quartile found significantly higher levels of NNRTI resistance (67%) compared with PI resistance mutations (13%).

The study team noted that because NNRTI-based regimens are associated with a relatively lower pill burden, they may be perceived as the regimens of choice for patients with adherence issues. However, the results from this study suggest that patients with suboptimal adherence may be at high risk for the development of drug resistance when placed on NNRTI-based regimens rather than PI-based regimens (Bangsberg et al. 2004). Because boosted PIs have greater potency than unboosted PIs, the superiority of NNRTIs to boosted PIs needs to be further defined.

Although NNRTI-based regimens are associated with superior virologic outcomes compared to some PI-based regimens, it is not clear whether this difference is due to the drug potency or better adherence to simpler regimens. Weiser and colleagues (2004) investigated this possibility in a study of homeless and marginally housed HIV-infected subjects. Adherence was again measured by unannounced visits for pill counts in 110 subjects over a mean period of 9.1 months. Even when controlling for adherence, the chances of achieving a plasma viral load below 50 copies/mL was 5.6 times greater among NNRTI users than among PI users (Weiser et al. 2004). Moreover, there was no statistically significant difference in adherence behavior between the two groups. A separate analysis of this cohort found viral suppression to levels below 400 copies/mL in patients with as low as 54% adherence to NNRTI regimens (Bangsberg et al. 2005). This finding led investigators to conclude that adherence rates of 95% may not be necessary for those using NNRTIs to achieve viral loads below 400 copies/mL, although near complete adherence does increase the likelihood of durable viral suppression regardless of regimen. The superiority of NNRTIs to PIs is possibly due to greater anti-HIV potency of the NNRTI class in general compared with the unboosted PIs used in this study. Another possibility is that the longer half-lives of the NNRTIs compared to the PIs resulted in the maintenance of effective levels of drug during periods of suboptimal adherence. However, caution in interpreting these data is advised because of the study's lack of randomization. Further research is needed with the currently preferred boosted PI combinations versus NNRTI-based regimens to confirm the possible difference between the 2 drug classes observed in both these analyses.

Adherence Counseling versus Medication Alarms

Mannheimer and colleagues (2004) conducted a randomized controlled trial of two adherence interventions: medication alarms and/or contact with staff members who provided individualized adherence counseling and support. All subjects were antiretroviral naive and were monitored for a median of 2.5 years. Among subjects who received individualized adherence support, the rate of first virologic failure was 14% lower than in subjects who used alarms only (Mannheimer et al. 2004). Not surprisingly, therefore, the research team found that subjects who received individualized counseling had greater increases in CD4 counts and more patients reporting 100% adherence.

Treatment Interruption

"Short-cycle" interruptions designed to minimize the risk of viral rebound while still providing some time off from daily pill taking are being explored. The FOTO study reported on 20, virally suppressed patients on continuous HAART. Subjects were enrolled and then given antiviral treatment for 5 consecutive days, with treatment interruptions on 2 consecutive days, usually on weekends (Cohen et al. 2004). In this open-label study, 10 participants were given efavirenz-based regimens, and 10 were given PI-based regimens (with lopinavir/ritonavir in

8 and nelfinavir in the remaining 2). After a median 42-week follow-up (range 8-48 weeks), the only 2 cases of virologic failure were reported in the PI arm, both at week 24 in patients taking lopinavir/ritonavir. Quality-of-life assessments suggest that participants preferred the FOTO regimen to standard schedules. The preliminary results from FOTO suggest that use of NNRTIs in very short but repeated treatment interruption may not be associated with the development of viral resistance in NNRTI-based regimens. Moreover, they highlight the possibility that after prolonged suppression, less-than-perfect adherence can still result in sustained benefit from therapy. Readers should bear in mind that this was a small study that lasted for only 1 year. Larger studies are need before further conclusions about the efficacy of this approach can be made.

See also Objective IV.29 on Treatment Interruptions in this Update.

Conclusions

All in all, treating patients with HIV/AIDS can be both challenging and rewarding. Ongoing, frank discussions between physicians and their patients help to identify any barriers to adherence. These discussions lay the foundation for collaboration between both parties to find solutions to these barriers (Chesney 2003).

Coping with HIV/AIDS treatment information can also be challenging to patients. Wu and colleagues (2002) note that these physician-patient discussions can help to engage and motivate patients to actively participate in their treatment and thereby help adherence. Although the therapy of patients with HIV/AIDS can at times be complex, the fact that morbidity and mortality due to AIDS-related complications have decreased since the introduction of HAART shows that it is possible for many patients and their doctors to successfully persevere in managing this disease and its many challenges.

References

Bangsberg DR, Charlebois ED, Grant RM, et al. High levels of adherence do not prevent accumulation of HIV drug resistance mutations. *AIDS*. **2003**;17:1925-1932.

Bangsberg DR, Guzman D, Riley ED, Clark R, Deeks SG. Nonnucleoside reverse transcriptase inhibitor (NNRTI) resistance occurs at lower levels of adherence than protease inhibitor (PI) resistance. In: Program and abstracts of the XV International Conference on AIDS, July 11-16, **2004**; Bangkok, Thailand. Abstract WePeB5820.

Bangsberg DR, Weiser S, Guzman D, Riley E. 95% adherence is not necessary for viral suppression to less than 400 copies/mL in the majority of individuals on NNRTI regimens. In: Program and abstracts of the 12th Conference on Retroviruses and Opportunistic Infections, February 22-25, **2005**; Boston, Massachusetts. Abstract 616.

Chesney M. Adherence to HAART regimens. *AIDS Patient Care STDs*. **2003**;17:169-177.

Cohen CJ, Morris A, Bazner S, et al. The FOTO Study: A pilot study of short-cycle treatment interruption, taking antiretroviral medications for Five days On, Two days Off (FOTO), for those with viral load suppression. In: Program and abstracts of the XV International AIDS Conference; July 11-16, **2004**; Bangkok, Thailand. Abstract TuPeB4575.

Department of Health and Human Services (DHHS). Guidelines for the Use of Antiretroviral Agents in HIV-1-Infected Adults and Adolescents. October 29, **2004**. Available at: http://www.aidsinfo.nih.gov/guidelines [accessed February 25, 2005].

Gross R, Bilker WB, Friedman HM, Strom BL. Effect of adherence to newly initiated antiretroviral therapy on plasma viral load. *AIDS*. **2001**;15:2109-2117.

King M, Brun S, Tschampa J, Moseley J, Kempf D. Relationship between adherence and the development of viral resistance in antiretroviral-naïve patients treated with either lopinavir/ritonavir (LPV/r) or nelfinavir (NFV). [Abstract 798.] *Antivir Ther.* **2003**;8(suppl.1):S407-S408.

Low-Beer S, Yip. B, O'Shaughnessy MV, et al. Adherence to triple therapy and viral load response [letter]. *J Acquir Immune Defic Syndr.* **2000**;23:360-361.

Mannheimer S, Morse E, Matts J, et al. Sustained benefit from a long-term antiretroviral (AR) adherence intervention: results of a large randomized clinical trial. In: Program and abstracts of the XV International Conference on AIDS, July 11-16, **2004**; Bangkok, Thailand. Abstract LbOrB15.

Murri R, Antinori A, Ammassari A, et al. Physician estimates of adherence and the patient-physician relationship. as a setting to improve adherence to antiretroviral therapy. *J Acquir Immune Defic Syndr.* **2002**;31:S158-S162.

Paterson DL, Swindells S, Mohr J, et al. Adherence to protease inhibitor therapy and outcomes in patients with HIV infection. *Ann Intern Med.* **2000**;133:21-30.

Rathbun R, Farmer K, Stephens J, Lockhart S. Impact of an adherence clinic on behavioral outcomes and virologic response: Results from a prospective, randomized, controlled pilot study. In: Program and abstracts of the 11th Conference on Retroviruses and Opportunistic Infections; February 8-11, **2004**; San Francisco, California. Abstract 562.

Starace F, Ammassari A, Trotta MP, et al. Depression is a risk factor for suboptimal adherence to highly active antiretroviral therapy. *J Acquir Immune Defic Syndr.* **2002**;31:S136-S139.

Weiser SD, Guzman D, Riley ED, Clark R, Bangsberg DR. Non-nucleoside reverse transcriptase inhibitors are more efficacious than protease inhibitors at suppressing viral load even after controlling for adherence. In: Program and abstracts of the XV International Conference on AIDS, July 11-16, **2004**; Bangkok, Thailand. Abstract WePeB5777.

Wu AW, Ammassari A, Antinori A. Adherence to antiretroviral therapy: where are we, and where do we go from here? *J Acquir Immune Defic Syndr.* **2002**;31:S95-S97.

(RLO-40)

IV.47. MORPHOLOGIC CHANGES

LEARNING OBJECTIVE: Describe morphologic changes (lipoatrophy and/or abnormal fat deposition) commonly observed in patients taking antiretroviral therapy and their association with antiretroviral agents.

Lipodystrophy is a general term that refers to abnormal fat distribution more frequently seen among HIV-infected patients since 1996 (see, e.g., Dong et al. 1999; Engelson et al. 1999; Carr et al. 1998a,b; Lo et al. 1998), although experts have not yet universally agreed on a definition of a syndrome, hampering research in this area.

Two common patterns of fat redistribution may occur separately or in combination:

1. Fat loss, or lipoatrophy, may be seen in the face because of loss of the buccal fat pads, leading to hollowing of the cheeks; in the arms and legs, due to loss of subcutaneous fat, resulting in prominent veins; and in the buttocks. Subcutaneous abdominal fat may also be lost but is less obvious.
2. Excessive central fat deposition (fat accumulation) may be seen within the abdomen (visceral vs. subcutaneous fat accumulation), at the base of the neck (dorsocervical fat pad, also called "buffalo hump") and sometimes all around the neck, resulting in a "bull neck." Suprapubic fat deposition and increased breast size are especially seen in women, though men also exhibit these conditions. Both lipoatrophy and fat deposition may occur in the same patient.

Prevalence

Because lipodystrophy has no standard case definition, it is not possible to determine its prevalence with certainty. Additionally, determination of the prevalence of morphologic changes is confounded by the varied methodologies used in clinical studies, such as differing patient populations, measures of body-shape change, duration of therapy and treatment regimens.

A cross-sectional analysis of the Multicenter AIDS Cohort found that 20% of men receiving combination antiretroviral therapy reported a combination syndrome of lipoatrophy and central fat accumulation, and that the prevalence of the fat changes plateaued within 2 years of starting combination antiretroviral therapy (Kingsley et al. 2001). A separate, prospective study of the Multicenter AIDS Cohort confirmed anthropometric differences, especially lipoatrophy, in 384 seropositive men receiving highly active antiretroviral therapy (HAART) compared with 314 seronegative men (Palella et al. 2004).

Etiology

The etiology of lipoatrophy and fat deposition in HIV-infected patients remains unclear. Recent studies have focused on lipoatrophy, and there is controversy as to whether it is a side effect of antiretroviral treatment, a manifestation of HIV disease itself, an epiphenomenon (e.g., associated with combination antiretroviral therapy-induced immune reconstitution) or a combination of any or all of these. Even less is currently known about the mechanism of fat deposition.

What's New

The Multicenter AIDS Cohort has provided additional data confirming the prevalence of lipoatrophy in men receiving HAART. The FDA has approved polylactic acid injections (Sculptra) for the treatment of HIV-associated facial lipoatrophy.

Key Points

- Lipodystrophy refers to abnormal fat distribution more frequently seen among HIV-infected patients since the introduction of combination antiretroviral therapy. Its cause, frequency and treatment remain unclear.
- Fat loss, or lipoatrophy, may be seen in the face, arms, legs and buttocks. Fat accumulation may be seen in the abdomen, neck and breasts — especially in women.
- Specific antiretroviral agents and antiretroviral combinations have been associated with peripheral fat loss.
- Additional risk factors for fat loss may include low CD4 count, white race and body mass index less than 24 kg/m^2.
- Attempts to reverse established lipodystrophy have had limited results. Prevention may be more effective, but prevention strategies remain highly speculative.

Evidence from prospective studies shows an increased risk of limb fat loss in patients treated with a combination of a protease inhibitor (PI) and nucleoside reverse transcriptase inhibitors (NRTIs) when compared with those who received dual PIs alone (Cohen et al. 2002). Other studies show an increased risk of limb fat loss in individuals who received stavudine and didanosine when compared with those who received zidovudine and lamivudine (Chene et al. 2002; Dubé et al. 2002), and in individuals who received stavudine rather than zidovudine (Joly et al. 2002; Nolan et al. 2002a). Greater fat loss has also been associated with nelfinavir treatment when compared with efavirenz (Dubé et al. 2002). As will be described, the substitution of abacavir for stavudine or zidovudine can modestly reverse peripheral lipoatrophy, supporting the relative contribution of these NRTIs to fat wasting.

Retrospective cross-sectional studies tend to reinforce the association of fat loss with stavudine (Mauss et al. 2002; Lichtenstein et al. 2001; Mallal et al. 2000a) and with more than 2 years of indinavir treatment (Lichtenstein et al. 2001). PI therapy may speed the onset of lipoatrophy when compared with dual-NRTI therapy, lending support to the view that the risk of lipoatrophy is elevated in patients receiving combined therapy with PIs and NRTIs (Mallal et al. 2000a). Mallal and colleagues studied the rate of fat wasting in 277 HIV-infected patients who were treated with NRTIs and/or PIs. They found that although NRTIs independently contributed to progressive fat wasting, the rate was slow relative to PIs. Combining the 2 drug classes appeared to synergistically accelerate fat wasting (Mallal et al. 2000a). More recent DEXA data from patients receiving the nonnucleoside reverse transcriptase inhibitor (NNRTI) efavirenz along with lamivudine and either stavudine or tenofovir suggest that significant fat loss can occur with stavudine therapy, even in a PI-sparing regimen (Staszewski et al. 2003). This finding is further supported by a randomized study of 237 antiretroviral-naive patients that compared stavudine with abacavir, both in combination with lamivudine/efavirenz (Podzamczer et al. 2004). Results showed a higher rate of lipoatrophy in patients in the stavudine arm by 48 weeks — 20% for stavudine and 2.7% for abacavir.

The mechanisms by which antiretroviral agents might cause lipodystrophy remain highly controversial. It was initially proposed that PIs, which are clearly associated with hyperlipidemia (see Objective IV.50 on Cardiovascular Disease in this Update), were the likely cause (Carr et al. 1998a,b), but lipodystrophy has also been observed among PI-naive patients (Engelson et al. 1999). Interactions between PIs and NRTIs at the cellular level, leading to disruption of the pathways governing adipocyte differentiation and apoptosis, have also been proposed as an underlying mechanism of the lipodystrophy syndrome (Caron et al. 2002a,b). Yet another theory is that NRTIs inhibit mitochondrial DNA (mtDNA) polymerase in fat cells, leading to death of fat cells and disruption of fat metabolism (Brinkman et al. 1999; Brinkman and Kakuda 2000; Carr et al. 2000; Mallal et al. 2000a). Suprailiac biopsies of adipose tissue from patients with lipodystrophy have revealed structural changes to adipocytes in NRTI-treated patients (Mallal et al. 2000b). Buttock fat biopsies conducted by another group found that NRTI-treated patients had mean mtDNA content 44% lower than untreated HIV-infected individuals. The same group also found that individuals with lipoatrophy had mean mtDNA content in subcutaneous buttock fat 39% lower than individuals without lipoatrophy (Walker et al. 2002). However, the relationship between measurements of mtDNA depletion, NRTI toxicity and lipoatrophy is hotly debated (e.g., Moyle 2001; Walker and Brinkman 2001). For example, Casula and colleagues (2002) found that mtDNA levels increased in peripheral blood mononuclear cells after commencing combination antiretroviral therapy despite the presence of stavudine in the regimen, which raises the possible issue of the tissue specificity of mtDNA assessment. There is currently no validated test of mtDNA content in peripheral blood or tissue commonly available to the practicing clinician.

Host factors have also been correlated with fat loss, including having had a CD4 nadir below 100 cells/mm^3, white race and body mass index below 24 kg/m^2 (Lichtenstein et al. 2001). Self-described lipoatrophy has been reported to be unusual in the absence of these non-drug-related factors (Lichtenstein et al. 2001). A polymorphism in the tumor necrosis factor alpha promoter gene at position 238 G/A has also been associated with faster onset of lipodystrophy, although no distinction was made between lipoatrophy and deposition (Nolan et al. 2002b). In addition, investigators have observed sex differences in the presentation of body fat changes. An Italian study of 2258 HIV-infected patients, 673 of whom were women, found that lipodystrophy was more frequent and more polymorphic in women than in men, raising the question of whether hormonal mechanisms play a role (Galli et al. 2003).

Management

In the absence of a proper understanding of the etiology of lipoatrophy and fat accumulation (studies have been short-term and in limited numbers of people), little in the way of effective treatment can be recommended:

- Several studies have shown that switching from stavudine to zidovudine or abacavir was associated with modest increases in peripheral fat as measured by highly sensitive technology (DEXA and CT scan) (McComsey et al. 2003; Carr et al. 2002; John et al. 2002). Although there was little or no correlation between changes noted on DEXA or CT scan and anthropometric measurements within 1 year of the switch from stavudine to zidovudine or abacavir, a lack of progression of fat wasting was noted following the switch (McComsey et al. 2003). Although the benefits of switching from stavudine have been somewhat limited, this is the first and only intervention, short of cosmetic procedures, that has been demonstrated to improve lipoatrophy. Recent data indicate that the benefits of switching may become more pronounced with longer follow-up. In one study, 104 weeks after the switch to abacavir from either zidovudine or stavudine, mean limb fat measured by DEXA scan had increased 1.26 kg (36%) in patients with moderate-to-severe lipodystrophy at baseline (Smith et al. 2003).
- With the approval of tenofovir, another alternative to stavudine – or zidovudine, the second thymidine analog – became available. A British study compared switching thymidine analogs to either abacavir or tenofovir during successful HAART (Moyle et al. 2005). Volunteers had moderate-to-severe lipoatrophy, and 71 were receiving stavudine while 34 took zidovudine. They were randomized to replace these drugs with standard doses of either abacavir or tenofovir. By week 48, limb fat had significantly increased by 0.5 kg with abacavir and 0.3 kg with tenofovir, though the difference in these increases was not statistically significant. The changes in visceral and subcutaneous abdominal fat were not significantly different either, though tenofovir produced a significantly better improvement in blood lipids.

- Another possibility would be to switch to a non-NRTI regimen. AACTG 5110 studied 101 patients with peripheral lipoatrophy and suppressed HIV. Study participants replaced their zidovudine or stavudine with abacavir, or to switched their entire regimen to lopinavir/ritonavir plus nevirapine (Murphy et al. 2005). By the end of 24 weeks, the lopinavir/ritonavir/nevirapine arm exhibited significantly greater changes in subcutaneous fat (+16.6% vs. +9.2%) and the ratio of visceral adipose tissue to total adipose tissue (-9.0% vs. -11.7%).

- A second AIDS Clinical Trials Group study, ACTG 5125s (a substudy of ACTG 5116), examined the effects of morphologic and metabolic effects of changing standard successful HAART regimens in patients with advanced HIV to just lopinavir/ritonavir (533/133 mg twice daily) plus efavirenz (600 mg twice daily) (Tebas et al. 2005). A comparator arm received efavirenz plus 2 NRTIs. Median baseline limb fat was 6 kg in the 62 trial participants. When evaluated at week 48, the NRTI-sparing arm had gained a median of 562 g, compared with a median loss of 246 g in the 2-NRTI arm. The difference became significant among the 46 participants evaluated after 104 weeks. The NRTI-sparing arm did have significantly higher total cholesterol and triglyceride levels at week 48. The parent trial, ACTG 5116, however, reported greater rates of treatment failure in the lopinavir/ritonavir/efavirenz arm due to increased toxicity and a trend toward excess virologic failure (Fischl et al. 2005).

- Metformin (Glucophage), gemfibrozil (Lopid) and rosiglitazone (Avandia) have not been found useful in small randomized studies (Martinez et al. 2002; Sutinen et al. 2002), although some studies report benefits from rosiglitazone (Avandia) (Gelato et al. 2002) and metformin (Glucophage)—most notably with metformin (Glucophage)—in patients with fat accumulation and insulin resistance (Hadigan et al. 2000). A 28-person trial (Hadigan et al. 2004) found that patients with fat loss and insulin resistance were treated with rosiglitazone (4 mg/day for 3 months) and appeared to benefit from both a reduction in insulin resistance and an improvement in fat loss. Adverse events included an elevation in mean total cholesterol level. In contrast, a 108-person, 48-week study of rosiglitazone (4 mg twice daily) observed no improvement in the patients' lipoatrophy despite significant decreases in 3 markers of insulin resistance (P = .01-.02) and plasma adiponectin levels (P < .0001) (Carr et al. 2004). A more recent 73-person study has confirmed the lack of benefit (Cavalcanti et al. 2005). The difference between study results may be due to the fact that Hadigan and colleagues included only patients with insulin resistance (Carr et al. 2004; Hadigan et al. 2004).

- Growth hormone has been shown in some small series to reduce fat accumulation in lipodystrophic patients (Lo et al. 2001; Mauss and Wolf 1999; Torres et al. 1999), but this effect is not sustained when treatment is discontinued, and there has been no improvement demonstrated for patients with fat atrophy. Also, it is extremely expensive and can precipitate glucose intolerance. In a study of 245 HIV-infected patients, excess trunk fat was reduced significantly (-8.6%, P <.001) from baseline at week 12 in 82 patients receiving growth hormone 4 mg/day, compared with 78 receiving placebo (-1% decrease) (Kotler et al. 2004b). In the induction/maintenance phase of this study, 145 patients received the 4-mg/day induction dose for 36 weeks, followed by a maintenance dose of 1 mg/day (Kotler et al. 2004a). The latest results showed that this maintenance dosage was associated with significant (P <.05) reductions in trunk fat from baseline at week 60.

- Exercise has been reported to be associated with reductions in abdominal fat (Jones et al. 2001; Roubenoff et al. 1999). In one study, patients exercised for 90 minutes 3 times each week for 10 weeks (Jones et al. 2001). The exercise regimen included 5 minutes of warm-up, 20 minutes of cycling at 70% peak heart rate, 60 minutes of resistance training and then a 5-minute cool down.

- No study using objective measures (DEXA, CT) has observed improvements in lipoatrophy after switching from PIs to an NNRTI- or abacavir-containing regimen. Some studies have shown a trend toward the reduction of central fat accumulation (Drechsler and Powderly 2002).

- An open-label, prospective study of niacin treatment (median, 3000 mg a day for over 24 weeks) in HIV-infected patients with fat redistribution syndrome, expanded intra-abdominal fat and hyperlipidemia found an association between niacin treatment and significant reductions in central fat accumulation as measured by CT scan (Fessel and Follansbee 2002). Additionally, reduction from baseline measures in central fat was associated with reduced total cholesterol and increased HDL cholesterol levels.

- Surgical and corrective interventions have been used to correct facial atrophy due to lipodystrophy. Interventions include liposuction, excision of buffalo humps and cheek implants (Serra 2002). One study that treated buffalo hump with liposuction or surgical removal found a lasting effect in 17 of 18 patients (14-36 months' follow-up) (Gervasoni et al. 2004). Another retrospective study of 10 patients treated for buffalo hump with ultrasound-assisted liposuction reported good cosmetic results for all patients, although relapse occurred in 5 patients (Piliero et al. 2003). A 96-week, 50-patient study of facial injections with polylactic acid (Sculptra) reported persistent enhancements in appearance and quality of life (Valantin et al. 2003). Nonvisible but palpable micronodules, noted in 44 % of patients after treatment, reduced spontaneously in 6 of these patients over the follow-up period.

Given that attempts at reversing established lipodystrophy have had limited benefit, prevention may be the most effective solution. However, because of a lack of prospective, randomized data, prevention strategies remain highly speculative. Despite this lack of data, some experts believe that prevention approaches might include avoiding certain NRTIs (e.g., stavudine, zidovudine and didanosine), which might reduce mitochondrial toxicity and thus lipoatrophy. Another suggested approach is to avoid PI-containing regimens because this may reduce the risk of fat accumulation, but data supporting this strategy are scant. Finally, switching treatment regimen at the earliest sign of lipodystrophy may stall its progression or allow for its reversal. Management of lipodystrophy remains highly speculative, controversial and requires more research.

See also Objectives II.10 and III.3 on Wasting in the AAHIVM 2003 Study Guide.

References

Brinkman K, Kakuda TN. Mitochondrial toxicity of nucleoside analogue reverse transcriptase inhibitors: a looming obstacle for long-term antiretroviral therapy? *Curr Opin Infect Dis*. **2000**;13:5-11.

Brinkman K, Smeitink JA, Romijn JA, Reiss P. Mitochondrial toxicity induced by nucleoside-analogue reverse-transcriptase inhibitors is a key factor in the pathogenesis of antiretroviral-therapy-related lipodystrophy. *Lancet.* **1999**;354:1112-1115.

Caron M, Auclair M, Kornprobst M, Capeau J. Indinavir-induced nuclear lamina alterations are correlated with adipocyte dysfunctions in cultured adipocytes [abstract]. *Antivir Ther.* **2002a**;7:L1.

Caron M, Auclair M, Kornprobst M, Capeau J. Stavudine and didanosine partly reversed the adverse effects of indinavir on cell differentiation and response to insulin but enhanced apoptosis of cultured adipocytes [abstract]. *Antivir Ther.* **2002b**;7:L6.

Carr A, Miller J, Law M, Cooper DA. A syndrome of lipoatrophy, lactic acidemia and liver dysfunction associated with HIV nucleoside analogue therapy: contribution to protease inhibitor-related lipodystrophy syndrome. *AIDS.* **2000**;14:F25-F32.

Carr A, Samaras K, Burton S, et al. A syndrome of peripheral lipodystrophy, hyperlipidemia, and insulin resistance in patients receiving HIV protease inhibitors. *AIDS.* **1998a**;12:F51-F58.

Carr A, Samaras K, Chisholm DJ, Cooper DA. Pathogenesis of HIV-1-protease inhibitor-associated peripheral lipodystrophy, hyperlipidemia, and insulin resistance. *Lancet.* **1998b**;351:1881-1883.

Carr A, Workman C, Rogers G, et al. No effect of rosiglitazone for the treatment of HIV-1 lipoatrophy: randomized, double-blind, placebo-controlled trial. *Lancet.* **2004**;363:429-438.

Carr A, Workman C, Smith D, et al. Abacavir substitution for nucleoside analogs in patients with HIV lipoatrophy. A randomized trial. *JAMA.* **2002**;288:207-215.

Casula M, de Baar MP, van Gemen B, et al. Therapy with efavirenz + ritonavir-boosted indinavir, with or without stavudine after 24 weeks does not increase mtDNA and mtRNA content of PBMC assessed by single-tube duplex real-time NASBA [abstract]. *Antivir Ther.* **2002**;7:L16.

Cavalcanti R, Kain K, Shen S, Raboud J, Walmsley S. A randomized placebo controlled trial of rosiglitazone for the treatment of HIV lipodystrophy. In: Program and abstracts of the 12th Conference on Retroviruses and Opportunistic Infections; February 22-25, **2005**; Boston, Massachusetts. Abstract 854.

Chene G, Angelini E, Cotte L, et al. Role of long-term nucleoside-analogue therapy in lipodystrophy and metabolic disorders in human immunodeficiency virus-infected patients. *Clin Infect Dis.* **2002**;34:649-657.

Cohen C, Shen Y, Rode R, et al. Effect of nucleoside (NRTI) intensification on prevalence of morphologic abnormalities (MoAs) at Year 5 of ritonavir (RTV) plus saquinavir (SQV) therapy in an HIV-infected cohort. In: Program and abstracts of the 9th Conference on Retroviruses and Opportunistic Infections; February 24-28, **2002**; Seattle, Washington. Abstract 683-T.

Dong K, Bausserman LL, Flynn MM, et al. Changes in body habitus and serum lipid abnormalities in HIV-positive women on highly active antiretroviral therapy. J Acquir Immunodefic Syndr. **1999**;21:107-113.

Drechsler H, Powderly WG. Switching effective antiretroviral therapy: a review. *Clin Infect Dis.* **2002**;35:1219-1230.

Dubé MP, Zackin R, Tebas P, et al. Prospective study of regional body composition in antiretroviral-naïve subjects randomized to receive zidovudine + lamivudine or didanosine + stavudine combined with nelfinavir, efavirenz, or both: A5005s, a substudy of ACTG 384 [abstract]. *Antivir Ther.* **2002**;7:L18.

Engelson EE, Kotler DP, Tan YX, Wang J, Pierson RN, Heymsfield SB. Fat distribution in HIV-infected patients reporting truncal enlargement quantified by whole-body magnetic resonance imaging. *Am J Clin Nutr.* **1999**;69:1162-1169.

Fessel J, Follansbee S. Effects of niacin upon fat expansion in HIV-positive patients who have the fat redistribution syndrome. In: Program and abstracts of the 9th Conference on Retroviruses and Opportunistic Infections; February 24-28, **2002**; Seattle, Washington. Abstract 703-T.

Fischl M, Bassett R, Collier A, et al. Randomized, controlled trial of lopinavir/ritonavir + efavirenz vs efavirenz + 2 nucleoside reverse transcriptase inhibitors following a first suppressive 3- or 4-drug regimen in advanced HIV disease. In: Program and abstracts of the 10th Conference on Retroviruses and Opportunistic Infections; February 22-25, **2005**; Boston, Massachusetts. Abstract 162.

Galli M, Veglia F, Angarano G, et al. Gender differences in antiviral drug–related adipose tissue alterations: women are at higher risk than men and develop particular lipodystrophy patterns. *J Acquir Immune Defic Syndr.* **2003**;34:58-61.

Gelato MC, Mynarcik DC, Quick JL, et al. Improved insulin sensitivity and body fat distribution in HIV-infected patients treated with rosiglitazone: a pilot study. *J Acquir Immune Defic Syndr.* **2002**;31:163-170.

Gervasoni C, Ridolfo AL, Vaccarezza M, et al. Long-term efficacy of the surgical treatment of buffalo hump in patients continuing antiretroviral therapy. *AIDS.* **2004**;18:574-576.

Hadigan C, Corcoran C, Basgoz N, Davis B, Sax P, Grinspoon S. Metformin in the treatment of HIV lipodystrophic syndrome: a randomized controlled trial. *JAMA.* **2000**;284c:472-477.

Hadigan C, Yawetz S, Thomas A, Havers F, Sax PE, Grinspoon S. Metabolic effects of rosiglitazone in HIV lipodystrophy: a randomized, controlled trial. *Ann Intern Med.* **2004**;140:786-794.

John M, James I, McKinnon E, et al. A randomised, controlled, open-label study of revision of antiretroviral regimens containing stavudine (d4T) and/or a protease inhibitor (PI) to zidovudine (ZDV)/lamivudine (3TC)/abacavir (ABC) to prevent or reverse lipoatrophy: 48-week data. In: Program and abstracts of the 9th Conference on Retroviruses and Opportunistic Infections; February 24-28, **2002**; Seattle, Washington. Abstract 700-T.

Joly V, Flandre P, Meiffredy V, et al. Increased risk of lipoatrophy under stavudine in HIV-1-infected patients: results of a substudy from a comparative trial. *AIDS.* **2002**;16:2447-2457.

Jones SP, Doran DA, Leatt PB, Maher B, Pirmohamed M. Short-term exercise training improves body composition and hyperlipidaemia in HIV-positive individuals with lipodystrophy. *AIDS.* **2001**;15:2049-2051.

Kingsley L, Smit E, Riddler S, et al. Prevalence of lipodystrophy and metabolic abnormalities in the Multicenter AIDS Cohort Studies (MACS). In: Program and abstracts of the 8th Conference on Retroviruses and Opportunistic Infections; February 4-8, **2001**; Chicago, Illinois. Abstract 538.

Kotler DP, Grunfeld C, Muurahainen N, et al. Low-dose maintenance therapy with recombinant human growth hormone sustains effects of previous r-hGH treatment in HIV+ patients with excess center fat: treatment results at 60 weeks. In: Program and abstracts of the 11th Conference on Retroviruses and Opportunistic Infections; February 8-11, **2004a**; San Francisco, California. Abstract 80.

Kotler DP, Muurahainen N, Grunfeld C, et al. Effects of growth hormone on abnormal visceral adipose tissue accumulation and dyslipidemia in HIV-infected patients. *J Acquir Immune Defic Syndr.* **2004b**;35:239-252.

Lichtenstein KA, Ward DJ, Moorman AC, et al. Clinical assessment of HIV-associated lipodystrophy in an ambulatory population. *AIDS.* **2001**;15:1389-1398.

Lo JC, Mulligan K, Noor MA, et al. The effects of recombinant human growth hormone on body composition and glucose metabolism in HIV-infected patients with fat accumulation. *J Clin Endocrinol Metab.* **2001**;86:3480-3487.

Lo JC, Mulligan K, Tai VW, Algren H, Schambelan M. "Buffalo hump" in men with HIV-1 infection. *Lancet.* **1998**;351:867-870.

Mallal SA, John M, Moore CB, James IR, McKinnon EJ. Contribution of nucleoside analogue reverse transcriptase inhibitors to subcutaneous fat wasting in patients with HIV infection. *AIDS.* **2000a**;14:1309-1316.

Mallal S, Nolan D. Light and electron microscopy findings in subcutaneous fat in antiretroviral-treated and naïve HIV-infected patients. In: Program and abstracts of the XIII International AIDS Conference; July **2000b**; Durban, South Africa. Abstract LbPeB7054.

Martinez E, Domingo P, Perz-Cuevas JB, et al. A randomized, double-blind, placebo-controlled, comparative study on the effects of metformin or gemfibrozil in lipodystrophic HIV-1 infected patients receiving protease inhibitors (PI). In: Program and abstracts of the 9th Conference on Retroviruses and Opportunistic Infections; February 24-28, **2002**; Seattle, Washington. Abstract 702-T.

Mauss S, Corzillius M, Wolf E, et al. Risk factors for HIV-associated lipodystrophy syndrome in a closed cohort of patients after 3 years of antiretroviral treatment. *HIV Med.* **2002**;3:49-55.

Mauss S, Wolf E. Reversal of protease inhibitor-related visceral abdominal fat accumulation with recombinant human growth hormone [letter]. *Ann Intern Med.* **1999**;131:313-314.

McComsey G, Williams V, Ward D, et al. Improvements in DEXA and CT scan values after a switch from stavudine to abacavir or zidovudine do not correlate with anthropometric measurements at 48 weeks. In: Program and abstracts of the 5th International Workshop on Adverse Drug Reactions and Lipodystrophy in HIV; July 8-11, **2003**; Paris, France. Abstract 90.

Moyle G. Mitochondrial toxicity hypothesis for lipoatrophy: a refutation. *AIDS.* **2001**;15:413-428.

Moyle G, Sabin C, Cartledge J, et al. A 48-week, randomized, open-label comparative study of tenofovir DF vs abacavir as substitutes for a thymidine analog in persons with lipoatrophy and sustained virological suppression on HAART. In: Program and abstracts of the 12th Conference on Retroviruses and Opportunistic Infections; February 22-25, **2005**; Boston, Massachusetts. Abstract 44LB.

Murphy R, Zhang R, Hafner R, et al. Switching to a thymidine analog-sparing or a nucleoside-sparing regimen improves lipoatrophy: 24-week results of a prospective randomized clinical trial, AACTG 5110. In: Program and abstracts of the 12th Conference on Retroviruses and Opportunistic Infections; February 22-25, **2005**; Boston, Massachusetts. Abstract 45LB.

Nolan D, James I, McKinnon E, et al. Effect of stavudine, zidovudine and HIV protease inhibitor therapy on subcutaneous leg fat wasting in HIV-infected males—a longitudinal study [abstract]. *Antivir Ther.* **2002a**;7:L18.

Nolan D, Moore C, Castley A, et al. Tumour necrosis factor alpha gene-238 G/A promoter polymorphism associated with more rapid onset of lipodystrophy [abstract]. *Antivir Ther.* **2002b**;7:L17.

Palella FJ Jr, Cole SR, Chmiel JS, et al. Anthropometrics and examiner-reported body habitus abnormalities in the Multicenter AIDS Cohort Study. *Clin Infect Dis.* **2004**:38:903-907.

Piliero PJ, Hubbard MJ, King J, Faragon JJ. Ultrasound-assisted liposuction of HIV-related buffalo humps. In: Program and abstracts of the 10th Conference on Retroviruses and Opportunistic Infections; February 10-14, **2003**; Boston, Massachusetts. Abstract 724.

Podzamczer D, Ferrer E, Sanchez P, et al. Toxicity and efficacy of 3TC/EFV associated with stavudine or abacavir in antiretroviral-naive patients: 48-week results of a randomized open and multicenter trial (ABCDE Study). In: Program and abstracts of the 11th Conference on Retroviruses and Opportunistic Infections; February 8-11, **2004**; San Francisco, California. Abstract 716.

Roubenoff R, Weiss L, McDermott A, et al. A pilot study of exercise training to reduce trunk fat in adults with HIV-associated fat redistribution. *AIDS.* **1999**;13:1373-1375.

Serra, M. Facial implants with polymethylmethacrylate (PMMA) for lipodystrophy correction: 36 month follow up. In: Program and abstracts of the XIV International AIDS Conference; July 7-12, **2002**; Barcelona, Spain. Abstract ThPeB7378.

Smith DE, Martin A, Carr A, et al. Continued recovery of subcutaneous fat wasting after switching from thymidine nucleoside analogues to abacavir. In: Program and abstracts of the 2nd IAS Conference on HIV Pathogenesis and Treatment; July 13-16, **2003**; Paris, France. Abstract LB18.

Staszewski S, Gallant JE, Pozniak AL, et al. Favourable metabolic profile for tenofovir disoproxil fumarate (TDF) versus stavudine (d4T) when used in combination with lamivudine and efavirenz in antiretroviral naïve patients: 96-week interim results. In: Program and abstracts of the 2nd IAS Conference on HIV Pathogenesis and Treatment; July 13-16, **2003**; Paris, France. Abstract 562.

Sutinen J, Hakkinen AM, Westerbacka S, et al. Rosiglitazone in the treatment of HAART-associated lipodystrophy (HAL): a randomized, double blind placebo-controlled study. In: Program and abstracts of the 9th Conference on Retroviruses and Opportunistic Infections; February 24-28, **2002**; Seattle, Washington. Abstract LB13.

Tebas P, Zhang J, Yarasheski K, et al. Switch to a protease inhibitor-containing/nucleoside reverse transcriptase inhibitor-sparing regimen increases appendicular fat and serum lipid levels without affecting glucose metabolism or bone mineral density. The results of a prospective randomized trial, ACTG 5125s. In: Program and abstracts of the 12th Conference on Retroviruses and Opportunistic Infections; February 22-25, **2005**; Boston, Massachusetts. Abstract 40.

Torres RA, Unger KW, Cadman JA, Kassous JY. Recombinant human growth hormone improves truncal adiposity and "buffalo humps" in HIV-positive patients on HAART. *AIDS.* **1999**;13:2479-2481.

Valantin M-A, Aubron-Olivier C, Ghosn J, et al. Polylactic acid implants (New-Fill)® to correct facial lipoatrophy in HIV-infected patients: results of the open-label study VEGA. *AIDS.* **2003**;17:2471-2477.

Walker U, Bickel M, Lutke Volksbeck SI, et al. Evidence of nucleoside analogue reverse transcriptase inhibitor-associated genetic and structural defects of mitochondria in adipose tissue of HIV-infected patients. *J Acquir Immune Defic Syndr.* **2002**;29:117-121.

Walker U, Brinkman K. An argument for mitochondrial toxicity in highly active antiretroviral therapy-induced lipoatrophy. *AIDS.* **2001**;15:1450-1452.

(RLO-41)

IV.49. METABOLIC COMPLICATIONS

LEARNING OBJECTIVE: Discuss the occurrence and management of metabolic complications of therapy, including but not limited to hyperlipidemia, insulin resistance and lactic acidosis.

Hyperlipidemia

Hyperlipidemia, including hypertrigylceridemia and hypercholesterolemia, has been noted among HIV-infected patients since the beginning of the epidemic but has become a much greater problem since the introduction of protease inhibitors (PIs). The exact mechanisms by which PIs raise blood lipids are unknown (Mulligan et al. 2000). In addition to PIs, the nucleoside reverse transcriptase inhibitor (NRTI) stavudine has been implicated in hyperlipidemia (Gallant et al. 2004; Moreno et al. 2003; Kumar et al. 2002). Nonnucleoside reverse transcriptase inhibitor (NNRTI)-based regimens have also been observed to increase total cholesterol (TC) and low-density lipoprotein cholesterol (LDL-c), but NNRTIs may also raise high-density lipoprotein cholesterol (HDL-c). The addition of enfuvirtide to an individualized regimen does not appear to have any adverse effect on fat distribution, lipids or glycemic laboratory parameters compared with patients treated with an optimized regimen only (Cooper et al. 2004).

Although many clinical trials of antiretroviral therapies have demonstrated treatment-related elevations in both triglycerides (TG) and LDL-c, recently reported data from the Multicenter AIDS Cohort Study suggest that some of the increases in TC and LDL-c seen after antiretroviral therapy initiation may be caused by removal of the lipid suppressive effects of the HIV infection itself (Riddler et al. 2003). Among this cohort of men, a drop in TC, LDL-c and HDL-c followed HIV infection. When commencing antiretroviral therapy, there was a rebound in TC and LDL-c levels to near baseline values. Lipid specimens in this study were obtained without regard to subjects' fasting status and thus, in this particular study, no conclusions can be drawn regarding the effect of HIV infection and treatment on HDL-c and TG levels. In a metabolic substudy of the ACTG 384 trial, which evaluated nelfinavir- and efavirenz-based antiretroviral regimens, lipid abnormalities were seen more frequently in those who started therapy with lower CD4 counts or higher viral loads (e.g., those delaying the initiation of antiretroviral therapy) (Dubé et al. 2004). In addition, efavirenz and nelfinavir were associated with similar increases in TG and TC levels, and TC levels increased more frequently in patients receiving a regimen with stavudine/didanosine compared with those receiving zidovudine/lamivudine. A prospective study conducted over 96 weeks examined metabolic parameters in treatment-naive patients receiving stavudine/lamivudine/nelfinavir, zidovudine/lamivudine/nelfinavir and zidovudine/lamivudine/abacavir (Kumar et al. 2004). Recipients of the first of these regimens had higher risk for elevated TC and LDL-c by 48 weeks.

Retrospective analyses of data from the D:A:D study have also shed light on the effect of different antiviral agents on plasma lipid levels (Fontas et al. 2004). This study demonstrated that patients receiving first-line regimens containing PIs had higher TC and total TG levels as well as higher TC:HDL-c ratios compared with treatment-naive patients, with the highest

What's New

New data have demonstrated key differences in the way different antiretroviral agents and classes of agents may affect lipid profiles, and point to several predictive factors for treatment-associated metabolic complications.

Key Points

- HIV infection itself is associated with decreased total cholesterol, high-density lipoprotein cholesterol and low-density lipoprotein cholesterol, and some of the increases that occur after initiation of HAART may be due to reversal of this lipid suppression.
- Recent data have shed light on the effect of different antiviral agents on plasma lipid levels in first-line regimens. Management options include dietary control and exercise, switching or discontinuing certain antiretrovirals, and treating with lipid-lowering agents.
- HIV-infected individuals are at increased risk for diabetes mellitus. Insulin resistance may develop with any protease inhibitor within a few weeks of therapy initiation.
- The reproducibility and predictive value of asymptomatic hyperlactatemia is as of yet unknown; as a result, there is no consensus regarding screening for hyperlactatemia in asymptomatic patients.
- Rarely, some patients do develop potentially fatal lactic acidosis, for which all antiretroviral therapy should be stopped immediately and supportive therapy initiated. When lactic acid levels have returned to normal and the acidosis has resolved, consideration should be given to restarting antiretroviral therapy, using medications that are less associated with lactic acidosis.

values occurring in patients receiving 2 PIs. Of the PI regimens, those containing ritonavir were associated with higher TC and TG levels and higher TC:HDL-c ratios than other PIs. Saquinavir was associated with the lowest TC:HDL-c ratios. Due to D:A:D's timing, it did not include regimens with atazanavir, although atazanavir is reputedly the most lipid-neutral PI (Squires et al. 2004; Haas et al. 2003). The NNRTI regimens were associated with higher levels of TC and LDL-c than those seen in treatment-naive patients (Fontas et al. 2004), but the increase in HDL-c associated with these regimens led to either an overall risk-lowering or risk-neutral effect.

Evaluation of hyperlipidemia in patients ready to initiate antiretroviral treatment begins with obtaining a fasting lipid profile before the start of treatment and then 3 to 6 months after initiating treatment (Dubé et al. 2003). The National Cholesterol Education Program's ATP III guidelines (Expert Panel 2001) advise determining a patient's coronary heart disease risk factors. If the patient has 2 or more risk factors, then his or her 10-year risk for myocardial infarction or cardiac death should be calculated. Modifiable nonlipid risk factors, such as cigarette smoking and exercise, should be addressed. If hyperlipidemia persists despite lifestyle changes, adjusting the patient's antiretroviral regimen or initiating lipid-altering agents should be considered.

Management of hyperlipidemia in patients with HIV infection consists of:

- Dietary control and exercise
- Treating the hyperlipidemia with lipid-lowering drugs, such as fibrates or statins
- Switching antiretroviral therapy to substitute other antiretrovirals for a suspect antiretroviral

Dietary measures should be stressed first when trying to lower lipid levels. If TG levels are high (over 500 mg/dL) and, particularly when other risk factors for cardiovascular disease are present, the fibrates gemfibrozil or fenofibrate are recommended (Dubé et al. 2003). Alternatives include niacin (the adverse effects of this agent, which include hyperglycemia, must be considered) and fish oils (omega-3-fatty acids) (Dubé et al. 2003). In a French randomized trial, a 1 g fish oil product (2 capsules three times daily) reduced hypertriglyceridemia in HAART patients by 25.5% after 8 weeks (versus a 1% increase in those assigned to the placebo) (De Truchis et al. 2005). TG reached normal levels in 22.4% of the fish oil arm compared with 6.5% of the placebo arm in this study.

When examining PIs, consideration should be given either to a PI-sparing regimen—if it is possible to do so while maintaining virologic control—or to a regimen containing atazanavir. Switching to PI-sparing regimens led to a marked metabolic improvement after 24 months of follow-up in one randomized study (Fisac et al. 2004). Results from a treatment trial of patients comparing atazanavir with either ritonavir or saquinavir versus a lopinavir/ritonavir combination suggest that, for treatment-experienced individuals, ritonavir-boosted atazanavir is associated with fewer effects on lipids than is lopinavir/ritonavir (Badaro et al. 2003). A week 12 interim analysis of a randomized trial in HIV-suppressed patients with elevated LDL-c found that switching to unboosted atazanavir from a previous PI resulted in a 15% reduction in LDL-c compared with remaining on the prior PI (Sension et al. 2005).

PIs may be the agents that clinicians most frequently associate with lipid perturbations, but the NRTI stavudine has also been shown to have an adverse impact on lipids (Moreno et al. 2003; Kumar et al. 2002). If switching off stavudine, consideration should be given to using another NRTI, such as tenofovir or abacavir. In a recent 3-year randomized trial, the combination of tenofovir DF, lamivudine and efavirenz provided HIV suppression comparable to stavudine, lamivudine and efavirenz in antiretroviral-naive patients and resulted in better lipid profiles and less lipodystrophy (Gallant et al. 2004). A separate study of 155 treatment-naive women comparing tenofovir DF versus stavudine in combination with lamivudine and efavirenz found similar results (De Ruiter et al. 2004).

Other switches may also be useful: A 48-week open-label randomized study of 30 HIV-infected individuals found that replacement a PI or an NNRTI with abacavir resulted in moderate improvements in both TC and LDL-c (Moyle et al. 2003). In the same trial, replacing stavudine with abacavir improved subcutaneous fat mass to a certain extent. A separate randomized, controlled, open-label study also found that switching from PI regimens to abacavir, nevirapine, adefovir and hydroxyurea resulted in improved lipid parameters (Carr et al. 2001).

Clinicians need to be aware of potential drug-drug interactions between cholesterol-lowering statins and PIs. PIs in general inhibit the cytochrome P450 3A4 enzyme, potentially leading to marked increases in statin levels. As a result, the statin of choice is pravastatin (Pravachol), which is not metabolized via this pathway; if treatment goals are not reached, low-dose atorvastatin (Lipitor) starting at a dose of 10 mg daily is an appropriate substitute (Dubé et al. 2003). There is less experience with fluvastatin (Lescol), but it is likely to be a reasonable alternative as well (Doser et al. 2002). Lovastatin (Mevacor) and simvastatin (Zocor) should not be used in order to avoid the risk of rhabdomyolysis secondary to extreme elevations in these statin levels by PIs (Dubé et al. 2003). For more information on these interactions, see Objective IV.9 on Antiretroviral Interactions With Non-Antiretroviral Drugs in this Update.

Recent data also suggest that concurrent statin therapy may blunt the CD4+ T-cell response in patients receiving HAART. One case-controlled study with 1:1 matching of 136 subjects found that patients receiving HAART experienced a blunted CD4 count elevation when starting statins. After 6 months, CD4 counts were up 24 cells/mm^3 with the concurrent statins compared with a rise of 68 cells/mm^3 without statins (Iloeje et al. 2004). Further study is needed to determine the clinical significance of this finding.

Insulin Resistance and Diabetes Mellitus

The onset of insulin resistance has been documented with several of the current PIs (Dubé et al. 2001; Mulligan et al. 2000; Walli et al. 1998), even within a few weeks of the initiation of therapy (Dubé et al. 2001). A minority of patients (~2%) develop insulin-dependent diabetes mellitus, which usually resolves if a patient stops the PI. New data from the Multicenter AIDS Cohort Study, which includes over 1100 men, have revealed that HIV-infected men receiving combination antiretroviral therapy are 3.1 times more likely to develop diabetes compared with an HIV-negative control group (Brown et al. 2004). Hyperglycemia was noted almost twice as frequently in treated HIV-infected men — not only in patients receiving PI-containing regimens but also in those treated with regimens containing stavudine or efavirenz. In small studies, both amprenavir and atazanavir did not appear to affect glucose transport or reduce insulin sensitivity (Noor et al. 2004; Dubé et al. 2002). These newer PIs might be considered as substitutes.

If discontinuation of the causative agent (e.g., the PI) is not an option or does not result in resolution of the diabetes mellitus, then the diabetes should be treated in the same manner as for HIV-negative patients.

Treatment of insulin resistance is not considered standard of care. Although insulin resistance is hypothesized to play a role in the development of lipodystrophy, it is uncertain whether its presence is related to the often coincident lipodystrophy.

Lactic Acidosis

Hyperlactatemia and lactic acidosis have been observed with all NRTIs. The risk is associated especially with stavudine and other dideoxy nucleosides (didanosine and zalcitabine) (Polo et al. 2003). Patients receiving ribavirin for hepatitis C should not take didanosine—the combination with ribavirin greatly increases the likelihood of lactic acidosis (Butt 2003; Glesby and Gerber 2003). Combining didanosine and stavudine, with or without hydroxyurea, also magnifies the risk (Moyle et al. 2002; Boubaker et al. 2001; Coghlan et al. 2001). The didanosine/stavudine combination should be avoided unless no other options are available and the potential benefits outweigh risks (DHHS 2004). Use of hydroxyurea with didanosine alone also increases the risk of lactic acidosis.

There are conflicting data regarding the prevalence of asymptomatic hyperlactatemia among patients receiving NRTI therapy, possibly due to inadequacies in collection technique (Wohl et al. 2004; Hocqueloux et al. 2003; Harris et al. 2002; McComsey et al. 2002; Boubaker et al. 2001; John et al. 2001). There are, as a result, no current recommendations for monitoring asymptomatic patients for hyperlactatemia.

Potentially life-threatening lactic acidosis associated with hepatic steatosis and sometimes pancreatitis is a rare, but rapidly fatal effect of NRTIs (DHHS 2004). Clinicians must be alert to the possibility of lactic acidosis in all NRTI-treated patients when fatigue, weight loss, nausea and anorexia occur. These can progress to respiratory distress, mental status declines and multiorgan failure. Therapy consists of discontinuing antiretroviral drugs and providing supportive care, such as rehydration, bicarbonate infusion and mechanical ventilation. There is some evidence that the use of vitamins and antioxidants (thymidine, riboflavin, coenzyme Q, thiamine, L-carnitine) might be helpful (Claessens et al. 2003; Gerard et al. 2003; Falcó et al. 2002; McComsey and Lederman 2002). Cautious reintroduction of the less toxic NRTIs should be considered after complete resolution of signs and symptoms of lactic acidosis (DHHS 2004). Use NRTIs with relatively low in vitro mitochondrial toxicity (abacavir, tenofovir, lamivudine, emtricitabine) (Lonergan et al. 2003) since such toxicity probably triggers lactic acidosis. NRTI-sparing regimens are another strategy worth considering (DHHS 2004).

For details on the potential effects of antiretroviral drugs in pregnant women, including an increased risk for lactic acidosis, see Objective IV.35 on Antiretroviral Agent Toxicity and Contraindication in Pregnancy in this Update.

References

Badaro R, DeJesus E, Lazzarin A, et al. Efficacy and safety of atazanavir (ATV) with ritonavir (RTV) or saquinavir (SQV) versus lopinavir/ritonavir (LPV/RTV) in combination with tenofovir (TFV) and one NRTI in patients who have experienced virologic failure to multiple HAART regimens: 16-week results from BMS AI424-045. In: Program and abstracts of the 2nd IAS Conference on HIV Pathogenesis and Treatment; July 13-16, **2003**; Paris, France. Abstract 118.

Boubaker K, Flepp M, Sudre P, et al. Hyperlactatemia and antiretroviral therapy: the Swiss HIV Cohort Study. *Clin Infect Dis*. **2001**;33:1931-1937.

Brown TT, Cole SR, Li X, et al. Prevalence and incidence of pre-diabetes and diabetes in the Multicenter AIDS Cohort Study. In: Program and abstracts of the 11th Conference on Retroviruses and Opportunistic Infections; February 8-11, **2004**; San Francisco, California. Abstract 73.

Butt AA. Fatal lactic acidosis and pancreatitis associated with ribavirin and didanosine therapy. *AIDS Read*. **2003**;13:344-348.

Carr A, Hudson J, Chuah J, et al. HIV protease inhibitor substitution in patients with lipodystrophy: a randomized, controlled, open-label multicentre study. *AIDS*. **2001**;15:1811-1822.

Claessens YE, Cariou A, Monchi M, et al. Detecting life-threatening lactic acidosis related to nucleoside-analog treatment of human immunodeficiency virus-infected patients, and treatment with L-carnitine. *Crit Care Med*. **2003**;31:1042-1047.

Coghlan ME, Sommadossi JP, Jhala NC, Many WJ, Saag MS, Johnson VA. Symptomatic lactic acidosis in hospitalized antiretroviral-treated patients with human immunodeficiency virus infection: a report of 12 cases. *Clin Infect Dis*. **2001**;33:1914-1921.

Cooper DA, Reiss P, Henry K, et al. The effects of enfuvirtide therapy on body composition and serum lipids through 48 weeks in the TORO trials. In: Program and abstracts of the 11th Conference on Retroviruses and Opportunistic Infections; February 8-11, **2004**; San Francisco, Caifornia. Abstract 715.

Department of Health and Human Services (DHHS). Guidelines for the Use of Antiretroviral Agents in HIV-1-Infected Adults and Adolescents. October 29, **2004** . Available at: http://AIDSinfo.nih.gov [accessed February 28, 2005].

De Ruiter A, Pozniak AL, Staszewski S, et al. Long-term safety and efficacy of tenofovir DF (TDF) versus stavudine (d4T) in combination with lamivudine (3TC) and efavirenz (EFV) in antiretroviral-naïve women: 144-week results. In: Program and abstracts of the XV International Conference on AIDS; July 11-16, **2004**; Bangkok, Thailand. Abstract MoOrB1083.

De Truchis P, Kirstetter M, Perier A, et al. Treatment of hypertriglyceridemia in HIV-infected patients under HAART, by (n-3)polyunsaturated fatty acids: a double-blind randomized prospective trial in 122 patients. In: Program and abstracts of the 12th Conference on Retroviruses and Opportunistic Infections; February 22-25, **2005**; Boston, Massachusetts. Abstract 39.

Doser N, Kübli S, Telenti A, et al. Efficacy and safety of fluvastatin in hyperlipidemic protease inhibitor-treated HIV-infected patients. *AIDS*. **2002**;16:1982-1983.

Dubé MP, Edmondson-Melancon H, Qian D, Aqeel R, Johnson D, Buchanan TA. Prospective evaluation of the effect of initiating indinavir-based therapy on insulin sensitivity and B-cell function in HIV-infected patients. *J Acquir Immune Defic Syndr*. **2001**;27:130-134.

Dubé MP, Qian D, Edmondson-Melancon H, et al. Prospective, intensive study of metabolic changes associated with 48 weeks of amprenavir-based antiretroviral therapy. *Clin Infect Dis*. **2002**;35:475-481.

Dubé MP, Stein JH, Aberg JA, et al. Guidelines for the evaluation and management of dyslipidemia in human immunodeficiency virus (HIV)–infected adults receiving antiretroviral therapy: recommendations of the HIV Medicine Association of the Infectious Disease Society of America and the Adult AIDS Clinical Trial Group. *Clin Infect Dis*. **2003**;33:613-627.

Dubé M, Zackin R, Parker R, et al. Prospective study of glucose and lipid metabolism in antiretroviral-naïve subjects randomized to receive nelfinavir, efavirenz, or both combined with zidovudine + lamivudine (ZDV + 3TC) or didanosine + stavudine: A5005s, a substudy of ACTG 384. In: Program and abstracts of the 11th Conference on Retroviruses and Opportunistic Infections; February 8-11, **2004**; San Francisco, California. Abstract 74.

Expert Panel on Detection, Evaluation, and Treatment of High Blood Cholesterol in Adults. Executive summary of the third report of the National Cholesterol Education Program (NCEP) Expert Panel on Detection, Evaluation, and Treatment of High Blood Cholesterol in Adults (Adult Treatment Panel III). *JAMA*. **2001**;285:2486-2497.

Falcó V, Rodríguez D, Ribera E, et al. Severe nucleoside-associated lactic acidosis in human immunodeficiency virus–infected patients: report of 12 cases and review of the literature. *Clin Infect Dis*. **2002**;34:838-846.

Fisac C, Fumero E, Crespo M, et al. Metabolic changes in patients switching from a protease inhibitor-containing regimen to abacavir, efavirenz, or nevirapine: 24-month results of a randomized study. In: Program and abstracts of the 11th Conference on Retroviruses and Opportunistic Infections; February 8-11, **2004**; San Francisco, California. Abstract 78.

Fontas E, van Leth F, Sabin CA, et al. Lipid profiles in HIV-infected patients receiving combination antiretroviral therapy: are different antiretroviral drugs associated with different lipid profiles? *J Infect Dis*. **2004**;189:1056-1074.

Gallant JE, Staszewski S, Pozniak AL, et al. Efficacy and safety of tenofovir DF vs stavudine in combination therapy in antiretroviral-naive patients: a 3-year randomized trial. *JAMA*. **2004**;292:191-201.

Gerard Y, Viget N, Yazdanpanah Y, et al. Hyperlactataemia during antiretroviral therapy: incidences, clinical data and treatment. *Therapie*. **2003**;58:153-158.

Glesby MJ, Gerber JG. Editorial comment: drug-drug interactions, hepatitis C, and mitochondrial toxicity. *AIDS Read*. **2003**;13:346-347.

Haas DW, Zala C, Schrader S, et al. Therapy with atazanavir plus saquinavir in patients failing highly active antiretroviral therapy: a randomized comparative pilot trial. *AIDS*. **2003**;17:1339-1349.

Harris M, Chan KJ, Tesiorowski A, et al. Random venous lactate levels among HIV-positive patients on antiretroviral therapy. *J Acquir Immune Defic Syndr*. **2002**;31:448-450.

Hocqueloux L, Alberti C, Feugeas J, et al. Prevalence, risk factors and outcome of hyperlactataemia in HIV-infected patients. *HIV Med*. **2003**;4:18-23.

Iloeje UH, Yuan Y, Moorman AC, Wood KC, Holmberg SD. Concurrent statin therapy blunts CD4+ cell gain in combination antiretroviral therapy (CART) treated HIV-infected patients. *Antivir Ther*. **2004**;9:L41.

John M, Moore CB, James IR, et al. Chronic hyperlactatemia in HIV-infected patients taking antiretroviral therapy. *AIDS*. **2001**;15:717-723.

Kumar P, Rodriguez-French A, Thompson M, et al. Prospective study of hyperlipidemia in ART-naive subjects taking Combivir/abacavir (COM/ABC), COM/nelfinavir (NFV), or stavudine (d4T)/lamivudine (3TC)/NFV (ESS40002). In: Program and abstracts of the 9th Conference on Retroviruses and Opportunistic Infections; February 24-28, **2002**; Seattle, Washington. Abstract 33.

Kumar P, Williams V, Tashima K, et al. Determinants of hyperlipidemia in ARV-naïve subjects treated with Trizivir (TZV), Combivir (COM)/nelfinavir (NFV), or stavudine (d4T)/lamivudine (3TC)/NFV. In: Program and abstracts of the 11th Conference on Retroviruses and Opportunistic Infections; February 8-11, **2004**; San Francisco, California. Abstract 713.

Lonergan JT, Barber ER, Mathews WC. Safety and efficacy of switching to alternative nucleoside analogues following symptomatic hyperlactatemia and lactic acidosis. *AIDS*. **2003**;17:2495-2499.

McComsey GA, Lederman MM. High doses of riboflavin and thiamine may help in secondary prevention of hyperlactatemia. *AIDS Read*. **2002**;12:222-224.

McComsey GA, Yau L, Southwell H, et al. Elevated lactate levels are uncommon, even in heavily pretreated HIV-infected subjects. In: Program and abstracts of the 9th Conference on Retroviruses and Opportunistic Infections; February 24-28, **2002**; Seattle, Washington. Abstract T-710.

Moreno S, Domingo P, Labarga P, et al. Dyslipidemia improvement in patients switching from d4T to Tenofovir. In: Program and abstracts of the 43rd Interscience Conference on Antimicrobial Agents and Chemotherapy; September 14-17, **2003**; Chicago, Illinois. Abstract H-855b.

Moyle GJ, Baldwin C, Langroudi B, Mandalia S, Gazzard BG. A 48-week, randomized, open-label comparison of three abacavir-based substitution approaches in the management of dyslipidemia and peripheral lipoatrophy. *J Acquir Immune Defic Syndr*. **2003**;33:22-28.

Moyle GJ, Datta D, Mandalia S, Morlese J, Asboe D, Gazzard BG. Hyperlactatemia and lactic acidosis during antiretroviral therapy: relevance, reproducibility and possible risk factors. *AIDS*. **2002**;16:1341-1349.

Mulligan K, Grunfeld C, Tai VW, et al. Hyperlipidemia and insulin resistance are induced by protease inhibitors independent of changes in body composition in patients with HIV infection. *J Acquir Immune Defic Syndr*. **2000**;23:35-43.

Noor MA, Parker RA, O'Mara E, et al. The effects of HIV protease inhibitors atazanavir and lopinavir/ritonavir on insulin sensitivity in HIV-seronegative health adults. *AIDS*. **2004**;18:2137-2144.

Polo R, Martinez S, Madrigal P, Gonzalez-Munoz M. Factors associated with mitochondrial dysfunction in circulating peripheral blood lymphocytes from HIV-infected people. *J Acquir Immun Defic Syndr.* **2003**;34:32-36.

Riddler SA, Smit E, Cole SR, et al. Impact of HIV infection and HAART on serum lipids in men. *JAMA.* **2003**;289:2978-2982.

Sension M, Grinsztejn B, Molina J, et al. AI424067: improvement in lipid profiles after 12 weeks of switching to atazanavir from boosted or unboosted protease inhibitors in patients with no previous PI virologic failure and hyperlipidemia at baseline. In: Program and abstracts of the 12th Conference on Retroviruses and Opportunistic Infections; February 22-25, **2005**; Boston, Massachusetts. Abstract 858.

Squires K, Lazzarin A, Gatell J, et al. Comparison of once-daily atazanavir with efavirenz, each in combination with fixed-dose zidovudine and lamivudine, as initial therapy for patients infected with HIV. *J Acquir Immune Defic Syndr.* **2004**;36:1011-1019.

Walli R, Herfort O, Michl GM, et al. Treatment with protease inhibitors associated with peripheral insulin resistance and impaired oral glucose tolerance in HIV-1 infected patients. *AIDS.* **1998**;12:F167-F173.

Wohl DA, Pilcher CD, Evans S, et al. Absence of sustained hyperlactatemia in HIV-infected patients with risk factors for mitochondrial toxicity. *J Acquir Immune Defic Syndr.* **2004**;35:274-278.

(RLO-42)

IV.50. CARDIOVASCULAR DISEASE

LEARNING OBJECTIVE: Discuss the risk of cardiovascular disease associated with HIV and its treatment, and compare this with risk due to smoking, hypertension, diabetes, family history and other cardiac risk factors.

Morbidity and mortality from HIV-related complications have decreased substantially since the introduction of highly active antiretroviral therapy (HAART) (Palella et al. 1998). At the same time, antiretroviral therapy appears to be linked to a number of metabolic abnormalities known to increase cardiovascular risk in the general population. Among these are increased levels of insulin resistance, total cholesterol (TC), low-density lipoprotein and triglycerides (Glesby 2001; Passalaris et al. 2000). Several important questions about HIV and the risk of coronary artery disease (CAD) may be raised:

1. Does HIV infection itself, independent of antiretroviral use, predispose to CAD?
2. Do the perturbations in glucose and lipid metabolism associated with antiretroviral therapy have the same implications for CAD risk as they do in the general population?
3. Does combination antiretroviral therapy increase CAD risk, and if so, can antiretroviral sequencing strategies minimize this risk without sacrificing efficacy?

At present, answers to these questions are incomplete, though results from the D:A:D study (discussed in the following section) shed light on the second two. Earlier, retrospective studies evaluating the impact of antiretroviral therapy came to conflicting conclusions, perhaps due to the populations or timeframe involved, the manner in which data were collected or the method of analysis. For example, a large retrospective study conducted in the Kaiser Permanente health system (Klein et al. 2002) found that CAD events were significantly higher in HIV-infected patients than in age-matched noninfected patients (6.5 versus 3.8 events/1000 person-years) but that rates in the HIV-infected patients were not associated with antiretroviral or protease inhibitor (PI) use. In the more recent Women's Interagency HIV Study (WIHS), investigators found no increase in self-reported incidence of angina, myocardial infraction, cerebrovascular accident or congestive heart failure over a 2-year period when comparing HIV-infected women taking PIs with those not taking PIs as well as with HIV-negative participants (Daftary et al. 2004).

In contrast, a nested case-control study following 2671 patients over 7330 person-years found that the incidence rates of coronary heart disease (myocardial infarction or unstable angina) in that cohort were about 2 to 3 times higher than expected (Moore et al. 2003). The higher event rates correlated not only with expected cardiovascular risk factors but also with antiretroviral drug use. Another study, from a large French cohort, found that the myocardial infarction rate in HIV-infected patients with less than 18 months of PI use was similar to the age-matched estimate in the general population (Mary-Krause et al. 2003). Additional follow-up found a trend to more myocardial infarctions with increasing treatment duration. The rate of myocardial infarction increased linearly with length of PI use, and the trend became significant in men with at least 30 months of PI exposure.

What's New

The D:A:D study has found that patients receiving antiretroviral therapy are at a higher risk for myocardial infarction as well as other cardiovascular events than are treatment-naive patients.

Key Points

- Some antiretroviral therapies is associated with increases in insulin resistance, total cholesterol, low-density lipoprotein and triglycerides. Recent studies have established that there are significant differences in the impact of antiretrovirals and antiretroviral regimens on these metabolic disturbances.
- In patients with clear indications for HIV treatment, the benefits of antiretroviral therapy outweigh the cardiovascular risks associated with therapy.
- Although past studies regarding the relationship between antiretroviral therapy and coronary artery disease (CAD) yielded conflicting results, the most conclusive evidence to date has identified an increase in myocardial infarction among patients on HAART.
- The D:A:D study indicated that cardiovascular risk increased with each additional year on HAART. Additional studies are necessary in order to confirm this finding.
- D:A:D did not find an association between hypertension and antiretroviral therapy.
- The impact of CAD risk reduction in HIV-infected patients has not yet been evaluated. Such interventions have been found effective in the general population. CAD risk reduction is therefore probably worthwhile in HIV-infected patients experiencing hyperlipidemia.

Key Points (cont.)

- Risk reduction includes recommending a healthy lifestyle; helping to establish exercise, weight loss, and other prevention programs; using lipid-lowering agents; and changing antiretroviral regimens to include more lipid-neutral agents.

The most definitive study to date, the D:A:D study, was a prospective observational study of 23,468 patients from 11 cohorts on 3 continents (Friis-Moller et al. 2003). This study found combination antiretroviral therapy to be an independent risk factor for CAD — with a 26% relative increase in the incidence of myocardial infarction for each year on combination antiretroviral therapy. In addition, the D:A:D study found that PIs, especially ritonavir, were more likely to cause significant lipid perturbations than were nonnucleoside reverse transcriptase inhibitors (NNRTIs). Patients receiving first-line regimens containing PIs had higher TC and triglyceride levels as well as higher TC:HDL-c ratios than did treatment-naive patients (Fontas et al. 2004). The highest levels appeared in those patients receiving 2 PIs. Patients receiving NNRTIs had higher TC and LDL-c levels than did treatment-naive patients, but the increase in HDL-c in these patients resulted in a neutral or favorable effect on the TC:HDL-c ratio.

Treatment-naive members of the D:A:D cohort had a myocardial infarction (MI) rate of 1.39 per 1000 patient-years (El-Sadr et al. 2005). Those with at least 6 years of therapy experienced an MI rate of 6.07 per 1000 patient-years. The risk of MI increased by 1.17-fold per year of HAART, and this increased risk was independent of sex and age, though adjusting for time-updated lipid levels did reduce the relative risk of treatment. Lipodystrophy did not affect MI risk.

The above data, while not definitive, demonstrate that antiretroviral therapy is likely to correlate with some increased risk of cardiovascular disease. It is important to put this risk into context given the overall marked improvement in HIV-related survival since the introduction of potent therapy.

A retrospective study including 1,463,227 patient-months of follow-up in HIV-infected U.S. veterans (Bozzette et al. 2003) provides perspective on this risk:benefit ratio. Over the preceding 8-year period, the rate of hospital admissions with cardio- or cerebrovascular diagnoses among HIV-infected patients remained essentially flat. Meanwhile, death from all causes dropped significantly with the widespread dissemination of PI-based antiretroviral regimens. Although this study was limited somewhat by its retrospective design and short follow-up, it clearly demonstrates that the benefits gained from using antiretroviral therapy in patients who need treatment greatly offset any increased risk accrued from cardiovascular disease.

No formal studies within HIV populations have been performed to evaluate the impact of CAD risk reduction; however, there is enough evidence suggesting the possibility of such a relationship to warrant the formation of guidelines on monitoring patients (Dubé et al. 2003).

Modifiable risk factors, such as hyperlipidemia, tobacco use, hypertension, diabetes mellitus and sedentary lifestyle, are as important in patients who have HIV infection as in those who do not. It is likely that the relative contribution of these is greater than any risk posed by antiretroviral therapy (Savès et al. 2003). A longitudinal analysis of blood pressure changes in the D:A:D study cohort found no evidence that antiretroviral therapy increased the risk of hypertension but that factors associated with elevated blood pressure in the general population predicted hypertension in this HIV-infected population (Thiébaut et al. 2004). A University of Washington study more recently reported the contrary result: NNRTIs and lopinavir/ritonavir (but not other PIs) increased the risk for hypertension, especially high systolic values (Crane et al. 2005).

Therefore, a standard part of the care of any HIV-infected patient should include an assessment for these risk factors and recommendations regarding a healthy lifestyle, and assistance to help the patient become involved in established prevention programs, such as smoking cessation, weight loss for obese patients, exercise, regulation of blood sugar for those with diabetes, and treatment of hypertension and dyslipidemia (Dubé et al. 2003; Savès et al. 2003; Sklar and Masur 2003).

References

Bozzette SA, Ake CF, Tam HK, Chang SW, Louis TA. Cardiovascular and cerebrovascular events in patients treated for human immunodeficiency virus infection. *N Engl J Med.* **2003**;348:702-710.

Crane H, Van Rompaey S, Kitahata M. The association between increasing blood pressure and use of NNRTI and lopinavir/ritonavir. In: Program and abstracts of the 12th Conference on Retroviruses and Opportunistic Infections; February 22-25, **2005**; Boston, Massachusetts. Abstract 873.

Daftary M, Dutta AP, Xue Z, et al. Women's Interagency HIV Study (WIHS): Cardiovascular outcomes in women on PI therapy. In: Program and abstracts of the XV International Conference on AIDS; July 11-16, **2004**; Bangkok, Thailand. Abstract MoPeC3592.

Dubé MP, Stein JH, Aberg JA, et al. Guidelines for the evaluation and management of dyslipidemia in human immunodeficiency virus (HIV)-infected adults receiving antiretroviral therapy: Recommendations of the HIV Medical Association of the Infectious Disease Society of America and the Adult AIDS Clinical Trial Group. *Clin Infect Dis.* **2003**;37:613-627.

El-Sadr W, Reiss P, De Wit S, et al. Relationship between prolonged exposure to combination ART and myocardial infarction: effect of sex, age, and lipid changes. In: Program and abstracts of the 12th Conference on Retroviruses and Opportunistic Infections; February 22-25, **2005**; Boston, Massachusetts. Abstract 42.

Fontas E, van Leth F, Sabin CA, et al. Lipid profiles in HIV-infected patients receiving combination antiretroviral therapy: are different antiretroviral drugs associated with different lipid profiles? *J Infect Dis.* **2004**;189:1056-1074.

Friis-Moller N, Sabin CA, Weber R, et al. Data Collection on Adverse Events of Anti-HIV Drugs (D:A:D) Study Group. Combination antiretroviral therapy and the risk of myocardial infarction. *N Engl J Med.* **2003**;349:1993-2003.

Glesby MJ. Metabolic complications of antiretroviral therapy: coronary artery disease risk. *Top HIV Med.* **2001**;9:14-20.

Klein D, Hurley LB, Quesenberry CP, et al. Do protease inhibitors increase the risk for coronary heart disease in patients with HIV-1 infection? *J Acquir Immune Defic Syndr.* **2002**;30:471-477.

Mary-Krause M, Cotte L, Simon A, Partisani M, Costagliola D, and the Clinical Epidemiology Group From the French Hospital Database. Increased risk of myocardial infarction with duration of protease inhibitor therapy in HIV-infected men. *AIDS.* **2003**;17:2479-2486.

Moore RD, Keruly JC, Lucas G. Increasing incidence of cardiovascular disease in HIV-infected persons in care. In: Program and abstracts of the 10th Conference on Retroviruses and Opportunistic Infections; February 10-14, **2003**; Boston, Massachusetts. Abstract 132.

Palella FJ, Delaney KM, Moorman AC, et al. Declining morbidity and mortality among patients with advanced human immunodeficiency virus infection. *N Engl J Med.* **1998**;338:853-860.

Passalaris J, Sepkowitz K, Glesby M. Coronary artery disease and human immunodeficiency virus infection. *Clin Infect Dis.* **2000**;31:787-797.

Savès M, Chene G, Ducimetière P, et al. Risk factors for coronary heart disease in patients treated for human immunodeficiency virus infection compared with the general population. *Clin Infect Dis.* **2003**;37:292-298.

Sklar P, Masur H. HIV infection and cardiovascular disease — is there really a link? [editorial]. *N Engl J Med.* **2003**;349:2065-2067.

Thiébaut R, El-Sadr W, Chenue G, et al. Predictors of hypertension and changes in blood pressure in HIV-infected patients in the D:A:D study. In: Program and abstracts of the 11th Conference on Retroviruses and Opportunistic Infections; February 8-11, **2004**; San Francisco, California. Abstract 75.

(RLO-43)

IV.51. IMMUNE RECONSTITUTION INFLAMMATORY SYNDROME

LEARNING OBJECTIVE: Discuss the clinical setting, manifestations and management of immune reconstitution inflammatory syndrome secondary to opportunistic infections and autoimmune disorders, including but not limited to MAC, TB, CMV, HBV, HCV, PML, HSV and VZV.

The widespread use of combination antiretroviral therapy has dramatically reduced HIV-associated mortality and the incidence of opportunistic infections (Palella et al. 1998). However, patients with advanced immunosuppression may remain at risk for opportunistic infections, particularly in the first few months of combination antiretroviral therapy (Ledergerber et al. 1999), and opportunistic infections encountered in the setting of combination antiretroviral therapy may have atypical features (DeSimone et al. 2000). In addition, patients may exhibit noninfectious autoimmune-mediated inflammatory reactions after beginning highly active antiretroviral therapy (HAART) even if they had not previously experienced such disorders (DeSimone et al. 2000).

A variety of terms have been used to describe atypical opportunistic infection manifestations as well as appearance or exacerbation of autoimmune disorders in the presence of combination antiretroviral therapy, including "immune reconstitution disease," "immune restoration disorder" and "paradoxical worsening." In general, immune reconstitution inflammatory syndrome (IRIS) occurs in one of several scenarios (reviewed in DeSimone et al. 2000):

- A patient receiving treatment for a known opportunistic infection or previously diagnosed autoimmune disorder subsequently initiates combination antiretroviral therapy
- Manifestations of a previously unrecognized opportunistic infection appear or are "unmasked" with the initiation of combination antiretroviral therapy
- Immune restoration occurring after the induction of combination antiretroviral therapy induces an immunopathologic response to an unknown antigen or antigens, thereby triggering an autoimmune reaction and subsequent disorder

Of note, clinicians in developing nations have described IRIS as access to HAART expands (Sungkanuparph et al. 2003).

This Objective discusses the manifestations, evaluation and potential therapy for IRIS due to a variety of opportunistic agents and immune-mediated reactions.

Tuberculosis

Enhanced inflammatory reactions during the treatment of tuberculosis (TB) are not unique to HIV-infected individuals or those receiving combination antiretroviral therapy. Paradoxical reactions in non-HIV-infected individuals initiating treatment for TB have been reported (Rodriguez-Bano et al. 1997; Chambers et al. 1984). The pathogenesis of paradoxical worsening is not well understood but has been hypothesized to result from increased expression of mycobacterial antigens during TB chemotherapy and/or from augmentation of

What's New

In addition to infectious immune reconstitution disorders, cases of autoimmune disorders (including systemic lupus erythematosus, sarcoidosis and Grave's disease) have either appeared or flared up after initiation of highly active antiretroviral therapy (HAART). Such incidents suggest that these disorders are manifestations of immune reconstitution inflammatory syndrome. The introduction of HAART in developing nations has led to descriptions of immune reconstitution inflammatory syndrome in these countries, too.

Key Points

- Immune reconstitution inflammatory syndrome (IRIS) occurs when a known or unknown opportunistic infection or autoimmune disorder flares or is "unmasked" with the initiation of combination antiretroviral therapy.
- Enhanced inflammatory reactions may be more likely in HIV-infected patients concurrently receiving combination antiretroviral therapy and anti-tuberculosis treatment.
- IRIS is a diagnosis of exclusion, and risk factors include greater post-HAART viral load reductions and extra-pulmonary TB at presentation. IRIS may occur in patients with or without significant CD4 cell deficiencies.
- Atypical presentations of MAC, immune recovery CMV uveitis and clinical and radiologic worsening and "unmasking" of known and subclinical PML can occur in HIV-infected patients who experience immune reconstitution on combination antiretroviral therapy.
- Differential diagnosis of hepatitis flares in HIV-infected patients coinfected with hepatitis B or C should include a second hepatitis viral infection, biliary disease and drug toxicity. Mild cases may be managed with observation, but antiretrovirals should be halted with severe changes.

Key Points (cont.)

- Autoimmune disorders, including pulmonary and nonpulmonary sarcoidosis, systemic lupus erythematosus, thyroiditis and Grave's disease, have also occurred in patients with restored immune function after HAART initiation.
- In the majority of HIV-infected patients, the benefits of HAART outweigh the risks, and concern about IRIS should not lead to the withholding of HAART from patients for whom it is indicated.

the host's immune response (Orlovic and Smego 2001). Because combination antiretroviral therapy is associated with improved antigen-specific CD4+ lymphocyte responsiveness (Wendland et al. 1999), concurrent use of combination antiretroviral therapy and TB chemotherapy might be anticipated to place patients at increased risk of IRIS. Case reports and case series have described a variety of manifestations of IRIS in HIV-infected patients receiving treatment for TB (Table IV.51-1), both without combination antiretroviral therapy (Hernandez-Albujar et al. 2000; Minguez et al. 2000; Orlovic and Smego 2001) and in conjunction with combination antiretroviral therapy (Orlovic and Smego 2001; Furrer and Malinverni 1999; Kunimoto et al. 1999; Crump et al. 1998).

Table IV.51-1. Manifestations and potential therapy for TB, MAC and CMV IRIS.

Opportunistic Infection	Manifestations of IRIS	Potential therapy
Tuberculosis	• New fever [1,2,3] • Weight loss [1,2] • Lymphadenitis ± drainage [2,4] • New or increased pulmonary infiltrates [3] • Expansion of intracranial tuberculomas [5] • Pleural effusion [2] • Ascites [2] • Hepatosplenomegaly [2] • Radiculomyelitis [6] • Breast abscess [4] • Psoas abscess [7] • Superior vena cava syndrome secondary to intrathoracic lymphadenopathy [1]	• Anti-TB therapy • Nonsteroidal anti-inflammatory drugs • Corticosteroids • Surgical lymph node resection • Incision and drainage of abscesses • In patients with known TB, consider delaying start of antiretroviral therapy until TB treated for 30 days [17]
Mycobacterium avium complex	• Fever [8,9] • Abdominal pain [8] • Lymphadenopathy (painful) - Peripheral ± drainage [10] - Intra-abdominal [8] • Vertebral/paraspinal mass [11] • Bone/joint infection [12] • Hepatosplenomegaly [9] • Pulmonary infiltrates [9] • Subcutaneous nodules [12,13] • Psoas abscess [14] • Leukocytosis [8,13]	• Anti-MAC therapy, in combination with corticosteroid if pain and lymphadenopathy continue (to be tapered based on clinical response) [18] • Surgical lymph node resection • Incision and drainage of abscesses
Cytomegalovirus retinitis (immune recovery uveitis)	• Symptoms [15,16] - Blurred vision - Floaters • Ophthalmologic exam [15,16] - Inactive CMV retinitis - Vitritis (≥1) - Cystoid macular edema - Epiretinal membrane	• Corticosteroids - Oral - Intraocular injection - Topical • Topical ketorolac

[1] Minguez et al. (2000)
[2] Furrer and Malinverni (1999)
[3] Kunimoto et al. (1999)
[4] Orlovic and Smego (2001)
[5] Crump et al. (1998)
[6] Hernandez-Albujar et al. (2000)
[7] Wendel et al. (2001)
[8] Race et al. (1998)
[9] Foudraine et al. (1999)
[10] Phillips et al. (1999)
[11] Currier et al. (2000)
[12] Zeller et al. (2002)
[13] Brown et al. (2001)
[14] Boyd and Brettle (1999)
[15] Karavellas et al. (1998)
[16] Nguyen et al. (2000)
[17] Rolla et al. (2003)
[18] DeSimone et al. (2003)

A small number of observational cohort studies have estimated the incidence of IRIS in HIV-infected patients treated for active TB (Narita et al. 1998; Dean et al. 2002; Navas et al. 2002). These data suggest that the incidence of IRIS in patients treated for TB is higher in HIV-infected patients treated concurrently with combination antiretroviral therapy than in HIV-infected patients not receiving combination antiretroviral therapy or in non-HIV-infected patients. Narita and colleagues (1998) prospectively evaluated the incidence of IRIS in 2 groups of patients (HIV-infected treated with combination antiretroviral therapy and non-HIV-infected) admitted to an inpatient TB treatment facility in 1996-97 and a historical control group of HIV-infected patients treated at the facility during 1986-87, before antiretrovirals were available. They reported a significantly higher incidence of IRIS in HIV-infected patients treated with both anti-TB therapy and combination antiretroviral therapy (12 of 33, 36%) compared with HIV-infected patients treated for TB alone (2 of 28, 7%, $P = .013$) or non-HIV-infected patients (1 of 55, 2%, $P < .001$). In this study, 7 of 8 combination antiretroviral therapy-treated patients with IRIS were anergic to purified protein derivative (PPD) before therapy, and 6 of the 7 became PPD-reactive during therapy. Similarly, a group in Spain (Navas et al. 2002) reported that 6 (35%) of 17 HIV-infected patients treated with both combination antiretroviral therapy and TB chemotherapy developed IRIS, compared with none of the HIV-infected patients treated for TB without combination antiretroviral therapy ($n = 59$, $P < .001$). Among 183 HIV-infected patients treated for TB at 12 centers in London, a lower incidence of IRIS was reported (5%), but IRIS was found to be more common when combination antiretroviral therapy was used in conjunction with TB therapy than when TB was treated in the absence of combination antiretroviral therapy (Dean et al. 2002). One small study (Wendel et al. 2001) found no significant difference in the incidence of IRIS in HIV-infected patients treated concurrently with combination antiretroviral therapy and TB chemotherapy (11%) compared with those treated with anti-TB therapy alone (7%), although IRIS was reportedly more severe in combination antiretroviral therapy-treated patients.

Reported risk factors for IRIS in patients treated with combination antiretroviral therapy and anti-TB therapy include a larger absolute decline in HIV viral loads after starting combination antiretroviral therapy (Navas et al. 2002; Narita et al. 1998) and extrapulmonary TB at presentation (Wendel et al. 2001). In 2 studies examining the issue, the magnitude of CD4 cell increase after beginning combination antiretroviral therapy was not significantly associated with IRIS (Navas et al. 2002; Narita et al. 1998).

In evaluating an HIV-infected patient with new signs or symptoms during TB treatment, IRIS should remain a diagnosis of exclusion, and other potential causes should be considered (CDC 2003). Other potential etiologies include failure of TB therapy (due to nonadherence, drug resistance, or poor absorption), MAC, disseminated fungal infections, *Pneumocystis* pneumonia, bacterial pneumonia or bacteremia, and lymphoma. Depending on the clinical findings, diagnostic evaluation may include expectorated or induced sputum, bronchoalveolar lavage, blood cultures, lymph node biopsy, abscess drainage, thoracentesis or abdominal paracentesis. When cultures from clinical specimens are positive for *Mycobacterium tuberculosis* in patients with a suspected IRIS, isolates should retain the same antimycobacterial susceptibility profile as the original specimen(s); otherwise, treatment failure cannot be excluded as a cause for new signs or symptoms.

No randomized clinical trial data or formal recommendations are available for treatment of TB IRIS in HIV-infected patients. Discontinuation and changes in anti-TB therapy or combination antiretroviral therapy are rarely indicated (CDC 2003). Watchful waiting or nonsteroidal anti-inflammatory drugs (NSAIDs) are appropriate for mild signs or symptoms. A short course of systemic corticosteroids has been used successfully with more severe manifestations (Navas et al. 2002; Furrer and Malinverni 1999; Kunimoto et al. 1999; Narita et al. 1998), and surgical management of suppurative lymph nodes or abscesses may also be indicated. One report suggests that in patients with known TB, delaying the start of combination antiretroviral therapy until the TB has been treated for 30 days may reduce the risk of IRIS in this setting (Rolla et al. 2003).

Mycobacterium avium Complex

The incidence of disseminated MAC infection in HIV-infected individuals, which is associated with profound immunosuppression, has declined sharply with the introduction of combination antiretroviral therapy (Palella et al. 1998). However, numerous reports have described atypical presentations of MAC in association with combination antiretroviral therapy (Zeller et al. 2002; Brown et al. 2001; Currier et al. 2000; Boyd and Brettle 1999; Foudraine et al. 1999; Phillips et al. 1999; Race et al. 1998). In contrast to TB-associated IRIS, in MAC-associated IRIS, MAC has most often been unrecognized and untreated before initiating combination antiretroviral therapy. Because MAC IRIS frequently occurs in close temporal association with combination antiretroviral therapy, researchers have hypothesized that IRIS represents an “unmasking” of subclinical MAC (Boyd and Brettle 1999; Foudraine et al. 1999; Phillips et al. 1999; Race et al. 1998). This hypothesis is supported by in vitro studies showing a rapid increase in MAC-specific immune reactivity in patients with advanced AIDS treated with combination antiretroviral therapy (Havlir et al. 2000; Foudraine et al. 1999).

The clinical presentation of MAC in the setting of combination antiretroviral therapy-mediated immune restoration is distinct from disease in patients with advanced AIDS who are not receiving combination antiretroviral therapy (see Objective III.4 on Opportunistic Infections: Presentation in the AAHIVM 2003 Study Guide). Disseminated infection (defined by positive cultures from blood or bone marrow aspirate) is less common in MAC IRIS than in typical infection. Phillips and colleagues (1999) compared MAC lymphadenitis in patients starting combination antiretroviral therapy within the previous 3 months with that in cases occurring in the setting of no or ineffective antiretroviral therapy and found disseminated MAC in 29% of the former group and 71% of the latter group.

In localized MAC infection, inflammatory reactions most commonly are localized to peripheral or intra-abdominal lymph nodes (Phillips et al. 1999; Race et al. 1998), although other sites have been reported (Table IV.51-1). Draining sinuses were reported in 6 of 12 combination antiretroviral therapy-associated mycobacterial lymphadenitis cases compared with none of 38 cases in which disease was diagnosed in the absence of effective antiretroviral therapy (Phillips et al. 1999). Histologic specimens from MAC IRIS patients often demonstrate evolving granulomas (Foudraine et al. 1999; Race et al. 1998), suggesting a partially effective immune response, whereas tissue reactions are often minimal in typical cases of MAC that occur in the absence of effective combination antiretroviral therapy.

In evaluating a suspected case of MAC IRIS, the differential diagnosis should include infectious and neoplastic diseases discussed earlier regarding IRIS with TB infection. If blood cultures and other minimally invasive tests are unrevealing, lymph node aspirate or biopsy for histopathology and cultures should be performed to secure the diagnosis. In reported cases of MAC IRIS, infection with MAC was often unrecognized before instituting combination antiretroviral therapy (Race et al. 1998; Boyd and Brettle 1999; Foudraine et al. 1999; Phillips et al. 1999).

Most MAC IRIS cases have been managed solely with multidrug MAC chemotherapy and continued combination antiretroviral therapy (Boyd and Brettle 1999; Foudraine et al. 1999; Phillips et al. 1999; Race et al. 1998). Physicians have prescribed an oral corticosteroid, tapered based on clinical response, in some situations (DeSimone et al. 2003; Brown et al. 2001), and incision and drainage of abscesses or large necrotic lymph nodes are appropriate.

In general, MAC chemotherapy should be continued indefinitely in patients failing to maintain immunologic reconstitution and good virologic control of HIV. The current U.S. Public Health Service guidelines on the prevention of opportunistic infections (CDC 2002) state that discontinuation of secondary prophylaxis for MAC may be considered when patients are asymptomatic from MAC disease, have completed 12 months of MAC therapy and have maintained a CD4 count over 100 cells/mm^3 for at least 6 months with combination antiretroviral therapy. Results from a retrospective study of 16 patients found that most (14 of 16) experienced complete resolution of symptoms after approximately 1 year of treatment for MAC (Riddell 2005). Patients who did not respond to MAC treatment, also had less substantial increases in CD4 counts in response to HAART. Seven of the 14 patients who responded completely to MAC-associated IRIS were able to discontinue treatment without recurrence of MAC-symptoms. In some cases (3 of 7), patients required additional treatment with oral corticosteroids for an average of 15 months.

Cytomegalovirus

Anti-CMV therapy has been safely discontinued in selected patients with CMV retinitis who have immune reconstitution with combination antiretroviral therapy (Whitcup et al. 1999). However, a vision-threatening syndrome, termed immune recovery uveitis (IRU) or immune recovery vitritis, has been described in patients with quiescent CMV retinitis who have experienced immune reconstitution on combination antiretroviral therapy (Nguyen et al. 2000; Karavellas et al. 1998). Clinically, patients with IRU present with painless visual blurring and "floaters" in the visual field (Nguyen et al. 2000; Karavellas et al. 1998). Vitreal inflammation and quiescent CMV retinitis are the hallmark findings on ophthalmologic exam, with cystoid macular edema and epiretinal membrane formation heralding more severe disease (Table IV.51-1) (Karavellas et al. 1998). Long-term complications of IRU may include proliferative vitreoretinopathy, posterior subcapsular cataracts and severe postoperative inflammation, which may permanently impair visual acuity (Karavellas et al. 2000).

The incidence of IRU in patients with CMV retinitis who have experienced immune reconstitution with combination antiretroviral therapy has been reported to be between 18% (Nguyen et al. 2000) and 63% (Karavellas et al. 1999). Twelve of 14 patients with treated CMV retinitis and a good immunologic response to combination antiretroviral therapy who were enrolled in a prospective trial of discontinuing anti-CMV therapy were reported to have evidence of IRU at enrollment (Whitcup et al. 1999). The extent of prior retinal involvement by CMV has been found to be a risk factor for IRU, with patients having 30% or more retinal involvement having a 4.5-fold risk (95% confidence interval, 1.1-18.3) of IRU compared with patients with 18% or less retinal involvement (Karavellas et al. 2001).

All patients with a history of CMV retinitis, regardless of response to combination antiretroviral therapy, should continue to be followed closely by an ophthalmologist experienced in ocular complications of HIV infection. Before making a diagnosis of IRU, other etiologies of vitritis should be considered, including drug reactions (notably cidofovir and rifabutin), syphilis or endophthalmitis (Karavellas et al. 2001; Nguyen et al. 2000). Oral, topical and intraocular injections of corticosteroids have been used in the treatment of IRU (Karavellas et al. 2001; Nguyen et al. 2000). One observational study reported significantly improved visual acuity outcomes in eyes treated with injected corticosteroids compared with eyes that were not treated, despite the fact that the former group had more severe visual impairment at baseline (Karavellas et al. 2001).

Hepatitis B Virus and Hepatitis C Virus

Because hepatitis B virus (HBV) and hepatitis C virus (HCV) share transmission risk factors with HIV, coinfection is a common clinical problem. Hepatitis, characterized by elevations in liver enzymes and clinical symptoms, including nausea, vomiting and tender hepatomegaly, is common in HIV-infected patients treated with combination antiretroviral therapy (Sulkowski et al. 2000).

In HIV-infected patients coinfected with HBV, the differential diagnosis of hepatitis flares associated with combination antiretroviral therapy is broad. IRIS has been proposed as a cause of hepatitis flares temporally associated with combination antiretroviral therapy in some HIV/HBV-coinfected patients (Velasco et al. 1999; Mastroianni et al. 1998; Carr and Cooper 1997). Patients presented with hepatitis flares within 1 to 3 months of starting combination antiretroviral therapy, and liver biopsies showed acute lobular hepatitis, without eosinophilic infiltrates (suggestive of drug hypersensitivity) or steatohepatitis (suggestive of nucleoside analogue toxicity) (Velasco et al. 1999; Mastroianni et al. 1998; Carr and Cooper 1997). In 2 of the reports, hepatitis flares after initiating combination antiretroviral therapy were associated with increased titers of antibodies directed against HBV, and clearance of the HBe antigen and HBV DNA from the serum, lending support to the hypothesis that the flare was caused by augmentation of the immune response against HBV (Velasco et al. 1999; Carr and Cooper 1997). In the cases reported above, the combination antiretroviral therapy regimens used did not include lamivudine or tenofovir, antiretroviral drugs with activity against HBV. Hepatitis flares have been reported in association with withdrawal of lamivudine from antiretroviral regimens (Bessesen et al. 1999), and emergence of lamivudine-resistant HBV isolates (Wolters et al. 2002; Bessesen et al. 1999). Acute infection with a second hepatitis virus (e.g., hepatitis A), biliary disease and drug toxicity should also be considered in the differential diagnosis of hepatitis flares in HIV/HBV-coinfected individuals treated with combination antiretroviral therapy.

IRIS has also been implicated in HIV/HCV-coinfected patients treated with combination antiretroviral therapy. Two patients with previously unrecognized HCV infection were reported who developed hepatitis flares and HCV seroconversion shortly after initiating combination antiretroviral therapy (John et al. 1998). In both cases, anti-HCV antibody, which had been negative before starting combination antiretroviral therapy, was detected during the evaluation of the hepatitis episode. The presence of HCV infection before combination antiretroviral therapy initiation was confirmed by detection of HCV RNA in stored serum samples. In other reports, initiation of combination antiretroviral therapy in HIV/HCV-coinfected patients was temporally associated with worsening hepatic pathology on biopsy and progression to decompensated liver disease (Vento et al. 1998; Zylberberg et al. 1998), as well as extrahepatic manifestations of HCV, including cutaneous porphyria (John et al. 1998) and cryoglobulinemia with polyarthritis (Monsuez et al. 1998). In prospective studies, initiation of combination antiretroviral therapy in HIV/HCV-coinfected patients has been associated with transient increases in HCV viral loads and variable changes in aminotransferase levels (Rutschmann et al. 1998; Vento et al. 1998).

At present, no guidelines are available for managing potential IRIS in HIV-infected patients coinfected with HBV or HCV. A thorough differential diagnosis should be considered, including infection with a new pathogen, other causes of hepatic disease (cholecystitis, etc.), drug toxicity, withdrawal of antiretroviral drugs with activity against HBV, and emergence of HBV resistance to lamivudine. Mild cases may be managed with observation; antiretroviral therapy should be halted with severe clinical or laboratory changes.

Progressive Multifocal Leukoencephalopathy

Combination antiretroviral therapy has produced dramatic improvement in the dismal prognosis of progressive multifocal leukoencephalopathy (PML). In one study, the median survival after PML diagnosis was 545 days for combination antiretroviral therapy recipients compared with 60 days in the pre-HAART era (Miralles et al. 1998). Combination antiretroviral therapy is also associated with clearance of JC virus DNA from cerebrospinal fluid in PML patients (Giudici et al. 2000), a phenomenon not observed in the pre-HAART era. However, clinical and radiologic worsening of known PML (Kotecha et al. 1998) and "unmasking" of previously subclinical PML (Mayo et al. 1998) have been reported in temporal association with institution of combination antiretroviral therapy. In one review, 5 of 27 PML patients diagnosed in the HAART era first manifested PML symptoms within 9 weeks of beginning combination antiretroviral therapy (Cinque et al. 2001). PML IRIS may be characterized by new or worsening neurologic symptoms and signs and/or radiologic progression. A key radiologic difference is that PML lesions in IRIS often demonstrate contrast enhancement (Collazos et al. 1999) or mass effect (Kotecha et al. 1998), features that are rarely seen with PML in untreated AIDS patients. In one case report, stereotactic brain biopsy from an enhancing area in a patient with PML IRIS showed prominent perivascular mononuclear inflammation with enlarged immunodendrocytes that were immunoreactive for papovavirus antigen (Kotecha et al. 1998). The differential diagnosis of PML IRIS should include other central nervous system processes, including toxoplasmosis, lymphoma, bacterial abscess and TB. Most cases of PML IRIS are mild and transient (Collazos et al. 1999; Kotecha et al. 1998) when combination antiretroviral therapy is continued, but there is scant published experience with managing more severe exacerbations.

Herpes Simplex and Varicella-Zoster Virus

Herpes simplex virus (HSV) has been implicated in IRIS only rarely. One article presented 3 patients with chronic, erosive lesions of the penis due to HSV after initiation of combination antiretroviral therapy (Fox et al. 1999). Immunohistochemistry was notable for an unusual prominence of plasma cell and eosinophils in the inflammatory infiltrate. In a skin lesion believed to be herpetic that is unresponsive to treatment, it is important to rule out acquired antiviral resistance (Safrin 1992), another pathogen, or malignancy.

HIV-infected patients appear to be at increased risk for herpes zoster in the first few months after initiation of combination antiretroviral therapy, suggesting an IRIS secondary to varicella zoster virus (VZV). Although HIV-associated zoster occurs most commonly at CD4 counts under 200 cells/mm^3 (Engels et al. 1999), observational studies have reported occurrences of zoster in around 8% of patients initiating combination antiretroviral therapy (Domingo et al. 2001; Martinez et al. 1998). In one cohort, 10 of 12 zoster cases diagnosed in 1997 were temporally associated with combination antiretroviral therapy initiation (Aldeen et al. 1998). Of note, studies have reported that a higher percentage of CD8+ lymphocytes at combination antiretroviral therapy initiation (Martinez et al. 1998) and a greater increase in CD8+ cells in the first weeks of combination antiretroviral therapy (Domingo et al. 2001; Martinez et al. 1998) were strongly associated with zoster risk. Zoster occurring as a potential IRIS does not appear to have any distinguishing clinical characteristics and generally responds well to standard antiviral therapy and pain management (Martinez et al. 1998).

Cryptococcal Meningitis

Anecdotal reports have described recurrent symptoms of cryptococcal meningitis (CM) in HIV-infected patients following initiation of HAART. A retrospective study reported that 12 of 52 (24%) patients who started HAART subsequent to receiving CM treatment experienced recurrent central nervous system symptoms; of these, half were attributed to IRIS (Solomon et al. 2005).

A second study reported similar results: Over an average follow-up period of 1.48 years, 18 of 59 (30.5%) patients were admitted with IRIS-related CM subsequent to starting HAART (Shelburne et al. 2005). Three of these had never before received a CM diagnosis whereas the others had undergone treatment in the past. Most patients developed symptoms within 30 days of initiating HAART. Patients with IRIS-related CM also were likely to have begun HAART within 30 days of their previous CM diagnosis. They had both higher initial cryptococcal antigen titers in their cerebrospinal fluid and higher intracranial pressure than patients with conventional AIDS-related CM. These observations suggest a high residual burden of fungal organisms or their remnants. Both types of patients received the same treatment (10-14 days of amphotericin followed by oral fluconazole), but there was a strong trend toward decreased mortality in those with IRIS (relative risk of 0.22, $P = .069$).

Researchers predict that cases of CM IRIS will increase in developing countries, where CM is common. At present, no particular recommendations can be made on management of CM IRIS (Solomon 2005).

Eosinophilic Folliculitis

Several recent reports describe cases of eosinophilic folliculitis (EF) that become evident after beginning HAART (Delfos et al. 2004; Aquilina et al. 2002; Bouscarat et al. 2000). It appears to be an inflammatory reaction to *Demodex folliculorum* mites, which are normal inhabitants of hair follicles. Researchers have long held that traditional HIV-associated eosinophilic folliculitis frequently arises from a hypersensitivity reaction to mites (Ellis and Scheinfeld 2004).

The clinical presentation of EF and response to treatment vary substantially between patients, making it difficult to differentiate between EF and drug toxicity. Most commonly, there are lesions on the face and/or upper trunk (Delfos et al. 2004; Aquilina et al. 2002; Bouscarat et al. 2000). Pruritus may (Delfos et al. 2004; Bouscarat et al. 2000) or may not (Aquilina et al. 2002) be present. In some but not all cases, there are coalescing lesions (Aquilina et al. 2002), which do not resemble the discrete follicular papules commonly seen with traditional HIV-associated EF (Ellis and Scheinfeld 2004). The time frame for the appearance of EF after initiation of HAART has varied from a few days (Delfos et al. 2004) to a few weeks (Delfos et al. 2004) to 2 months (Aquilina et al. 2002). For definitive diagnosis, Delfos and coworkers (2004) recommend staining skin scrapings with 10% potassium hydroxide and using a 10x-20x magnification as the easiest way to observe the mites; they note that histologic assessment of skin biopsy is less sensitive.

In some cases, there has been spontaneous regression of the skin condition within 3 months (Bouscarat et al. 2000). Therapies considered effective in at least some patients include topical corticosteroid cream (betamethasone dipropionate 0.05%) (Bouscarat et al. 2000), a topical antiparasitic such as permethrin (Nix) (Aquilina et al. 2002) and topical metronidazole cream (Metrocream) (Delfos et al. 2004). Note, however, that some authors doubt the effectiveness of metronidazole, a treatment for rosacea, for this condition (Aquilina et al. 2002).

Physicians have reported a dramatic 2- to 3-week recovery from a single dose (200 mcg/kg body weight) of oral ivermectin (Stromectol) in patients who have failed topical therapies (Delfos et al. 2004; Aquilina et al. 2002). To prevent reinfestation, follow-up therapy was instituted with either weekly topical permethrin (Nix) (Aquilina et al. 2002) or topical metronidazole (Delfos et al. 2004).

There are no data on possible interactions between ivermectin and antiretroviral drugs. Still, it is important to recall that ivermectin, protease inhibitors and NNRTIs are all substrates of the P-glycoprotein drug transporters on cell membranes, raising concerns about drug-drug interactions (Delfos et al. 2004). The physicians in one case report were faced with a patient on lopinavir/ritonavir (Delfos et al. 2004). They chose to switch that individual to a triple-NRTI regimen (Trizivir) in order to prevent any interaction with ivermectin.

Autoimmune Disorders

Autoimmune disorders are another type of condition that can emerge or reactivate after HAART initiation (DeSimone et al. 2000). Peyronie's disease (Rogers and French 2004), Guillain-Barré syndrome (Piliero et al. 2003) and Reiter's syndrome (Neumann et al. 2003) have been described in case reports as manifestations of IRIS. Clinicians treating patients who present with immune-mediated conditions after initiation of HAART should suspect IRIS. They must be able to rapidly differentiate between infectious and noninfectious disorders in order to prescribe appropriate treatment (DeSimone 2000).

Systemic lupus erythematosus and sarcoidosis

Both systemic lupus erythematosus (SLE) and sarcoidosis have a lower incidence in HIV-infected individuals compared with the general population (Diri et al. 2000; Mirmirani et al. 1999). This suggests that the immunosuppressive effect of HIV inhibits the development of CD4-cell-mediated autoimmune complexes (Diri et al. 2000; Mirmirani et al. 1999). With the introduction of HAART, case reports implicate IRIS in the development or reemergence of SLE and pulmonary and nonpulmonary sarcoidosis in patients with HIV infection or AIDS who have initiated suppressive antiretroviral therapy (Mirmirani et al. 1999; Diri et al. 2000).

Diri et al. (2000) and Calza et al. (2003) describe women who developed SLE and, in one instance, discoid lupus erythematosus (Calza et al. 2003) within several months of starting HAART. In a report by Naccache et al. (1999), 2 patients developed sarcoidosis or sarcoid-like pulmonary disorders after receiving HAART. Clinical and radiographic presentation did not differ from that of non-HIV-infected patients with sarcoidosis. Patients were either asymptomatic or complained of exertional dyspnea, and chest x-rays revealed diffuse interstitial micronodular lesions, which were confirmed by CT scan. These patients did not require systemic corticosteroids. They were managed conservatively and without discontinuing HAART.

A retrospective analysis of the radiographic and clinical findings of 10 HIV-infected patients newly diagnosed with pulmonary sarcoidosis found that 2 of these 10 patients were diagnosed within 5 months of experiencing dramatic increases in CD4 cell counts subsequent to HAART (Haramati et al. 2001). A third patient experienced a flare-up of previously diagnosed sarcoidosis (manifested as acute ear swelling) that coincided with a HAART-induced leap in CD4 count from 194 to 541 cells/mm^3.

As is the case with non-HIV-infected patients, sarcoidosis and SLE are diagnoses of exclusion; causative infectious agents must be ruled out before the appropriate immunologic diagnosis is made. Clinicians should monitor their patients receiving HAART for signs and symptoms of rheumatologic conditions (which may be either new presentations or flare-ups of previously diagnosed autoimmune disorders), particularly after increases in CD4 cell counts are noted.

Thyroiditis and Grave's disease

Onset and exacerbation of autoimmune thyroiditis have been attributed to IRIS in a number of cases. Rosenfeld and Calabrese (1999) describe an HIV-infected patient who experienced progression from euthyroid Hashimoto's thyroiditis to hypothyroidism after initiation of HAART.

Another report describes 5 individuals (4 men and 1 woman) who developed Grave's disease after suppression of viral load to undetectable levels and recovery of CD4 counts with HAART (Jubault et al. 2000). None of these individuals had a personal or family history of thyroid disease or was taking medications that might disrupt thyroid function, and all developed clinically apparent hyperthyroidism within 14 to 22 months of starting HAART. Most notably, laboratory results for these patients revealed antithyroid antibodies after immune restoration, whereas pre-HAART screening for such antibodies was negative. Such findings indicate IRIS-associated new-onset Grave's disease as opposed to an exacerbation of preexisting autoimmune thyroid disease.

In mild cases, treatment for Grave's disease consists of managing hyperthyroid symptoms, generally with beta-blockers, until the patient becomes euthyroid (Weetman 2000). Severe cases require suppression of the hyperthyroidism with antithyroid drugs, radioactive iodine or thyroidectomy. Lifelong hypothyroidism, treated with replacement therapy, is a possible consequence.

References

Aldeen T, Hay P, Davidson F, et al. Herpes zoster infection in HIV-seropositive patients associated with highly active antiretroviral therapy. *AIDS*. **1998**;12:1719-1720.

Aquilina C, Viraben R, Sire S. Ivermectin-responsive *Demodex* infestation during human immunodeficiency virus infection. A case report and literature review. *Dermatology*. **2002**;205:394-397.

Bessesen M, Ives D, Condreay L, et al. Chronic active hepatitis B exacerbations in human immunodeficiency virus-infected patients following development of resistance to or withdrawal of lamivudine. *Clin Infect Dis.* **1999**;28:1032-1035.

Bouscarat F, Maubec E, Matheron S, Descamps V. Immune recovery inflammatory folliculitis [letter]. *AIDS.* **2000**;14:617-618.

Boyd AE, Brettle RP. Localized *Mycobacterium avium* intracellulare psoas abscess in patients with AIDS after antiretroviral therapy [letter]. *AIDS.* **1999**;13:2185-2186.

Brown M, Williams IG, Miller RF. Deterioration of disseminated cutaneous *Mycobacterium avium* complex infection with a leukaemoid reaction following institution of highly active antiretroviral therapy [letter]. *Sex Transm Infect.* **2001**;77:149-150.

Calza L, Manfredi R, Colangeli V, D'Antuono A, Passarini B, Chiodo F. Systemic and discoid lupus erythematosus in HIV-infected patients treated with highly active antiretroviral therapy. *Int J STD AIDS.* **2003**;14:356-359.

Carr A, Cooper DA. Restoration of immunity to chronic hepatitis B infection in HIV-infected patient on protease inhibitor. *Lancet.* **1997**;349:995-996.

Centers for Disease Control and Prevention (CDC). Guidelines for preventing opportunistic infections among HIV-infected persons — 2002 recommendations of the U.S. Public Health Service and the Infectious Diseases Society of America. *MMWR Morb Mortal Wkly Rep.* **2002**;51(RR-8).

Centers for Disease Control and Prevention (CDC). Treatment of tuberculosis. *MMWR Morb Mortal Wkly Rep.* **2003**;52(RR-11):1-77.

Chambers ST, Hendrickse WA, Record C, Rudge P, Smith H. Paradoxical expansion of intracranial tuberculomas during chemotherapy. *Lancet.* **1984**;2:181-184.

Cinque P, Pierotti C, Vigano MG, et al. The good and evil of HAART in HIV-related progressive multifocal leukoencephalopathy. *J Neurovirol.* **2001**;7:358-363.

Collazos J, Mayo J, Martinez E, et al. Contrast-enhancing progressive multifocal leukoencephalopathy as an immune reconstitution event in AIDS patients. *AIDS.* **1999**;13:1426-1428.

Crump JA, Tyrer MJ, Lloyd-Owen SJ, Han LY, Lipman MC, Johnson MA. Military tuberculosis with paradoxical expansion of intracranial tuberculomas complicating human immunodeficiency virus infection in a patient receiving highly active antiretroviral therapy. *Clin Infect Dis.* **1998**;26:1008-1009.

Currier JS, Williams PL, Koletar SL, et al. Discontinuation of *Mycobacterium avium* complex prophylaxis in patients with antiretroviral therapy-induced increases in CD4+ cell count. A randomized, double-blind, placebo-controlled trial. AIDS Clinical Trials Group 362 Study Team. *Ann Intern Med.* **2000**;133:493-503.

Dean GL, Edwards SG, Ives NJ, et al. Treatment of tuberculosis in HIV-infected persons in the era of highly active antiretroviral therapy. *AIDS.* **2002**;16:75-83.

Delfos NM, Collen AFS, Kroon FP. *Demodex* folliculitis: a skin manifestation of immune reconstitution disease [letter]. *AIDS.* **2004**;18:701-702.

DeSimone JA, Babinchak TJ, Kaulback KR, Pomerantz RJ. Treatment of *Mycobacterium avium* complex immune reconstitution disease in HIV-1–infected individuals. *AIDS Patient Care STDs.* **2003**;17:617-622.

DeSimone JA, Pomerantz RJ, Babinchak TJ. Inflammatory reactions in HIV-1-infected persons after initiation of highly active antiretroviral therapy. *Ann Intern Med.* **2000**;133:447-454.

Diri E, Lipsky PE, Berggren RE. Emergence of systemic lupus erythematosus after initiation of highly active antiretroviral therapy for human immunodeficiency virus infection. *J Rheumatol.* **2000**;27: 2711-2714.

Domingo P, Torres OH, Ris J, et al. Herpes zoster as an immune reconstitution disease after initiation of combination antiretroviral therapy in patients with human immunodeficiency virus type-1 infection. *Am J Med.* **2001**;110:605-609.

Ellis E, Scheinfeld N. Eosinophilic pustular folliculitis: a comprehensive review of treatment options. *Am J Clin Dermatol.* **2004**;5:189-197.

Engels EA, Rosenberg PS, Biggar RJ. Zoster incidence in human immunodeficiency virus-infected hemophiliacs and homosexual men, 1984-1997. *J Infect Dis.* **1999**;180:1784-1789.

Fox PA, Barton SE, Francis N, et al. Chronic erosive herpes simplex virus infection of the penis, a possible immune reconstitution disease. *HIV Med.* **1999**;1:10-18.

Furrer H, Malinverni R. Systemic inflammatory reaction after starting highly active antiretroviral therapy in AIDS patients treated for extrapulmonary tuberculosis. *Am J Med.* **1999**;106:371-372.

Giudici B, Vaz B, Bossolasco S, et al. Highly active antiretroviral therapy and progressive multifocal leukoencephalopathy: effects on cerebrospinal fluid markers of JC virus replication and immune response. *Clin Infect Dis.* **2000**;30:95-99.

Haramati LB, Lee G, Singh A, Molina PL, White CS. Newly diagnosed pulmonary sarcoidosis in HIV-infected patients. *Radiology*. **2001**;218: 242-246.

Havlir DV, Schrier RD, Torriani FJ, Chervenak K, Hwang JY, Boom WH. Effect of potent antiretroviral therapy on immune responses to *Mycobacterium avium* in human immunodeficiency virus-infected subjects. *J Infect Dis*. **2000**;182:1658-1663.

Hernandez-Albujar S, Arribas JR, Royo A, Gonzalez-Garcia JJ, Pena JM, Vazquez JJ. Tuberculous radiculomyelitis complicating tuberculous meningitis: case report and review. *Clin Infect Dis*. **2000**;30:915-921.

John M, Flexman J, French MA. Hepatitis C virus-associated hepatitis following treatment of HIV-infected patients with HIV protease inhibitors: an immune restoration disease? *AIDS*. **1998**;12:2289-2293.

Jubault V, Penfornis A, Schillo F, et al. Sequential occurrence of thyroid autoantibodies and Grave's disease after immune restoration in severely immunocompromised human immunodeficiency virus-1-infected patients. *J Clin Endocrinol Metab*. **2000**;85:4254-4257.

Karavellas MP, Azen SP, MacDonald JC, et al. Immune recovery vitritis and uveitis in AIDS: clinical predictors, sequelae, and treatment outcomes. *Retina*. **2001**;21:1-9.

Karavellas MP, Lowder CY, Macdonald C, Avila CP Jr, Freeman WR. Immune recovery vitritis associated with inactive cytomegalovirus retinitis: a new syndrome. *Arch Ophthalmol*. **1998**;116:169-175.

Karavellas MP, Plummer DJ, MacDonald JC, et al. Incidence of immune recovery vitritis in cytomegalovirus retinitis patients following institution of successful highly active antiretroviral therapy. *J Infect Dis*. **1999**;179:697-700.

Karavellas MP, Song M, MacDonald JC, Freeman WR. Long-term posterior and anterior segment complications of immune recovery uveitis associated with cytomegalovirus retinitis. *Am J Ophthalmol*. **2000**;130:57-64.

Kotecha N, George MJ, Smith TW, et al. Enhancing progressive multifocal leukoencephalopathy: an indicator of improved immune status? *Am J Med*. **1998**;105:541-543.

Kunimoto DY, Chui L, Nobert E, Houston S. Immune mediated "HAART" attack during treatment for tuberculosis. Highly active antiretroviral therapy. *Int J Tuberc Lung Dis*. **1999**;3:944-947.

Ledergerber B, Egger M, Erard V, et al. AIDS-related opportunistic illnesses occurring after initiation of potent antiretroviral therapy: the Swiss HIV Cohort Study. *JAMA*. **1999**;282:2220-2226.

Martinez E, Gatell J, Moran Y, et al. High incidence of herpes zoster in patients with AIDS soon after therapy with protease inhibitors. *Clin Infect Dis*. **1998**;27:1510-1513.

Mastroianni CM, Trinchieri V, Santopadre P, et al. Acute clinical hepatitis in an HIV-seropositive hepatitis B carrier receiving protease inhibitor therapy. *AIDS*. **1998**;12:1939-1940.

Mayo J, Collazos J, Martinez E. Progressive multifocal leukoencephalopathy following initiation of highly active antiretroviral therapy. *AIDS*. **1998**;12:1720-1722.

Minguez C, Roca B, Gonzalez-Mino C, Simon E. Superior vena cava syndrome during the treatment of pulmonary tuberculosis in an HIV-1 infected patient [case report]. *J Infect*. **2000**;40:187-189.

Miralles P, Berenguer J, Garcia de Viedma D, et al. Treatment of AIDS-associated progressive multifocal leukoencephalopathy with highly active antiretroviral therapy. *AIDS*. **1998**;12:2467-2472.

Mirmirani P, Maurer TA, Herndier B, McGrath M, Weinstein MD, Berger TG. Sarcoidosis in a patient with AIDS: a manifestation of immune restoration syndrome. *J Am Acad Dermatol*. **1999**;41:285-286.

Monsuez JJ, Vittecoq D, Musset L, et al. Arthralgias and cryoglobulinemia during protease inhibitor therapy in patient infected with human immunodeficiency virus and hepatitis C virus. *Arthritis Rheum*. **1998**;41:740-743.

Naccache J-M, Antoine M, Wislez M, et al. Sarcoid-like pulmonary disorder in human immunodeficiency virus-infected patients receiving antiretroviral therapy. *Am J Respir Crit Care Med*. **1999**;159: 2009-2013.

Narita M, Ashkin D, Hollender ES, Pitchenik AE. Paradoxical worsening of tuberculosis following antiretroviral therapy in patients with AIDS. *Am J Respir Crit Care Med*. **1998**;158:157-161.

Navas E, Martin-Davila P, Moreno L, et al. Paradoxical reactions of tuberculosis in patients with the acquired immunodeficiency syndrome who are treated with highly active antiretroviral therapy. *Arch Intern Med*. **2002**;162:97-99.

Neumann S, Kreth F, Schubert S, Mossner J, Caca K. Reiter's syndrome as a manifestation of an immune reconstitution syndrome in an HIV-infected patient: successful treatment with doxycycline [letter]. *Clin Infect Dis*. **2003**;36:1628-1629.

Nguyen QD, Kempen JH, Bolton SG, Dunn JP, Jabs DA. Immune recovery uveitis in patients with AIDS and cytomegalovirus retinitis after highly active antiretroviral therapy. *Am J Ophthalmol*. **2000**;129:634-639.

Orlovic D, Smego RA Jr. Paradoxical tuberculous reactions in HIV-infected patients. *Int J Tuberc Lung Dis.* **2001**;5:370-375.

Palella FJ Jr, Delaney KM, Moorman AC, et al. Declining morbidity and mortality among patients with advanced human immunodeficiency virus infection. HIV Outpatient Study Investigators. *N Engl J Med.* **1998**;338:853-860.

Phillips P, Kwiatkowski MB, Copland M, Craib K, Montaner J. Mycobacterial lymphadenitis associated with the initiation of combination antiretroviral therapy. *J Acquir Immune Defic Syndr Hum Retrovirol.* **1999**;20:122-128.

Piliero PJ, Fish DG, Preston S, et al. Guillain-Barré syndrome associated with immune reconstitution. *Clin Infect Dis.* **2003**;36:e111-e114.

Race EM, Adelson-Mitty J, Kriegel GR, et al. Focal mycobacterial lymphadenitis following initiation of protease-inhibitor therapy in patients with advanced HIV-1 disease. *Lancet.* **1998**;351:252-255.

Riddell J, Kaul D, Mitty J, Kazanjian P. *Mycobacterium avium* complex immune reconstitution inflammatory syndrome: long-term outcomes. In: Program and abstracts of the 12th Conference on Retroviruses and Opportunistic Infections; February 22-25, **2005**; Boston, Massachusetts. Abstract 883.

Rodriguez-Bano J, Muniain MA, Aznar J, Perez-Cano R, Corral JL. Systemic paradoxical response to antituberculous drugs: resolution with corticosteroid therapy. *Clin Infect Dis.* **1997**;24:517-519.

Rogers GD, French MA. Peyronie's disease in men with HIV responding to highly active antiretroviral therapy. *HIV Med.* **2004**;5:185-186.

Rolla V, Vieira A, Marinho F, Lourenco MC, Morgado MG. Phase IV clinical trial to access [sic] the efficacy and safety of antiretroviral treatment with ritonavir and saquinavir (400 mg-400 mg) concomitant with rifampicin in tuberculosis and AIDS patients. In: Program and abstracts of the 2nd IAS Conference on HIV Pathogenesis and Treatment; July 13-16, **2003**; Paris, France. Abstract 882.

Rosenfeld CR, Calabrese LH. Progression of autoimmune thyroiditis in an HIV-infected woman on HAART. *AIDS Read.* **1999**;9:393-397.

Rutschmann OT, Negro F, Hirschel B, et al. Impact of treatment with human immunodeficiency virus (HIV) protease inhibitors on hepatitis C viremia in patients coinfected with HIV. *J Infect Dis.* **1998**;177:783-785.

Safrin S. Treatment of acyclovir-resistant herpes simplex virus infections in patients with AIDS. *J Acquir Immune Defic Syndr.* **1992**;5(suppl 1):S29-S32.

Shelburne SA, Darcourt J, White AC, et al. The role of immune reconstitution inflammatory syndrome in AIDS-related *Cryptococcus neoformans* disease in the era of highly active antiretroviral therapy. *Clin Inf Dis.* **2005**; 40:1049-1052.

Solomon C, Masliah A, Mathews C, McCutchan A. Recurrent meningeal symptoms during HAART in patients with prior cryptococcal meningitis. In: Program and abstracts of the 12th Conference on Retroviruses and Opportunistic Infections; February 22-25, **2005**; Boston, Massachusetts. Abstract 880.

Sulkowski MS, Thomas DL, Chaisson RE, et al. Hepatotoxicity associated with antiretroviral therapy in adults infected with human immunodeficiency virus and the role of hepatitis C or B virus infection. *JAMA.* **2000**;283:74-80.

Sungkanuparph S, Vibhagool A, Mootsikapun P, Chetchotisakd P, Tansuphaswaswadikul S, Bowonwatanuwong C. Opportunistic infections after the initiation of highly active antiretroviral therapy in advanced AIDS patients in an area with a high prevalence of tuberculosis [letter]. *AIDS.* **2003**;17: 2129-2131.

Velasco M, Moran A, Tellez MJ. Resolution of chronic hepatitis B after ritonavir treatment in an HIV-infected patient. *N Engl J Med.* **1999**;340:1765-1766.

Vento S, Garofano T, Renzini C, et al. Enhancement of hepatitis C virus replication and liver damage in HIV-coinfected patients on antiretroviral combination therapy. *AIDS.* **1998**;12:167-168.

Weetman AP. Grave's disease. *N Engl J Med.* **2000**;343:1236-1248.

Wendel KA, Alwood KS, Gachuhi R, Chaisson RE, Bishai WR, Sterling TR. Paradoxical worsening of tuberculosis in HIV-infected persons. *Chest.* **2001**;120:193-197.

Wendland T, Furrer H, Vernazza PL, et al. HAART in HIV-infected patients: restoration of antigen-specific CD4 T-cell responses in vitro is correlated with CD4 memory T-cell reconstitution, whereas improvement in delayed type hypersensitivity is related to a decrease in viraemia. *AIDS.* **1999**;13:1857-1862.

Whitcup SM, Fortin E, Lindblad AS, et al. Discontinuation of anticytomegalovirus therapy in patients with HIV infection and cytomegalovirus retinitis. *JAMA.* **1999**;282:1633-1637.

Wolters LMM, Niesters HGM, Hansen BE, et al. Development of hepatitis B virus resistance for lamivudine in chronic hepatitis B patients co-infected with the human immunodeficiency virus in a Dutch cohort. *J Clin Virol.* **2002**;24:173-181.

Zeller V, Truffot C, Agher R, et al. Discontinuation of secondary prophylaxis against disseminated *Mycobacterium avium* complex infection and toxoplasmic encephalitis. *Clin Infect Dis*. **2002**;34:662-667.

Zylberberg H, Pialoux G, Carnot F, et al. Rapidly evolving hepatitis C virus-related cirrhosis in a human immunodeficiency virus-infected patient receiving triple antiretroviral therapy. *Clin Infect Dis*. **1998**;27:1255-1258.

■

(RLO-44)

IV.52. OCCUPATIONAL POSTEXPOSURE PROPHYLAXIS

LEARNING OBJECTIVE: Discuss the efficacy data and protocol of postexposure antiretroviral prophylaxis for occupational percutaneous and mucocutaneous exposure to HIV according to current CDC, Occupational Safety & Health Administration (OSHA), and local guidelines.

In 1991, the Occupational Safety & Health Administration (OSHA 2004a), a division of the U.S. Department of Labor, issued the Bloodborne Pathogens Standard (No. 1910.1030) to protect workers from the risk of exposure to bloodborne pathogens. In 2001, OSHA revised these guidelines in response to the Needlestick Safety and Prevention Act. The revised standards clarify that employers must use safer needle devices and involve employees in selecting these devices. The updated standard also requires employers to maintain a log of injuries from contaminated sharps. Additionally, 26 states and U.S. territories have approved State Occupational Safety and Health Plans (OSHA 2004b). Employers in these states must comply with state-specific requirements (OSHA 2004c). Employers in states without State OSHA Plans should establish postexposure prophylaxis (PEP) policies and programs within the context of current approaches to HIV treatment and review them periodically.

Risk of Seroconversion

Studies indicate that the risk for seroconversion after needle-stick exposure to HIV-infected blood is between 0.1% and 0.5% (Bell 1997; Ippolito et al. 1993). The level of risk associated with exposure of mucous membranes may be greater. The risk associated with exposure of nonintact skin is very low (Ippolito et al. 1993).

The following factors have been associated with an increased risk of seroconversion after an occupational exposure (Cardo et al. 1997):

- Injury from a device visibly contaminated with the patient's blood
- Injury during a procedure that involved a needle being placed directly in a vein or artery
- Deep injuries
- Advanced HIV disease in the source patient

In a retrospective case-control study (Cardo et al. 1997), after controlling for other risk factors for HIV transmission, use of zidovudine monotherapy for PEP was associated with an 81% reduction in the risk of acquiring HIV infection. Animal studies also support the potential efficacy of PEP. However, there are no definitive data from prospective studies (CDC 2001a).

PEP Therapy Recommendations

In general, five basic principles should govern PEP management following occupational exposures to HIV (Henderson 2001):

- Treatment should be available immediately
- Exposure should be confirmed (consult HIV experts, if necessary)

What's New

OSHA updated the Bloodborne Pathogens Standard to better protect workers from needle-stick injuries. Many states have State OSHA Plans. Postexposure prophylaxis regimens should consist of either a two- or three-drug antiretroviral combination, based on the risk level of the exposure and tolerability of the treatment. Postexposure prophylaxis regimens without protease inhibitors may be better tolerated.

Key Points

- Although the general risk of HIV seroconversion after needle-stick is low, other factors can increase that risk.
- Data from retrospective studies strongly indicate that use of post-exposure prophylaxis (PEP) does significantly reduce the risk of transmission from occupational exposure.
- Existing protocols should be followed carefully, and exposed health care workers should be monitored for side effects and adherence.
- Recent studies show that a protease inhibitor-sparing PEP regimen is better tolerated than one that includes a protease inhibitor.

- A PEP regimen with the best likelihood for adherence should be selected (considering therapy and viral level of source patient)
- Side effects should be anticipated and treated prophylactically
- Adherence and adverse effects should be monitored

Following exposure, the exposed person should be evaluated and tested for HIV within hours after exposure. If the source person is found to be HIV-negative, further follow-up of the exposed person is usually not necessary (CDC 2001a).

The CDC currently recommends that when PEP is indicated, therapy should consist of either a two- or three-drug antiretroviral combination, depending on the level of risk involved in the exposure (Table IV.52-1) (Bassett et al. 2004; CDC 2001a).

Table IV.52-1. U.S. Public Health Service guidelines: empirical postexposure prophylaxis.

	HIV status of source patient			
	HIV+		Unknown	HIV-
Exposure type	Asymptomatic[1]	Symptomatic[2]		
Percutaneous injury				
Less severe	2-drug regimen	3-drug regimen	None[3]	None
Severe	3-drug regimen	3-drug regimen	None[3]	None
MM/nonintact skin				
Small volume	2-drug regimen	2-drug regimen	None[3]	None
Large volume	3-drug regimen	3-drug regimen	None[3]	None

MM = mucous membranes

[1] Includes HIV RNA load below 1500 copies/mL.

[2] Includes AIDS, acute seroconversion, or high viral load.

[3] 2-drug regimen if source patient is likely HIV-positive; treatment should be discontinued if source determined later to be HIV-negative.

Reproduced with permission from Bassett et al. 2004.

Bassett and colleagues (2004) constructed a decision model for PEP. Using data from the medical literature, the model predicted an HIV transmission rate of 105 cases/100,000 high-risk needle-sticks with a two-drug regimen compared with 108 cases/100,000 high-risk needle-sticks with a three-drug regimen. The transmission rate with no PEP following high-risk needle-sticks was 300 cases/100,000.

Zidovudine/lamivudine is a commonly used nucleoside reverse transcriptase inhibitor (NRTI) backbone, although use of alternative agents should also be considered, especially when resistance to zidovudine and/or lamivudine is high in the local setting. If known, results of resistance testing and history of current and past antiretroviral therapy of the source patient should also be taken into account when attempting to select active antiretroviral agents (El-Far et al. 2003). If a third agent is used, indinavir, nelfinavir, efavirenz or abacavir should be considered; other agents may also be considered with expert consultation (CDC 2001a). When used in PEP regimens, nevirapine has been associated with severe adverse events, including cases of life-threatening hepatotoxicity, leading the CDC to advise that "in many circumstances, the risks associated with [nevirapine] as part of a PEP regimen outweigh the anticipated benefits" (CDC 2001b).

The incidence of side effects and discontinuation of PEP have been shown to increase with the number of agents included in the treatment. A review of PEP studies found that two-drug regimens had 59% toxicity and 21% discontinuation rates compared with 66% and 28%, respectively, for three-drug regimens (reviewed in Bassett et al. 2004). However, three-drug regimens should be considered in areas where drug resistance is common (Bassett et al. 2004) A previous PEP study in France found that treatment modification or discontinuation due to side effects occurred in 27% of individuals who received a four-drug regimen, compared with 17% on a three-drug regimen that included nelfinavir, and 7% on triple-NRTI regimens (Larsen et al. 2003).

Two recent studies indicate that PEP regimens without protease inhibitors are better tolerated than those including protease inhibitors. A tolerability study comparing three regimens — zidovudine plus lamivudine (ZDV-3TC) coformulation (Combivir) (n = 38), ZDV-3TC plus nelfinavir (n = 223), and stavudine (d4T) and lamivudine (3TC) plus tenofovir (n = 155) — found that fewer patients discontinued the d4T + 3TC + tenofovir regimen (1.4%) because of intolerance compared with patients receiving either the ZDV-3TC (7.9%) or ZDV-3TC + nelfinavir (5.4%) regimen (Winston et al. 2004). Overall, a significant proportion of patients receiving the ZDV-3TC (23.7%) and ZDV-3TC + nelfinavir regimens (18.4%) did not complete the 28-day treatment because of intolerance or they were lost to follow-up, compared with patients receiving the d4T + 3TC + tenofovir regimen (6.4%, P = .001).

A multicenter, prospective study comparing the tolerability of ZDV-3TC + nelfinavir (n = 301), ZDV-3TC + lopinavir/ritonavir (Kaletra) (n = 139), and ZDV-3TC + tenofovir (n = 148) found that fewer patients receiving the ZDV-3TC + tenofovir regimen (18.5%) discontinued due to adverse events, compared with patients receiving the ZDV-3TC + nelfinavir (34.5%) and ZDV-3TC + lopinavir/ritonavir (22.5%) regimens (Rabaud et al. 2004). Additionally, more patients completed the 28-day ZDV-3TC + tenofovir regimen without side effects (44.5%) than did patients receiving the ZDV-3TC + lopinavir/ritonavir (41.0%) and ZDV-3TC + nelfinavir (20.5%) regimens; however, there was no significant between-group difference for the incidence of side effects.

Preclinical studies of such agents as tenofovir (Van Rompay et al. 2001, 2000) and CCR5-binding molecules (Golding et al. 2003) have demonstrated the efficacy of prophylactic treatment immediately following exposure to HIV. Tenofovir has been combined with ZDV-3TC in a prospective French study of 171 people that included 49 occupationally exposed health care workers (Valle et al. 2004). Of people receiving PEP, 82% completed the 28-day treatment, which was well tolerated by 55%. Clinical PEP studies using investigational CCR-binding molecules have not yet been published.

PEP should be administered for 4 weeks, and adherence to the treatment regimen should be emphasized. Two reports found that many health care workers discontinued at least one of the drugs early because of side effects (Parkin et al. 2000; Puro 2000). Another anecdotal report of clinical experience estimates that 4-week adherence could be a mere 10% to 30% (Nadler 2001).

References

Bassett IV, Freedberg KA, Walensky RP. Two drugs or three? Balancing efficacy, toxicity, and resistance in postexposure prophylaxis for occupational exposure to HIV. *Clin Infect Dis.* **2004**;39:395-401.

Bell DM. Occupational risk of human immunodeficiency virus infection in healthcare workers: an overview. *Am J Med.* **1997**;102(suppl 5B):9-15.

Cardo DM, Culver DH, Ciesielski CA, et al. A case-control study of HIV seroconversion in health care workers after percutaneous exposure. *N Engl J Med.* **1997**;337:1485-1490.

Centers for Disease Control and Prevention (CDC). Updated U.S. Public Health Service guidelines for the management of occupational exposures to HBV, HCV, and HIV and recommendations for postexposure prophylaxis. MMWR Recommendations and Reports **2001a**;50(RR-11):1-42.

Centers for Disease Control and Prevention (CDC). Serious adverse events attributed to nevirapine regimens for postexposure prophylaxis after HIV exposures — worldwide, 1997-2000. *MMWR Morb Mortal Wkly Rep.* **2001b**;49:1153-1156.

El-Far F, Diaz RS, Gasparoto CT, Medeiros EAS. Postexposure prophylaxis with antiretroviral: are we doing it right? Are we thinking about the sensibility profile of antiretroviral? In: Program and abstracts of the 2nd International AIDS Society Conference on HIV Pathogenesis and Treatment; July 13-16, **2003**, Paris, France. Abstract 1172.

Golding H, Aliberti J, King LR et al. Inhibition of HIV-1 infection by a CCR5-binding cyclophilin from Toxoplasma gondii. *Blood.* **2003**;102:3280-3286.

Henderson DK. HIV postexposure prophylaxis in the 21st century. *Emerg Infect Dis.* **2001**;7:254-258.

Ippolito G, Puro V, De Carli G. The risk of occupational human immunodeficiency virus in health care workers. The Italian Study Group on Occupational Risk of HIV Infection. *Arch Intern Med.* **1993**;153:1451-1458.

Larsen C, Lot F, Basselier B, Semaille C. Prescription and toxicity of post-exposure prophylaxis for occupational and non-occupational exposures to HIV in France. In: Program and abstracts of the 2nd International AIDS Society Conference on HIV Pathogenesis and Treatment; July 13-16, **2003**, Paris, France. Abstract 1169.

Nadler J. Editorial comment in: Proia LA, Kessler HA. Rationale and recommendations for HIV postexposure prophylaxis. *Infect Med.* **2001**;18:428-438.

Occupational Safety & Health Administration (OSHA). Bloodborne pathogens and needlestick prevention [US Dept. of Labor]. **2004a**. Available at: http://www.osha.gov/SLTC/bloodbornepathogens/index.html [accessed February 14, 2005].

Occupational Safety & Health Administration (OSHA). State occupational safety and health plans. [US Dept. of Labor]. **2004b**. Available at: http://www.osha.gov/fso/osp/index.html [accessed February 14, 2005].

Occupational Safety & Health Administration (OSHA). Bloodborne pathogens and needlestick prevention. OSHA standards [US Dept. of Labor]. **2004c**. Available at: http://www.osha.gov/SLTC/bloodbornepathogens/compliance.html [accessed February 14, 2005].

Parkin JM, Murphy M, Anderson J, El-Gadi S, Forster G, Pinching AJ. Tolerability and side-effects of post-exposure prophylaxis for HIV infection. *Lancet.* **2000**;355:722-723.

Puro V. Post-exposure prophylaxis for HIV infection [letter]. *Lancet.* **2000**;355:1556-1557.

Rabaud C, Burty C, Valle C, et al. Post-exposure prophylaxis of HIV infection: Comparison of the tolerability of 3 PEP regimens. In: Program and abstracts of the International AIDS Conference; July 11-14, **2004**; Bangkok, Thailand. Abstract TuPeB4651.

Valle C, Prazuck T, Christian B, et al. Tolerability of post-exposure prophylaxis of HIV infection with the combination of zidovudine/lamivudine + tenofovir. In: Program and abstracts of the International AIDS Conference; July 11-4, **2004**; Bangkok, Thailand. Abstract TuPeB4647.

Van Rompay KK, McChesney MB, Aguirre NL, Schmidt KA, Bischofberger N, Marthas ML. Two low doses of tenofovir protect newborn macaques against oral simian immunodeficiency virus. *J Infect Dis.* **2001**;184:429-438.

Van Rompay KK, Miller MD, Marthas ML, et al. Prophylactic and therapeutic benefits of short-term 9-[2-(R)-(Ph osphonomethoxy)Propyl]Adenine (PMPA) administration to newborn macaques following oral inoculation with simian immunodeficiency virus with reduced susceptibility to PMPA. *J Virol.* **2000**;74:1767-1774.

Winston A, McAllister J, Cooper D, Carr A. The use of triple nucleoside and nucleotide regimen for non-occupational HIV post exposure prophylaxis. In: Program and abstracts of the International AIDS Conference; July 11-14, **2004**; Bangkok, Thailand. Abstract TuPeB4658.

(RLO-45)

IV.53. NONOCCUPATIONAL EXPOSURE PROPHYLAXIS

LEARNING OBJECTIVE: Discuss the use of pre- and postexposure antiretroviral prophylaxis for nonoccupational settings, including sexual exposure or rape.

Postexposure Prophylaxis

Recent data in humans demonstrate that postexposure prophylaxis (PEP) may afford protection from HIV infection after nonoccupational exposures, such as sexual contact or intravenous-drug use. A review of 700 PEP recipients in San Francisco found 7 seroconverters by week 12 (Roland et al. 2004). These PEP "failures" were marked by either late commencement of drugs, poor adherence, or possible further HIV exposures before or after PEP.

On the basis of data from animal transmission models, perinatal clinical trials, and observational nonoccupational PEP (nPEP) studies, the U.S. Department of Health and Human Services (DHHS) has recently established guidelines for nPEP for persons with a substantial risk of HIV exposure (CDC 2005a). The guidelines exclude exposures to workers in health care, sanitation, public safety, and laboratory settings; perinatal situations are also excluded. The nPEP guidelines are based on the risk of transmission:

High-risk situations

- HIV-infected source
- Exposure to mucous membrane, nonintact skin, or percutaneous contact with blood, semen, vaginal or rectal secretions, breast milk, or any body fluid that is visibly contaminated with blood
- Patient seeks care within 72 hours of exposure

Recommendation: Initiate a 28-day nPEP regimen with highly active antiretroviral therapy (HAART) within 72 hours (CDC 2005a).

Unknown-risk situations

- HIV status is unknown

  and/or

- Patient seeks care after 72 hours of exposure

Recommendation: nPEP is not recommended when the transmission risk is considered negligible or when patients seek care more than 72 hours after a substantial exposure. However, nPEP may be prescribed if the exposure was substantial and the diminished potential benefit of nPEP outweighs the potential risk for adverse events from antiretroviral medications (CDC 2005).

Table IV.53-1 displays the DHHS recommendations for antiretroviral regimens for nPEP (CDC 2005).

What's New

The U.S. Department of Health and Human Services (DHHS) has established guidelines for nonoccupational postexposure prophylaxis (nPEP). New data indicate a substantially increased risk of sexual transmission from a partner with acute HIV infection.

Key Points

- Postexposure prophylaxis (PEP) may protect against HIV infection after nonoccupational exposure if initiated within 72 hours of exposure and maintained for 28 days.
- Sexual exposure to highly transmissible acute HIV infections may be an indication for administration of PEP.
- Tenofovir-based preexposure prophylaxis is now undergoing clinical trials.

Table IV.53-1. Antiretroviral regimens for nonoccupational postexposure prophylaxis of HIV infection (CDC 2005a).

Preferred regimens	
NNRTI-based	Efavirenz[1] plus (lamivudine or emtricitabine) plus (zidovudine or tenofovir)
PI-based	Lopinavir/ritonavir (Kaletra) plus lamivudine or emtricitabine plus zidovudine
Alternative regimens	
NNRTI-based	Efavirenz plus (lamivudine or emtricitabine) plus (abacavir or didanosine or stavudine[2])
PI-based	Atazanavir plus (lamivudine or emtricitabine) plus (zidovudine or stavudine or abacavir or didanosine) or (tenofovir plus ritonavir [100 mg/day])
	Fosamprenavir plus (lamivudine or emtricitabine) plus (zidovudine or stavudine or abacavir or tenofovir or didanosine)
	Fosamprenavir/ritonavir[3] plus (lamivudine or emtricitabine) plus (zidovudine or stavudine or abacavir or tenofovir or didanosine)
	Indinavir/ritonavir[3,4] plus (lamivudine or emtricitabine) plus (zidovudine or stavudine or abacavir or tenofovir or didanosine)
	Lopinavir/ritonavir (Kaletra) plus (lamivudine or emtricitabine) plus (stavudine or abacavir or tenofovir or didanosine)
	Nelfinavir plus (lamivudine or emtricitabine) plus (zidovudine or stavudine or abacavir or tenofovir or didanosine)
	Saquinavir (hgc or sgc)/ritonavir plus (lamivudine or emtricitabine) plus (zidovudine or stavudine or abacavir or tenofovir or didanosine)
Triple-NRTI	Abacavir plus lamivudine plus zidovudine (only when an NNRTI- or PI-based regimen cannot or should not be used)

NNRTI = nonnucleoside reverse transcriptase inhibitor; PI = protease inhibitor; hgc = hard-gel saquinavir capsule; sgc = soft-gel capsule; NRTI = nucleoside reverse transcriptase.

1 Efavirenz should be avoided in pregnant women and women of childbearing potential.

2 Higher incidence of lipoatrophy, hyperlipidemia, and mitochondrial toxicities associated with stavudine vs. other NRTIs.

3 Low-dose (100-400 mg) ritonavir.

4 Use of ritonavir with indinavir might increase risk for renal adverse events.

nPEP may be especially important following exposure to sexual partners experiencing acute infection. A study of men with acute HIV infection, but no other STDs, found that changes in semen HIV-1 concentrations paralleled those in plasma concentrations (Pilcher et al. 2004). Using predictive modeling of viral dynamics, high HIV-1 semen concentrations were estimated to increase transmission during heterosexual sex by 8-10 fold between 20 and 54 days after infection. Postexposure prophylaxis should be considered for people exposed to acute HIV infections during sexual activity.

In situations where exposure is due to sexual assault, clinicians should ensure appropriate counseling and assistance to the survivor in all cases (CDC 1998). New York State guidelines urge a more aggressive approach, recommending that clinicians offer nPEP to survivors regardless of suspicions about the perpetrator's potential HIV status or risk (NYSDOH 2001). The rational selection of drugs for use in this setting is hampered by the limited data available on the pharmacokinetics and pharmacodynamics of antiretroviral agents in the genital tract. However, as with occupational PEP, if source patient information about resistance testing and history of current and past antiretroviral therapy is available, this should be taken into account when attempting to select active antiretroviral agents (El-Far et al. 2003).

Because of the challenges of providing nPEP after nonoccupational exposure, the San Francisco PEP Study was conducted to explore the characteristics of those seeking nPEP after sexual or intravenous-drug use exposure to HIV. Participants received dual-NRTI therapy, and 78% completed the 4-week treatment (a remarkably higher rate than among those with occupational exposure. (See Objective IV.52 on Occupational Postexposure Prophylaxis in this Update.) A second course of nPEP was provided to 12% who had repeat exposures (Kahn et al. 2001).

Contacting and offering HIV testing to source patients could decrease unnecessary use of PEP (Greub et al. 2002).

Preexposure Prophylaxis

There is increasing interest in utilizing existing antiretrovirals for preexposure prophylaxis (PREP) (Youle and Wainberg 2003; Hosseinipour et al. 2002). PREP can help protect high-risk populations unable to use condoms, including sex workers and women in general, as well as men who have sex with men. A leading drug candidate is tenofovir, which is relatively potent, stable, in the body, low in toxicity, and less likely to generate resistant virus. The CDC is conducting phase II/III trials with tenofovir in the United States, Botswana and Thailand, while Family Health International is engaged in similar trials in 4 other African countries (CDC 2005b).

References

Centers for Disease Control and Prevention (CDC). Antiretroviral postexposure prophylaxis after sexual, injection-drug use, or other nonoccupational exposure to HIV in the United States: recommendations from the U.S. Department of Health and Human Services. *MMWR Morb Mortal Wkly Rep*. **2005a**;54(RR-2):1-28.

Centers for Disease Control and Prevention (CDC). CDC trials of oral tenofovir for preventing HIV infection [fact sheet]. January 3, **2005b**. Available at: http://www.cdc.gov/hiv/PUBS/TenofovirFactSheet.htm [accessed April 26, 2005].

Centers for Disease Control and Prevention (CDC). Management of possible sexual, injecting-drug-use, or other nonoccupational exposure to HIV, including considerations related to antiretroviral therapy: Public Health Service statement. *MMWR Morb Mortal Wkly Rep*. **1998**;47(RR-17):1-17.

El-Far F, Diaz RS, Gasparoto CT, Medeiros EAS. Postexposure prophylaxis with antiretroviral: Are we doing it right? Are we thinking about the sensibility profile of antiretroviral? In: Program and abstracts of the 2nd IAS Conference on HIV Pathogenesis and Treatment; July 13-16, **2003**; Paris, France. Abstract 1172.

Greub G, Gallant S, Zurn P, et al. Spare nonoccupational HIV postexposure prophylaxis by active contacting and testing of the source person. *AIDS*. **2002**; 16:1171-1176.

Hosseinipour M, Cohen MS, Vernazza PL, Kashuba AD. Can antiretroviral therapy be used to prevent sexual transmission of human immunodeficiency virus type 1? *Clin Infect Dis*. **2002**;34:1391-1395.

Kahn JO, Martin JN, Roland ME, et al. Feasibility of postexposure prophylaxis (PEP) against human immunodeficiency virus infection after sexual or injection drug use exposure: the San Francisco PEP Study. J Infect Dis. **2001**;183:707-714.

New York State Department of Health. HIV prophylaxis following sexual assault: guidelines for adults and adolescents. Criteria for the Medical Care of Adults with HIV Infection. New York State Department of Health AIDS Institute; July **2001**. Available at: http://www.hivguidelines.org/public_html/center/clinical-guidelines/pep_guidelines/pep_card.pdf [accessed February 21, 2005].

Pilcher CD, Tien HC, Eron JJ, et al. Brief but efficient: acute HIV infection and the sexual transmission of HIV. *J Infect Dis*. **2004**;189:1785-1792.

Roland M, Coates T, Tapia J, Krone M, Neilands T, Hecht F. Seroconversion following non-occupational post-exposure prophylaxis. In: Program and abstracts of the 11th Conference on Retroviruses and Opportunistic Infections; February 8-11, **2004**; San Francisco, California. Abstract 888.

Youle M, Wainberg MA. Pre-exposure chemoprophylaxis (PREP) as an HIV prevention strategy. *J Int Assoc Physicians AIDS Care*. **2003**;2(3):102-105.

(RLO-46)

IV.57. GENETIC APPROACHES TO HIV THERAPY

LEARNING OBJECTIVE: Describe new genetic approaches in research to find new treatments for HIV, such as gene therapy and RNA interference.

There is a need for novel treatment strategies given the limitations of HAART: the emergence of drug resistance and toxicities, the burdensome life-long dosing and, ultimately, the persistence of viral reservoirs beyond the reach of current agents.

Gene therapy, occasionally referred to as "intracellular immunization," is a treatment process that involves inserting protective genes into cells either mechanically or by viral vectors. The goal of therapy is to have target cells produce the gene products for as long as the cells live, spreading the genes as they multiply.

There are several challenges in the development of gene therapy. To begin with, it is difficult to insert genes into sufficient numbers of the intended cells, a process usually performed ex vivo. The body contains over 100 billion cells infectible by HIV. Once transfused into the body, the bioengineered cells must then express the new genes at protective levels without eliciting a host immune response. The cells have to exhibit a survival advantage to persist and, optimally, multiply further. Immune responses to the new gene products (or the viral vector used to transfect cells in vivo) can be severe enough to defeat the therapy or even cause serious illness on their own. There is also the possibility of malignancy if gene therapy counteracts natural cellular controls. For attempts at antiretroviral therapy, targeting highly specific HIV genetic sequences has the drawback of facilitating resistance through simple mutation.

Ribozymes

Ribozymes are small RNA molecules that lyse specific RNA sequences on target molecules. Since the HIV genome is constructed from RNA, ribozymes can inhibit multiple steps in the HIV life cycle at once (Ngok et al. 2004). Initially, they protect uninfected cells by attacking the viral RNA of invading HIV. Later, they can break up short messenger RNA from the viral genes, and finally, they can halt HIV replication by destroying the full-length RNA emanating from infected cells' nuclei. As RNA molecules, the ribozymes are less likely to elicit an immune response than gene therapy that causes the cells to produce new proteins.

A phase I study inserted a ribozyme sequence targeting both the *tat* and *vpr* HIV genes into CD34+ hematopoietic progenitor cells extracted from 10 HIV-infected patients (Amado et al. 2004). Investigators employed a viral vector for the ex vivo transduction, with the control and active vector used in an equal number of cells. The cells were monitored for persistence after reinfusion. The number of cells transduced ranged from approximately 1-10 x 10^6/kg of body weight. Transduction efficiency in the first three patients was low (less than 1%-4%). Nonetheless the ribozyme sequence was detected in progeny leukocytes 6 to 12 months after infusion. Transduction efficiencies in the rest of the cohort were improved (7%-57%), and persistence was detected for 12 to 36 months. The proportion of progeny cells within the total population was small, from 0.01% to 0.001%.

What's New

This learning objective is new to the AAHIVM Core Curriculum. See Key Points below for information highlights.

Key Points

- Gene therapy may overcome many of the drawbacks to drug treatment by making cells inherently immune to HIV.
- Gene therapy has many hurdles of its own that are slowing development, including delivery of the genes to sufficient number of cells, adequate gene expression and immune responses against viral vectors and new gene products.
- Ribozymes are RNA-based enzymes. They can break up specific RNA sequences that HIV produces at various points in its life cycle.
- An alternative method is RNA interference, a natural cellular process that can silence gene expression as well as degrade the HIV RNA genome after cell entry.
- Another promising approach involves viral vectors that impart cells with the ability to create their own antiretroviral agents, such as an enfuvirtide-like compound able to block virus-cell fusion.

All of the trial participants were receiving antiretroviral therapy. Changes in viremia and CD4 count responded to changes in drug therapy and were not dependent on gene persistence or expression in any particular cell type. Investigators concluded that future trials should involve a larger number of transduced cells. A controlled phase II trial is under way and will compare viral load dynamics when antiretroviral therapy is halted 40 weeks after the ribozymes or control cells are infused (NIH 2005).

RNA Interference

RNA interference (RNAi) acts by "silencing" the messenger RNA transcribed from HIV (or other) genes. It is a primary antiviral defense mechanism of plants and lower animals but recently has been found in mammals, too (Kitabwalla and Ruprecht 2002). The mammalian form is dependent on the presence of short lengths of double-stranded RNA (lengths longer than 30 base pairs spark the production of interferon alpha in mammalian cells). The "small interfering RNA" (siRNA) forms a complex with a nuclease and helicase, and the strands are separated. They can then link up with single RNA strands with the complementary sequence. At this point, the attached nuclease destroys the linked RNA.

In plants and invertebrates, copies of a given siRNA are amplified into many copies by the cells for repeated cycles of gene silencing. The siRNA can even spread to other cells. Such amplification may not happen in mammals, but this highly sequence-specific defense is still easily triggered and takes advantage of established natural, nonimmunogenic processes.

As with ribozymes, HIV is potentially vulnerable to RNAi at several points in its life cycle. University of Massachusetts researchers constructed siRNA that targeted the HIV genes *vif* and *nef* as well as the long terminal repeat at the ends of the genome (Jacque et al. 2002). When these siRNA and a homologous HIV clone were introduced together into cells, virus production 24 hours later was 30- to 50-fold less than that of cells without the siRNA. siRNA with even a single nucleotide mismatch was markedly less suppressive. The siRNA could also attack the full-length HIV genome as it infected new cells. The investigators transfected a cell line with the siRNA 20 hours before exposing it to homologous HIV. One hour after infection, viral RNA could not be detected in cells with the siRNA sequences. After 36 hours, the level of cyclic DNA—an intermediate form between the invading HIV RNA genome and the proviral DNA integrated into cellular genes—was dramatically lower in the cells with siRNAs. Again, singly mismatched siRNA was only partially suppressive at both timepoints.

RNAi can also "knock down" cellular genes whose products are needed by HIV. (Gene silencing to shape cellular development may be RNAi's main purpose in higher animals.) This is accomplished by degrading the messenger RNA that genes express. Given RNAi's exquisite sensitivity, it could be highly vulnerable to HIV escape mutants. Attacking cellular genes is a way around this issue.

The same University of Massachusetts team looked at ways to inhibit the transcription of the proviral HIV genome, a vital step in HIV replication that involves the HIV *tat* gene plus a cellular cyclin/CDK9 complex (Chiu et al. 2004). The group impaired cyclin and CDK9 production with siRNA. The strategy correlated well with inhibited *tat* transactivation and HIV replication in the cultured cells. In another case, siRNA that targeted the chemokine receptor CXCR4 was introduced into cells in culture. These cells then did not produce CXCR4 and were protected against CXCR4-tropic, but not CCR5-tropic, HIV (Zhou et al. 2004). A third recent study used siRNA to block PARP-1, a nuclear enzyme needed to activate the HIV genome (Kameoka et al. 2004). The siRNA suppression of PARP-1 resulted in strong suppression of HIV replicative capacity, although the HIV DNA within the cellular genomes remained unaffected.

Transduction of gene plasmids for the desired siRNA offers several advantages over inserting the siRNA itself. Cells could then regularly produce the needed siRNA on their own, subject to the control of inducible promoter regions included in the genes (Jacque et al. 2002). Plasmids with genes for siRNA that silence HIV's *vif* gene proved highly effective. They reduced viral production 20- to 30-fold in cell cultures relative to nontransfected cells, inhibiting viral production in primary lymphocytes.

Fusion Inhibition

RNAi and ribozymes can only degrade existing molecules; they cannot create new protective molecular forms. A recent report (Egelhofer et al. 2004) focused on inducing cells to produce their own version of enfuvirtide.

Enfuvirtide locks onto a complementary portion of HIV gp41 envelope protein to block virus-cell fusion. A protein itself (and derived from a portion of gp41), enfuvirtide suffers from a lack of oral availability, site reactions when injected into subcutaneous fat and rapid breakdown when it enters the bloodstream (Fuzeon 2004). All of this would be obviated if cells themselves produced a similar-acting compound and attached it to their membranes. But the immunogenicity of such a membrane component is a potential pitfall: The engineered cells might be rapidly eliminated by the immune system.

The challenge was studied with a new gp41-derived fusion inhibitor, C46, which contains 10 amino acids beyond the enfuvirtide sequence. It was introduced into cells by means of a retroviral vector (Egelhofer et al. 2004) that included accessory genes whose products anchored the C46 on cell membranes. The vector also sometimes contained a genetic sequence for the HIV Rev response element (RRE). The RRE sequence acts as a decoy for HIV Rev, a protein that shepherds transcripted HIV RNA genomes out of the cell nucleus (a late step in viral replication). The result was a form of combination therapy meant to counteract resistance to the fusion inhibitor.

A cell-to-cell fusion assay (involving test lymphocytes that express HIV envelope protein) found a fourfold reduction in this activity, indicating a similar mode of action as with enfuvirtide). Transfected primary lymphocytes with or without the added RRE exhibited a 1- to 2-log reduction in p24 antigen reduction over 12 days. (Note that the cultured cells were selected for C46 expression.) In these experiments, additional activity attributable to the RRE sequence was detectable.

Preclinical studies in macaque monkeys found no evidence of toxicity or immunogenicity (Egelhofer et al. 2004). Human trials are in preparation.

References

Amado RG, Mitsuyasu RT, Rosenblatt JD, et al. Anti-human immunodeficiency virus hematopoietic progenitor cell-delivered ribozyme in a phase I study: myeloid and lymphoid reconstitution in human immunodeficiency virus type-1-infected patients. *Hum Gene Ther.* **2004**;15:251-262.

Chiu YL, Cao H, Jacque JM, Stevenson M, Rana TM. Inhibition of human immunodeficiency virus type 1 replication by RNA interference directed against human transcription elongation factor P-TEFb (CDK9/CyclinT1). *J Virol.* **2004**;78:2517-2529.

Egelhofer M, Brandenburg G, Martinius H, et al. Inhibition of human immunodeficiency virus type 1 entry in cells expressing gp41-derived peptides. *J Virol.* **2004**;78:568-575.

Fuzeon (enfuvirtide) [prescribing information]. Nutley, NJ: Roche Pharmaceuticals; October **2004**.

Jacque JM, Triques K, Stevenson M. Modulation of HIV-1 replication by RNA interference. *Nature.* **2002**;418:435-438.

Kameoka M, Nukuzuma S, Itaya A, et al. RNA interference directed against Poly(ADP-Ribose) polymerase 1 efficiently suppresses human immunodeficiency virus type 1 replication in human cells. *J Virol.* **2004**;78:8931-8934.

Kitabwalla M, Ruprecht RM. RNA interference – a new weapon against HIV and beyond. *N Engl J Med.* **2002**;347:1364-1367.

National Institutes of Health (NIH). Genetic Modification Clinical Information System. A Randomize Phase II, Double Blind, Controlled Trial to Evaluate the Safety and Efficacy of Autologous CD34+ Hematopoietic Progenitor Cells Transduced with Placebo or an anti-HIV-1 Ribozyme (OZ1) in Patients with HIV-1 Infection. Available at: http://www.gemcris.od.nih.gov/Contents/GC_CLIN_TRIAL_RPT_VIEW.asp?WIN_TYPE=R&CTID=95 [accessed February 6, **2005**].

Ngok FK, Mitsuyasu RT, Macpherson JL, Boyd MP, Symonds GP, Amado RG. Clinical gene therapy research utilizing ribozymes: application to the treatment of HIV/AIDS. *Methods Mol Biol.* **2004**;252:581-598.

Zhou N, Fang J, Mukhtar M, Acheampong E, Pomerantz RJ. Inhibition of HIV-1 fusion with small interfering RNAs targeting the chemokine coreceptor CXCR4. *Gene Ther.* **2004**;11:1703-1712.

■

POST-TEST

The 2005 Update to the *HIV Medicine Self-Directed Study Guide* is designed for use by physicians, physician assistants, nurse practitioners, registered nurses and pharmacists specializing in care for patients with HIV/AIDS throughout the United States.

CONTINUING EDUCATION CREDIT APPLICATION INSTRUCTIONS

1. Keep a record of the time required to complete each section.
2. Review the post-test at the end of this volume.
3. Complete application, activity evaluation, and post-test online at the AAHIVM Website at http://www.aahivm.org (click on "Study Guide") before the activity expiration date (June 30, 2006). You must score at least 70% to pass the post-test.

Computer System Requirements

Your web browser must support the following technologies:

- Cookies are enabled
- Support JavaScript
- Allow Popup Windows

You must be using the latest version of any of the following web browsers:

- Mozilla Firefox
- Internet Explorer
- Opera
- Safari

(Links are provided for free browser program upgrades if needed.)

Note: There is an application fee of $50 per submission. Certificates will be mailed by Medical Education Collaborative within 6 weeks of receiving your payment with successfully completed application, evaluation and post-test.

For questions regarding the accreditation of this program, please contact Medical Education Collaborative at (303) 420-3252.

ACCME

This activity has been planned and implemented in accordance with the Essential Areas and Policies of the Accreditation Council for Continuing Medical Education (ACCME) through the joint sponsorship of Medical Education Collaborative, Inc. (MEC) and the American Academy of HIV Medicine (AAHIVM). MEC is accredited by the ACCME to provide continuing medical education for physicians. MEC designates this educational activity for a maximum of 17.25 category 1 credits towards the AMA Physician's Recognition Award. Each physician should claim only those credit hours that he/she actually spent in the activity.

AANP

This program has been approved for 20.7 contact hours of continuing education by the American Academy of Nurse Practitioners (AANP). Program ID 0504191.

ANCC

This program qualifies for 20.7 contact hours. This activity is cosponsored with Medical Education Collaborative, Inc. (MEC) and the American Academy of HIV Medicine (AAHIVM). MEC is accredited as a provider of continuing nursing education by the American Nurses Credentialing Center's (ANCC) Commission on Accreditation. Provider approved by the California Board of Registered Nursing, Provider Number CEP 12990, for 20.7 contact hours.

ACPE

17.25 contact hours (1.725 CEUs) of credit for pharmacists. Approval of this course for pharmacists is under a cosponsorship agreement between Medical Education Collaborative, Inc. (MEC) and the American Academy of HIV Medicine (AAHIVM). MEC is approved by the American Council on Pharmaceutical Education (ACPE) as a provider of continuing pharmaceutical education. ACPE# 815-999-05-041-H01. The program is designed for all pharmacists.

POST-TEST

1. **Which of the following statements is true about HIV epidemiology and transmission in the United States:**

   A. Although sexually transmitted diseases (STDs) are increasing, they have not been found to increase the risk for HIV infection.

   B. HIV infection is increasing in men who have sex with men (MSM), with young African American men appearing to be at greatest risk.

   C. Among women, HIV disproportionately affects white intravenous-drug users.

   D. Transmission of resistant virus is rapidly decreasing.

   E. Resistance testing is not indicated in newly infected individuals.

2. **Which of the following statements is true regarding the global epidemiology of HIV infection:**

   A. Subtype B is the predominant type of HIV-1 throughout the world.

   B. Non-subtype B virus has not yet become established in the Western Hemisphere.

   C. Group O HIV-1 is the most common worldwide.

   D. The emergence of antiretroviral drug resistance may differ among subtypes of HIV-1.

   E. Most of the HIV infection in women is from regions outside of sub-Saharan Africa.

3. **On the basis of currently available information, which of the following factors is associated with increased risk of progression to AIDS:**

   A. Mutation in CCR5 promoter.

   B. Deletion in CCR5.

   C. HLA B57.

   D. Co-infection with hepatitis G (GBV-C).

   E. Lower *pol* replication capacity.

4. **Which one of the following statements concerning superinfection is true:**

   A. The emergence of genetically distinct virus in a patient with known previous genotype is evidence of superinfection.

   B. Evidence concerning superinfection is not yet sufficient to include information about the possibility of reinfection when counseling patients about risk reduction.

   C. The presence of circulating recombinant viruses along with animal data argues for the possibility of superinfection.

   D. The immune response to the primary HIV infection protects against subsequent infection with other HIV strains.

   E. Superinfecting strains of HIV are likely to be drug-resistant.

5. **Which of the following statements regarding rapid HIV antibody testing is true:**

   A. The assay can be used for diagnostic purposes in all persons, regardless of age.

   B. Some rapid assays can be used outside of a traditional laboratory.

   C. The test performed using a urine specimen is as sensitive as the test with a blood specimen.

   D. The test should be avoided during pregnancy.

   E. The test can determine whether someone has been infected for less than 6 months.

6. **Which of the following statements regarding the incidence of large-joint pain, osteoporosis and bone fractures among HIV-infected persons is true:**

   A. The decreased incidence of reactive arthritis is due to the decreased incidence of gonorrhea infection.

   B. Low bone mineral density (BMD) is not associated with tenofovir and abacavir treatment.

   C. The incidence of age-related diseases, such as osteoporosis, has decreased in the HIV-infected population.

   D. The hip joint is more commonly affected by avascular necrosis (AVN) than is the spine.

   E. A small percentage of HIV-infected patients with AVN possess one or more traditional AVN risk factors, including corticosteroid use, hyperlipidemia, hypercoagulability, alcoholism and smoking.

7. Which of the following statements about human papillomavirus (HPV)-related complications in patients with HIV/AIDS is true:

A. Persons with HIV/AIDS are at decreased risk for anal cancer compared with the general, HIV-negative population.

B. Regular screening with high-resolution anoscopy is not needed to confirm anal Pap smear results.

C. The use of HAART has improved immunity to many infections but does not appear to restore immunity to HPV.

D. Patients should return for follow-up in 6 months if a Pap smear uncovers low-grade intraepithelial lesions or cells of undetermined significance.

E. The tolerability of the treatment options for anal cancer is similar in HIV-positive and HIV-negative patients.

8. Acute HIV infection may be an important issue for transmission of HIV infection because:

A. It is a time when viral load is very high.

B. Absence of HIV antibodies with subsequent negative HIV test may facilitate high-risk sexual behavior.

C. Acute HIV infection is not frequently diagnosed.

D. Diagnosing acute HIV-infection allows earlier risk-reduction counseling.

E. All of the above.

9. The approach to developing a preventive vaccine for HIV infection is hampered by which of the following:

A. Poor enrollment in clinical trials.

B. Insufficient commitment from funding agencies.

C. Lack of a suitable population in which to do vaccine research trials.

D. Uncertainty about what the correlates are for protective immunity.

E. Unwillingness to use attenuated live virus vaccine approaches.

10. The Health Insurance Portability and Accountability Act of 1996 (HIPAA) stipulates that:

A. Clinicians cannot release confidential information for treatment and payment purposes, even if this information is handled or transmitted in a secure fashion.

B. Providers must give patients a written description of their privacy practices and must also document that their patients have received this.

C. Providers must meet certain privacy and security standards, but only if the provider deems it financially feasible to do so.

D. Failure to comply with HIPAA may lead to civil actions and fines but not to criminal penalties.

E. Disclosure of confidential information without a patient's consent is prohibited, even in special circumstances, such as domestic violence and/or sexual assault.

11. It would generally be considered safe to discontinue prophylaxis in which of the following patients:

A. A patient with a history of histoplasmosis in whom HAART has yielded a sustained CD4 count of over 100 cells/mm^3.

B. A patient with a history of coccidioidomycosis in whom combination antiretroviral therapy has yielded CD4 count increases to over 150 cells/mm^3 for longer than 3 months.

C. A patient who has never experienced *Pneumocystis jiroveci* pneumonia and has had combination antiretroviral therapy-induced increases in CD4 count to over 200 cells/mm^3 for at least 3 months.

D. An asymptomatic patient with a history of toxoplasmosis encephalitis whose CD4+ T cells have increased with combination antiretroviral therapy to over 150 cells/mm^3 for at least 6 months.

E. A patient who has never developed *Mycobacterium avium* complex and who has had HAART-induced increases in CD4 count to over 75 cells/mm^3 for at least 3 months.

12. Which of the following statements regarding methicillin-resistant *Staphylococcus aureus* (MRSA) skin disease is true:

A. MRSA can manifest clinically as pustular folliculitis, abscesses or infected lacerations.

B. MRSA is a hospital-acquired infection and is uncommon in the community setting.

C. MRSA cannot be transmitted from casual, skin-to-skin contact.

D. Penicillin and first-generation cephalosporins are the treatment of choice for MRSA.

E. Cultures are not necessary in the presence of symptomatic MRSA infections.

13. Which of the following statements regarding available treatments for hepatitis B virus (HBV) and hepatitis C virus (HCV) in patients coinfected with HIV is true:

A. Pegylated interferon alfa plus ribavirin successfully manages HCV within the context of HIV coinfection.

B. The experimental HBV nucleoside analog LdT has shown synergistic anti-HBV activity with the approved nucleoside analog lamivudine.

C. The combination of ribavirin and didanosine is effective against HIV infection because they act synergistically with few adverse reactions.

D. The decision on when to start HCV therapy should include weighing the possible benefits of improving tolerance to antiretrovirals in those given hepatitis C treatment first against the risks of a CD4 count decline while on interferon in those not yet given antiretrovirals.

E. HCV genotype-1 infection is associated with a better response to pegylated interferon alfa plus ribavirin.

14. Which of the following statements regarding the most recent course of the syphilis epidemic in the United States is most true:

A. Most cases of early syphilis are being diagnosed in pregnant women who are screened for prenatal care.

B. Syphilis is slowly declining in incidence in the United States.

C. A significant number of new syphilis cases are occurring in women.

D. The distribution of new syphilis cases is essentially identical to the demographics and population distribution in the country.

E. Syphilis rates among young men who have sex with men (MSM) have risen dramatically and many cases are linked to sexual relationships established over the Internet.

15. Which of the following statements regarding the treatment of acute HIV infection is true:

A. It has been shown to minimize or prevent the establishment of reservoirs of HIV-infected cells.

B. Data from clinical trials have not been encouraging, and such treatment is not considered the standard of care.

C. Treatment of primary HIV infection consistently allows for viral control once therapy is discontinued.

D. The possibility of infection with drug-resistant virus should not affect the choice of therapy when treatment is initiated at this stage.

E. Early treatment has no effect on HIV-specific immunity.

16. Which of the following reflects recommendations in the antiretroviral guidelines from both the Department of Health and Human Services (DHHS) and the International AIDS Society-USA Panel (IAS-USA):

A. Treatment should be deferred in asymptomatic patients with CD4 counts above 350 cells/mm^3.

B. Treatment can be deferred in symptomatic patients with low levels of HIV-RNA.

C. Viral load is not as strong a factor as CD4 count in making treatment decisions.

D. Treatment should be initiated for asymptomatic patients with HIV-RNA over 100,000 copies/mL.

E. Treatment can be delayed for all patients with CD4 count over 200 cells/mm^3.

17. The best time to commence antiretroviral therapy in an HIV-infected patient is:

A. When the patient's CD4 count falls below 200 cells/mm^3.

B. When the patient's viral load rises above 100,000 copies/mL.

C. When the patient appears ready to adhere to dosing schedules.

D. Determined by balancing the risks and benefits for the individual patient.

E. As soon as the patient is diagnosed – "hit hard, hit early."

18. Which of the following antiretrovirals can be prescribed at the usual dose in patients with hepatic failure:

A. Atazanavir.

B. Fosamprenavir.

C. Indinavir.

D. Enfuvirtide.

E. All of the above.

19. Genetic variability among which of the following can clinically affect agents commonly used to treat HIV:

A. Immune characteristics, drug metabolizing enzymes, targets and transporters.

B. Drug targets and transporters.

C. Immune characteristics and drug metabolizing enzymes.

D. Drug metabolizing enzymes.

E. Immune characteristics.

20. Which of the following regarding nevirapine hepatotoxicity is true:

A. Hepatotoxicity is more common in patients with CD4 counts below 200 cells/mm^3.

B. The risk for hepatotoxicity increases more in women than in men.

C. The risk for hepatotoxicity is almost exclusively within the first 4 to 6 weeks of therapy.

D. Pregnancy appears to have a protective effect against the development of hepatotoxicity.

E. Nevirapine can be restarted once rash resolves and liver enzyme levels normalize.

21. Which of the following statements regarding methadone is true:

A. Protease inhibitors (PIs), but not nonnucleoside reverse transcriptase inhibitors (NNRTIs), cause a reduction in methadone levels.

B. Withdrawal symptoms, if they appear, happen at least 6 to 8 weeks after starting antiretroviral therapy.

C. Withdrawal symptoms may be precipitated by stopping antiretrovirals.

D. Nucleoside reverse transcriptase inhibitors (NRTIs) do not appear to significantly alter methadone levels, with the exception of abacavir.

E. Indinavir has the most significant interaction with methadone compared with the other PIs.

22. JF started therapy 9 months ago with tenofovir/lamivudine/lopinavir/ritonavir. He presents to the clinic and his viral load, which was undetectable, is now measurable at 1000 copies/mL. You order a resistance test that detects M184V alone. Which of the following statements is true:

A. Protease inhibitor resistance actually exists but is not detected upon genotypic resistance testing.

B. The M184V mutation alone prohibits future didanosine use.

C. Emtricitabine is active versus the M184V mutation.

D. Continued viral replication on the current antiretroviral regimen could select for the K65R mutation.

E. The M184V limits the response to efavirenz in future treatment.

23. Which of the following is currently (as of March 2005) FDA-approved for once-daily dosing:

A. Lopinavir/ritonavir.

B. Saquinavir/ritonavir.

C. Atazanavir.

D. Nevirapine.

E. Indinavir/ritonavir.

24. Questions of individual patient characteristics and drug resistance aside, which of the following antiretroviral combinations has the best established efficacy as an initial regimen for a 28-year-old man with a CD4 count of 150 cells/mm^3, a viral load of 50,000 copies/mL, and no history of opportunistic infections, according to the current Department of Health and Human Services (DHHS) Guidelines:

A. Abacavir/lamivudine/tenofovir (all once daily).

B. Lamivudine/tenofovir/efavirenz.

C. Tenofovir/emtricitabine/delavirdine.

D. Lopinavir/ritonavir (coformulation)/stavudine/didanosine.

E. Stavudine/lamivudine/indinavir.

25. Which of the following is a coformulation containing a new antiretroviral agent:

A. Combivir.

B. Truvada.

C. Kaletra.

D. Epzicom.

E. All of the above.

26. Which of the following combinations of agents requires a change in dosing:

A. Lopinavir/ritonavir 400 mg/100 mg twice daily in combination with fosamprenavir 700 mg twice daily.

B. Efavirenz 600 mg once daily plus fosamprenavir/ritonavir (1400/300 mg) once daily.

C. Tenofovir 300 mg once daily plus lopinavir/ritonavir 400 mg/100 mg twice daily.

D. Tenofovir 300 mg once daily plus atazanavir 400 mg once daily.

E. Efavirenz 600 mg once daily plus lopinavir/ritonavir (533/133 mg) twice daily.

27. Which of the following regarding pharmacokinetic enhancement of protease inhibitors with ritonavir is true:

A. The addition of ritonavir increases the overall daily pill burden.

B. Doses of ritonavir less than 200 mg should be avoided because of insufficient cytochrome P450 inhibition.

C. Treatment-naive patients on atazanavir/ritonavir once daily have exhibited significant improvements in lipid profiles compared with lopinavir/ritonavir.

D. When atazanavir is taken with efavirenz, it is recommended that atazanavir be combined with low-dose ritonavir.

E. The optimal dose of lopinavir/ritonavir/fosamprenavir is 400/200/700 mg twice daily.

28. Which of the following HAART (highly active antiretroviral therapy) regimens is inadvisable:

A. Tenofovir, lamivudine and efavirenz.

B. Abacavir, lamivudine and efavirenz.

C. Tenofovir, lamivudine and abacavir.

D. Zidovudine, lamivudine and nevirapine.

E. Tenofovir, emtricitabine, abacavir and lopinavir/ritonavir.

29. Which patient would be the best candidate for resistance testing:

A. A person on initial therapy with a viral load of 600 copies/mL after 4 weeks of treatment.

B. A woman with no known medical history who comes to the hospital in labor and tests HIV-positive with a rapid enzyme-linked immunosorbent assay (ELISA).

C. A patient not yet on therapy who seroconverted 5 years ago.

D. A patient on a second regimen of tenofovir/lamivudine/lopinavir/ritonavir and a viral load of 60,000 copies/mL.

E. A patient who stopped therapy 6 months ago and wants to resume.

30. Which of the following situations describes a potential cause of regimen failure:

A. A patient reports difficulty remembering to take medication every day, forgetting to take antiretrovirals at least three days a week.

B. A patient on his first antiretroviral regimen finds efavirenz intolerable because of disturbing dreams but asks to be switched to a protease inhibitor-based regimen before the toxicity affects his adherence.

C. A patient with a consistent undetectable viral load asks to be switched to an antiretroviral regimen that is taken only once a day.

D. A highly treatment-experienced patient whose first regimen was AZT monotherapy is now on combination therapy and still maintains an undetectable viral load.

E. A newly infected patient is put on a starting antiretroviral regimen containing efavirenz and has an undetectable viral load after 30 weeks on treatment.

31. Which of the following statements regarding the K65R mutation is true:

A. The presence of L74V prevents the emergence of HIV with K65R.

B. K65R does not cause resistance to thymidine analogs.

C. The use of a thymidine analog in an antiretroviral regimen appears to decrease the incidence of K65R.

D. Treatment options following development of K65R have been well described.

E. The presence of L74V combined with K65R always results in HIV with a very low replicative capacity.

32. Which of the following is TRUE about use of the replication capacity test:

A. In studies, results of the replication capacity assay have provided insights into why there may be a disconnect between CD4 counts and HIV levels.

B. In treatment-naive patients, a low replication capacity has been shown to support the decision to delay the initiation of treatment.

C. Patients found to have an HIV isolate with a low replication capacity are unlikely to transmit their virus to another person.

D. When a patient is experiencing virologic failure with an increasing HIV RNA level, results of the replication capacity assay have been shown to be helpful in choosing the next regimen.

E. There is a single method to measure viral fitness.

33. Treatment interruptions have been proven to be clinically useful in which of the following settings:

A. Treatment of acute HIV infection to allow patients to stop their antiretroviral therapy after achieving high-level suppression.

B. In salvage therapy to allow for the return of drug-sensitive virus and more effective use of the next regimen.

C. As a means to decrease cost and toxicity through short on-and-off cycles.

D. In chronically infected patients with low CD4 counts to reduce toxicity.

E. None of the above.

34. An HIV-infected woman not on therapy presents with a viral load of 14,000 copies/mL and a CD4 count of 810 cells/mm^3 and is 6 weeks pregnant. She is placed on initial therapy of zidovudine + lamivudine (Combivir) and nelfinavir and, after 8 weeks, achieves a plasma viral load below 50 copies/mL. She maintains this level of viral suppression throughout pregnancy and after successful delivery wishes to stop therapy. You accept her choice but counsel her that there is some risk for the development of resistance to one or more of the drugs that she is taking. To which drug(s) is her virus most likely to develop resistance if she stops this combination:

A. Zidovudine.

B. Lamivudine.

C. Nelfinavir.

D. Both zidovudine and lamivudine.

E. All three drugs.

35. Which of the following classes of investigational agents has raised concerns about inducing rapid progression of HIV disease:

A. Fusion blockers.

B. Coreceptor antagonists.

C. Integrase inhibitors.

D. Maturation inhibitors.

E. Anti-CD4 antibodies.

36. Which of the following statements regarding investigational strategies with approved antiretrovirals is true:

A. Induction/maintenance strategies attempt to decrease antiretroviral exposure and, hence, side effects and cost.

B. Boosted double-protease inhibitor (PI) regimens are superior to single boosted PI regimens in PI-experienced patients.

C. Nucleoside reverse transcriptase inhibitor (NRTI)-sparing regimens using lopinavir/ritonavir have proved effective, unlike combinations with other PIs.

D. The strategies outlined in this Study Guide represent creative solutions to intractable treatment problems and should be instituted on a widespread basis.

E. Quadruple drug combinations are definitely superior to triple-drug combinations as initial therapy.

37. Which of the following drugs is contraindicated as part of antiretroviral therapy in HIV-infected pregnant women:

A. Ritonavir.

B. Enfuvirtide.

C. Tenofovir.

D. Efavirenz.

E. Zidovudine.

38. When prescribing protease inhibitors to pregnant women, which of the following is the best course of action:

A. Use nevirapine exclusively.

B. Increase the recommended dosage.

C. Boost with ritonavir.

D. Closely monitor for indications of viral breakthrough and drug toxicities.

E. Apply the latest research findings on pharmacokinetics during pregnancy.

39. One of your patients has a viral load of 5000 copies/mL and a CD4 count of 250 cells/mm^3 after a year on therapy. Pretreatment, the patient's viral load was 50,000 copies/mL, and his CD4 count was 180 cells/mm^3. Genotyping finds no new mutations, but counseling reveals that the patient's adherence to the dosing schedule is slipping. Which of the following is the most appropriate next step:

A. Do nothing. Someone with a viral load this low will have a stable or increasing CD4 count.

B. Give the patient a drug holiday so that he does not waste drugs by letting drug-resistant HIV arise.

C. Talk to the patient about his lifestyle and habits; see if adjustments can be made or find a simpler regimen.

D. Switch immediately to a salvage therapy with a different resistance profile.

E. Order a phenotype test to further check on resistance patterns.

40. Which of the following statements regarding lipodystrophy in patients taking antiretroviral therapy is true:

A. Small randomized trials of several oral antihyperglycemic agents, including metformin (Glucophage), have demonstrated that these agents significantly reduce the incidence of lipodystrophy in patients receiving antiretroviral therapy.

B. Stavudine has been implicated in the development of lipoatrophy, but only in patients receiving concomitant protease inhibitor therapy.

C. Techniques currently employed in the management of lipodystrophy in patients receiving antiretroviral therapy include treatment with niacin, metformin (Glucophage) and growth hormone as well as exercise and surgical intervention.

D. Although the etiology of lipoatrophy is well understood, the mechanisms behind fat accumulation require further investigation.

E. Research has shown that injections with polylactic acid (Sculptra) have successfully improved facial appearance in patients with treatment-associated facial lipoatrophy but that treated patients reported high levels of anxiety and depression even after treatment.

41. Which one of the following statements regarding metabolic complications of antiretroviral therapy is true:

A. The statin of choice for patients requiring pharmacologic treatment of hyperlipidemia is simvastatin.

B. After diagnosis of lactic acidosis is made, a patient's NRTIs should be discontinued, while other agents in her or his regimen should be continued and supportive therapy provided.

C. First-line regimens containing protease inhibitors, except atazanavir, have been shown to have more deleterious effects on LDL-c and TC in comparison to other regimens.

D. Because asymptomatic hyperlactatemia may indicate impending lactic acidosis, periodic monitoring of lactate levels should be performed in patients taking NRTIs.

E. NNRTI-based regimens have been observed to increase total and LDL cholesterol while decreasing HDL-c levels.

42. Recent data on antiretroviral therapy and cardiovascular disease have indicated that:

A. Patients receiving first-line HAART regimens containing 2 protease inhibitors have similar elevations in TC and triglyceride levels as patients receiving HAART regimens containing a single protease inhibitor.

B. For treatment-naive patients with a family history of coronary artery disease, the risks of HAART generally outweigh the benefits.

C. Patients receiving NNRTIs have higher TC and LDL-c levels than do treatment-naive patients; in addition, the decrease in HDL-c in these patients results in a detrimental effect on the TC:HDL-c ratio.

D. Antiretroviral therapy with any class of agents results in a 2-fold increased risk of hypertension.

E. HAART results in a 26% relative increase in the incidence of myocardial infarction for each year on combination antiretroviral therapy.

43. Which one of the following statements regarding the autoimmune manifestations of immune reconstitution inflammatory syndrome (IRIS), as discussed in this Study Guide, is most true:

A. IRIS-associated autoimmune disorders generally represent immune-mediated conditions that have an increased incidence in HIV-infected individuals compared with the general population.

B. Autoimmune manifestations of IRIS always represent "unmasking" or flare-ups of disorders that were present before HAART was initiated.

C. Eosinophilic folliculitis (EF) is a highly variable skin eruption.

D. Autoimmune-related IRIS is generally a diagnosis of exclusion. It requires careful investigation in order to rule out causative infectious agents.

E. Clinical presentations of autoimmune disorders arising from immune reconstitution vary greatly from those seen in HIV-negative individuals.

44. Which of the following 28-day regimens is most likely to be completed after an occupational exposure:

A. Two-drug regimen.

B. Three-drug regimen with a protease inhibitor.

C. Three-drug regimen without a protease inhibitor.

D. Four-drug regimen.

E. The number of drugs per regimen has no bearing on the compliance.

45. Which of the following is a hurdle to establishing more reliable guidelines for nonoccupational postexposure prophylaxis (nPEP):

A. The probability of sexual transmission is highly variable but is substantially increased when a partner is undergoing acute HIV infection.

B. An uncontrolled cohort study demonstrated that nPEP failures often delayed the initiation of therapy or failed to take therapy reliably.

C. Available antiretroviral agents have side effects.

D. Drug pharmacokinetics in the genital tract do not necessarily mirror those in the blood.

E. A remarkably high rate of treatment completion has been recorded.

46. Which of the following regarding the current status of gene therapy is most true:

A. It is forging ahead and will soon replace HAART.

B. RNA interference (RNAi) has established a clear advantage in this field.

C. A focus on cellular targets is the preferred way to overcome HIV resistance.

D. There are a number of promising early studies but serious challenges remain.

E. Safety has been clearly demonstrated in human beings.

APPENDIX: THE 2005 CORE CURRICULUM LEARNING OBJECTIVES

PART I: OVERVIEW OF HIV INFECTION

PART II: APPROACH TO THE PATIENT WITH HIV

PART III: CLINICAL MANIFESTATIONS OF HIV INFECTION AND ASSOCIATED CONDITIONS

PART IV: PRINCIPLES OF ANTIRETROVIRAL THERAPY

PART V: RESEARCH ISSUES

PART I: OVERVIEW OF HIV

CHAPTER 1: EPIDEMIOLOGY AND CLASSIFICATION

➔ I.1	U.S. EPIDEMIOLOGY	Describe current demographic trends in HIV disease in the United States, especially regarding gender, sexuality, race/ethnicity, age, injection-drug use, socioeconomic status, emerging subtypes and transmission of resistant virus.
➔ I.2	GLOBAL VIROLOGY	Discuss the global prevalence and geographic distribution of HIV-1 and HIV-2 infection, including HIV-1 classes/clades/recombinant forms, and the implications for therapy.
I.3	AIDS DEFINITION	Describe the CDC classification system for HIV and the case definition for AIDS.

CHAPTER 2: BASIC SCIENCE AND PATHOGENESIS

I.4	BASIC HIV VIROLOGY	Demonstrate a knowledge of basic HIV virology, including the HIV intracellular life-cycle stages that are used as pharmacologic targets.
➔ I.5	PREDICTIVE FACTORS FOR HIV DISEASE PROGRESSION	Demonstrate knowledge of the factors predictive of HIV disease progression, including host factors that can result in differences in progression, and how to communicate this concept to patients.
I.6	VIRAL REPLICATION	Discuss the HIV life cycle in the human body and the CD4+ T cell, monitoring of CD4 count and HIV viral load, and HIV replication kinetics, for patient and community education settings.
I.7	IMMUNE RESPONSE TO HIV	Describe the immune response to HIV and the interaction between the virus and the immune system.

CHAPTER 3: TRANSMISSION

I.8	MODES	Explain the modes of sexual and nonsexual transmission of HIV and their relative risks, including the impact of untreated STDs, in a manner appropriate for educating patients and the community about HIV risk and prevention.
I.9	UNSUBSTANTIATED MODES	Describe the evidence against unsubstantiated HIV transmission modes (e.g., mosquito-borne transmission).
➔ I.10	SUPERINFECTION	Discuss the data regarding HIV co-infection and superinfection/reinfection, and the implications for patient education/management.

CHAPTER 4: DETECTION AND DIAGNOSIS

I.11	FALSE-POSITIVE AND FALSE-NEGATIVE TEST RESULTS	Discuss the problem of false-positive and false-negative results when testing populations of high versus low HIV prevalence, and the problems associated with the window period.
I.12	TEST SENSITIVITIES AND SPECIFICITIES	Discuss the sensitivity and specificity of enzyme immunoassay (EIA) and Western blot HIV antibody tests.
➔ I.13	TESTING METHODS	Describe the benefits, limitations, appropriate use, interpretation and confirmation of available testing methods for HIV-1 and its various clades, and for HIV-2.
I.14	DIAGNOSIS OF PRIMARY INFECTION	Describe the approach to the diagnosis of the acute retroviral syndrome (primary HIV infection), including use of HIV viral load.

PART II: APPROACH TO THE PATIENT WITH HIV

CHAPTER 5: HISTORY

II.1 TAKING PATIENT HISTORIES
Describe proper history taking in an HIV-infected patient, including an appropriate systems review for both an initial visit and a routine follow-up visit.

II.2 TAKING SENSITIVE HISTORIES
Describe methods for nonjudgmentally screening HIV-positive patients for behaviors associated with transmission of HIV and other STDs.

CHAPTER 6: PHYSICAL EXAMINATION AND LAB EVALUATION

II.3 KEY COMPONENTS OF PHYSICAL EXAMINATION
Describe key components of the physical examination and evaluation of the HIV-infected patient.

II.4 BASELINE LABORATORY EVALUATIONS
Identify important baseline laboratory evaluations for the new patient with HIV infection.

II.5 PROPHYLAXIS INDICATIONS
Discuss laboratory indications for specific prophylaxis of opportunistic infections.

CHAPTER 7: SYMPTOMS/SYSTEM EVALUATION

II.6 RESPIRATORY SYMPTOMS
Discuss the differential diagnosis of the following respiratory symptoms in HIV-infected patients:
- (a) shortness of breath;
- (b) chest pain;
- (c) cough.

II.7 GASTROINTESTINAL SYMPTOMS
Discuss the differential diagnosis of the following gastrointestinal symptoms in HIV-infected patients:
- (a) diarrhea;
- (b) odynophagia/dysphagia;
- (c) abdominal pain;
- (d) rectal pain or mass.

II.8 NEUROLOGIC SYMPTOMS
Discuss the differential diagnosis according to disease stage of the following neurologic symptoms in HIV-infected patients:
- (a) headache;
- (b) seizure;
- (c) painful feet;
- (d) paraplegia;
- (e) hemiparesis;
- (f) altered mental status.

II.9 VISUAL SYMPTOMS
Discuss the differential diagnosis of abnormal visual symptoms in HIV-infected patients.

II.10 DERMATOLOGIC PRESENTATIONS
Discuss the most common skin eruptions seen in HIV-infected patients.

→ **II.11 LARGE-JOINT PAIN, OSTEOPOROSIS, AND BONE FRACTURES**
Discuss the evaluation of hip and other large-joint pain in HIV-infected patients.

II.12 FATIGUE
Discuss the differential diagnosis of fatigue in HIV-infected patients.

II.13 WASTING — Discuss the differential diagnosis of wasting in HIV-infected patients.

II.14 FEVER — Discuss the differential diagnosis of fever in HIV-infected patients.

II.15 SLEEP DISORDERS — Discuss the differential diagnosis of insomnia and other sleep disturbances in HIV-infected patients.

CHAPTER 8: HIV TESTING AND COUNSELING

II.16 CONFIDENTIAL AND ANONYMOUS TESTING — Discuss confidential and anonymous HIV testing, pre- and posttest counseling, consent for HIV testing, implications and follow-up of rapid test results, and prenatal/neonatal HIV antibody testing.

II.17 PATIENT EDUCATION ESSENTIALS — Outline the basic information needed (including antiretroviral therapy, adherence and treatment complications) and its appropriate sequencing for a newly diagnosed HIV-infected patient.

CHAPTER 9: HEALTH MAINTENANCE

II.18 CONTRAINDICATED COMMON VACCINES — Identify any commonly used vaccines that are contraindicated or require special considerations when used in HIV-infected patients.

II.19 RECOMMENDED VACCINES — Discuss the use of pneumococcal vaccine, hepatitis A and B vaccines, tetanus vaccine and influenza vaccines in HIV-infected patients, and their efficacy according to disease stage.

→**II.20 PAP SMEARS** — Discuss the recommended frequency and specimen collection technique, and cite indications for specialist referral for colposcopy or high-resolution anoscopy or biopsy, for the following:

(a) genital tract Pap smears in HIV-infected women;
(b) anal Pap smears in HIV-infected men and women.

II.21 FAMILY PLANNING AND PRECONCEPTION CARE — Discuss family planning and preconception care considerations in serodiscordant and seropositive couples, including:

(a) preconception counseling about HIV, pregnancy and prevention of perinatal transmission;
(b) preconception care, including techniques that have been developed to achieve conception without transmission of infection in serodiscordant couples;
(c) the prevalence and management of infertility;
(d) prevention of unintended pregnancy and use of dual protection methods (ways to prevent both pregnancy and transmission/acquisition of sexually transmitted infection).

II.22 TUBERCULOSIS SCREENING AND ASSESSMENT — Describe tuberculosis screening indications (including exposure history) and assessment methods (including selection, interpretation and limitations of screening test in HIV-infected patients).

II.23 DENTAL CARE — Discuss the importance of routine dental care for HIV-infected patients and essential information to be included in the treating physician's written referral.

II.24 NUTRITIONAL CARE — Discuss indications for nutritional supplements in HIV-infected patients and essential information to be included in the treating physician's written referral.

II.25 SMOKING CESSATION — Describe the special risks posed by smoking for HIV-infected patients.

II.26 EXERCISE AND FITNESS — Discuss the importance of exercise in routine health maintenance of the HIV-infected patient.

→ **Denotes Recent Learning Objectives**

CHAPTER 10: HIV TRANSMISSION PREVENTION

→ II.27	**HIV TRANSMISSION RISK ASSESSMENT AND RISK-REDUCTION COUNSELING**	Describe appropriate and comprehensive HIV and STD risk assessment and risk reduction/behavioral intervention counseling for patients, in accordance with current CDC guidelines, with special attention to "prevention for positives (HIV-infected patients)" and high-risk groups of HIV-positive patients; and identify where to find information and materials to assist in these HIV prevention efforts.
II.28	**PATIENT MISCONCEPTIONS ABOUT TRANSMISSION**	Describe misconceptions that patients often have about HIV transmission and prevention, including the risk for transmission associated with specific sexual behaviors, the effect of antiretroviral therapy on risk for transmission and the effectiveness of postexposure prophylaxis for nonoccupational exposure to HIV.
II.29	**PARTNER COUNSELING AND NOTIFICATION**	Explain the rationale and current CDC recommendations for providing partner counseling and referral services (PCRS) to HIV-positive patients and their partners; describe the basic steps involved in PCRS and partner notification; and identify where to find information and materials to assist in this process.
II.30	**HYGIENE AND INFECTION-CONTROL COUNSELING**	Discuss information that should be conveyed to HIV-infected patients and their household contacts to enhance hygiene and infection control in the home.
II.31	**MOTHER-TO-CHILD TRANSMISSION PREVENTION (MTCTP)**	Discuss issues relating to MTCTP in HIV-infected women.
II.32	**INJECTION-DRUG USE**	Describe HIV prevention messages that should be communicated to HIV-infected injection-drug users who continue to inject.
II.33	**BREAST-FEEDING**	Discuss issues surrounding breast-feeding by HIV-infected women in the developed-world setting.
II.34	**PUBLIC HEALTH INTERVENTIONS**	Describe major features of CDC guidelines for implementing HIV prevention, including increased screening and testing for HIV.
II.35	**TUBERCULOSIS PREVENTION**	Describe the rationale and essential components of tuberculosis prevention in the context of HIV prevention, detection and management.
→ II.36	**PREVENTIVE HIV VACCINE RESEARCH**	Discuss current research on the development of vaccines to prevent HIV infection.

CHAPTER 11: CARE SETTINGS/MODALITIES

II.37	**UNIVERSAL PRECAUTIONS**	Describe the scientific rationale and specific components of universal precautions in health care settings for preventing transmission of bloodborne pathogens (i.e., HIV, HBV, HCV).
II.38	**HIV-INFECTED HEALTH CARE WORKERS**	Discuss appropriate infection-control measures and local requirements for an HIV-infected health care worker.
II.39	**PULMONARY TUBERCULOSIS AND INFECTION CONTROL**	Describe proper infection-control procedures for patients with proven or suspected pulmonary tuberculosis.
II.40	**OCCUPATIONAL EXPOSURE MANAGEMENT**	Identify critical elements in the management of occupational needle-stick exposures.

II.41 ANTIRETROVIRALS DURING AND AFTER HOSPITALIZATION	Discuss issues in determining the relative priority of initiating and/or maintaining antiretroviral therapy in the context of the hospitalized HIV patient with significant comorbid conditions, as well as issues of continuity of care after the inpatient setting.
II.42 PERIOPERATIVE CARE	Describe important considerations in the perioperative care of an HIV-infected patient.
II.43 AIDS-RELATED DEMENTIA AND IN-HOME CARE	Identify key elements of a discussion with the family of a person with AIDS-related dementia regarding in-home care.
II.44 TRANSPLANTATION	Describe indications and outcomes for organ transplantation in HIV-infected patients.

CHAPTER 12: PAIN MANAGEMENT

II.45 PRINCIPLES OF PAIN MANAGEMENT	Discuss the principles of pain management and the use of NSAIDs, opiates, anticonvulsants, and antidepressants, and describe the pyramid of pain management from weakest to strongest analgesic.
II.46 OPIOID AGENTS	Describe the characteristics of different opioid agents, including efficacy and side effects.
II.47 PAIN MANAGEMENT IN CURRENT AND PAST SUBSTANCE USERS	Describe the special considerations involved in pain management for HIV-infected patients with current or past substance use.

CHAPTER 13: SPECIAL POPULATIONS

II.48 DIVERSITY AWARENESS	Recognize the impact and importance of culture, ethnicity, immigration status, sexual orientation, religion, gender, drug use/injection-drug use, disability and age on the care of HIV patients.
II.49 ISSUES OF PROVIDER DISTRUST	Describe causes and implications of provider distrust among HIV-infected patients.
II.50 APPROACH TO HIV DENIALIST VIEWS	Summarize the views of those who believe that AIDS is not caused by HIV, and the approach to patients who raise questions about these views.
II.51 CARING FOR HIV-INFECTED WOMEN	Discuss the following specific issues in the management of HIV-infected women: (a) differentiation in the natural history of HIV disease in women compared with that in men; (b) differences in viral load and implications for initiation of antiretroviral therapy; (c) important considerations in the use of hormonal contraceptives; (d) sex-specific presentation of medication side effects (e.g., lipodystrophy).
II.52 CARING FOR HIV-INFECTED CHILDREN	Identify similarities and differences in the diagnosis, laboratory markers, vaccinations, spectrum of disease manifestations, antiretroviral treatment and opportunistic infection prophylaxis in HIV-infected prepubertal children compared with HIV-infected adults.
II.53 CARING FOR HIV-INFECTED ADOLESCENTS	Describe the potential for physiologic and cognitive development in an HIV-infected adolescent to affect treatment adherence and secondary prevention.
II.54 CARING FOR OLDER HIV-INFECTED PATIENTS	Describe how the diagnosis and management of HIV-infected patients who are 50 years or older differs from that of younger adult patients.
II.55 CARING FOR TRANSGENDER HIV-INFECTED PATIENTS	Describe the management of transgender HIV-infected patients, including routine health maintenance and use of hormone therapy.
II.56 DRUG-USE TERMS	Define terminology commonly used in the context of substance use.

II.57	**HOMELESS POPULATIONS**	Describe special considerations affecting medical management of homeless individuals.
II.58	**INCARCERATED POPULATIONS**	Recognize important medical and social problems that can occur for HIV-infected patients during incarceration and upon release.
II.59	**RURAL POPULATIONS**	Describe obstacles to optimal HIV care for patients in rural settings.
II.60	**MIGRATING POPULATIONS**	Discuss limitations in HIV care and special needs among migrant populations or patients with undocumented citizenship.
II.61	**SUBSTANCE USE IN HIV-INFECTED PATIENTS**	Discuss the importance of identifying and treating substance use and dependence in HIV-infected patients and the impact on HIV transmission, antiretroviral adherence and overall medical care outcomes.

CHAPTER 14: PSYCHOSOCIAL AND ECONOMIC ISSUES

II.62	**MANAGING DIFFICULT PATIENTS**	Describe the professional approach to HIV-infected patients with personality and other behavioral disorders.
II.63	**ETHICAL ISSUES**	Discuss the following issues in HIV and ethics: (a) confidentiality and right to privacy; (b) duty to report communicable diseases; (c) death with dignity; (d) patient-provider relationship boundaries.
II.64	**DISCLOSURE**	Discuss the potential risks, benefits and ethical dimensions of disclosing HIV diagnosis to family, friends, sexual partners and employers.
II.65	**PSYCHOSOCIAL AND ECONOMIC PROBLEMS**	Describe psychosocial and economic problems that commonly affect the lives and care of HIV-infected patients, including family ostracism, job loss, lack of insurance, loss of disability benefits, etc.
II.66	**DOMESTIC VIOLENCE**	Discuss the association of HIV and domestic violence and describe appropriate interventions.

CHAPTER 15: COMPLEMENTARY AND ALTERNATIVE MEDICINE APPROACHES

II.67	**HERBAL REMEDIES/ VITAMIN SUPPLEMENTS/ OTHER NUTRIENTS**	Discuss known interactions between herbal remedies/vitamin supplements/other nutrients and antiretroviral agents, and describe appropriate advice to HIV-infected patients who intend to self-medicate with these agents, with or without antiretroviral therapy.
II.68	**PSYCHOLOGICAL/ PSYCHOIMMUNOLOGIC BENEFITS**	List possible psychological/psychoimmunologic benefits that patients may derive from complementary and alternative therapy interventions.

CHAPTER 16: SYSTEMS-BASED PRACTICE

II.69	**AFTER-HOURS/WEEKEND CARE**	Describe the appropriate responsibilities for the HIV clinician regarding care after hours and during weekends.
II.70	**COORDINATION WITH HEALTH CARE MANAGERS AND INTERDISCIPLINARY TEAMS**	Describe when and how to coordinate care effectively with health care managers and interdisciplinary teams.

II.71	**STRATEGIES FOR SUCCESSFUL REFERRAL**	Describe strategies that clinicians can use to increase the likelihood that referrals will be completed successfully.
II.72	**HIV CARE IN DIFFERENT REIMBURSEMENT SETTINGS**	Review the various methods for reimbursement of HIV-related health care services in the United States.
II.73	**PUBLIC POLICY ISSUES AND ACCESSING FINANCIAL ASSISTANCE PROGRAMS**	Recognize key public policy issues related to the financing and delivery of health care and related services for people with and at risk for HIV infection, and define and describe how to access the following: (a) the federal Ryan White CARE Act and its ADAP program; (b) compassionate access/medication assistance program supported by pharmaceutical companies.
II.74	**CPT CODES AND REIMBURSEMENT**	Describe the principles and importance of appropriate CPT codes used for HIV and related conditions.
II.75	**COSTS OF CARE**	Describe recent trends in the inpatient and outpatient costs of HIV care in the United States and explain the role of the health care provider in cost-conscious utilization of limited resources.

CHAPTER 17: PALLIATIVE CARE AND END-OF-LIFE SUPPORT

II.76	**CARING FOR THE TERMINALLY ILL PATIENT**	Discuss the clinician's responsibilities in caring for the terminally ill person with HIV.
II.77	**HOSPICE CARE**	Identify the role of hospice care and discuss: (a) HIV-related conditions for which hospice care is a frequent alternative; (b) advantages to the patient, family and loved ones of hospice care for a terminally ill person with HIV disease; (c) the pros and cons of in-patient versus at-home hospice care.
II.78	**PALLIATIVE CARE**	Discuss palliative care for common symptoms in end-stage HIV-infected patients, including but not limited to fatigue, sleep disturbance, pruritus, dyspnea, hiccups and dry mouth.

CHAPTER 18: LEGAL ISSUES

II.79	**DISEASE REPORTING SYSTEM**	Discuss the system of disease reporting in the United States and identify reportable conditions relevant to HIV care.
II.80	**PARTNER NOTIFICATION**	Describe the rationale for partner notification practices in HIV disease.
II.81	**ISSUES IN NONDISCLOSURE**	Discuss the physician's ethical and legal responsibilities to HIV-infected patients who do not disclose their HIV status to sexual and needle-sharing partners.
II.82	**TREATING MINORS**	Describe legal issues related to treatment of minors with HIV infection.
→ II.83	**CONFIDENTIALITY**	Discuss legal issues related to confidentiality and HIV, including health information protected under HIPAA's Privacy Rule and HIPAA's impact on communicating a patient's personal health information.
II.84	**ADVANCE PLANNING**	Discuss the use of advance directives, durable power of attorney and health proxy for HIV-infected patients.

PART III: CLINICAL MANIFESTATIONS OF HIV INFECTION AND ASSOCIATED CONDITIONS

CHAPTER 19: HIV-SPECIFIC MANIFESTATIONS

III.1	SYMPTOMS AND SIGNS OF ACUTE HIV INFECTION	Describe the symptoms and signs of the clinical presentation of acute HIV infection.
III.2	SYMPTOMS AND SIGNS OF CHRONIC HIV INFECTION	Describe constitutional symptoms and clinical signs of chronic HIV infection.
III.3	HIV WASTING SYNDROME	Describe the presentation and management of wasting due to HIV disease, and define the HIV wasting syndrome.

CHAPTER 20: OPPORTUNISTIC INFECTIONS

III.4	PRESENTATION	Describe the relative frequencies and various clinical presentations of common opportunistic infections: (a) bacterial infections; (b) fungal infections; (c) mycobacterial infections; (d) protozoan/parasitic infections; (e) viral infections.
III.5	DIAGNOSTIC LAB PROCEDURES	Identify the appropriate procedures and laboratory investigations required to make a diagnosis for each of the opportunistic infections indicated in Objective III.4.
III.6	PREFERRED AND ALTERNATIVE TREATMENTS	Cite the preferred and alternative treatment regimens for each of the opportunistic infections indicated in Objective III.4.
III.7	DRUG TOXICITY MANAGEMENT	Describe common toxicities and their management for each of the medications used to treat opportunistic infections.
→ III.8	PROPHYLAXIS	List the recommended prophylactic regimens for PCP, MAC, fungal infections, toxoplasmosis and herpesvirus infections (including CMV), citing the guidelines for initiation of prophylaxis (including co-trimoxazole desensitization) and discontinuation of prophylaxis.
III.9	ENVIRONMENTAL PROTECTION STRATEGIES	Describe environmental protection strategies that minimize the risk of acquiring specific opportunistic infections.

CHAPTER 21: MALIGNANCIES AND NEOPLASMS

III.10	NEWLY HIV-ASSOCIATED CANCERS	Cite data regarding an increase among HIV-infected patients in frequency of malignancies not previously associated with HIV infection, and describe appropriate cancer screening.
III.11	KAPOSI'S SARCOMA	Describe the screening, presentation, diagnosis, treatment, prognostic indicators and appropriate specialist referral for Kaposi's sarcoma (KS).

III.12 LYMPHOMA — Describe the screening, presentation, diagnosis, treatment, prognostic indicators and appropriate specialist referral for lymphoma.

III.13 CASTLEMAN'S DISEASE — Describe Castleman's disease, including clinical manifestations, histopathology, chemotherapy, prognosis and the role of the appropriate specialist referral.

III.14 HHV-8 — Discuss the etiologic role of HHV-8 in Castleman's disease and in body-cavity (effusion) lymphoma.

III.15 HUMAN PAPILLOMAVIRUS — Discuss the prevalence and role of human papillomavirus involving the lower genital tract, and anal canal dysplasia and carcinoma.

III.16 LOWER GENITAL TRACT DYSPLASIA — Describe guidelines for screening of lower genital tract dysplasia in HIV-infected women and indications for specialist referral for appropriate evaluation and management of abnormal screening.

III.17 ANAL DYSPLASIA — Discuss current considerations in the evaluation and management of anal dysplasia and neoplasia.

CHAPTER 22: DERMATOLOGIC COMPLICATIONS

III.18 PRESENTATION AND TREATMENT — Describe the presentation and therapy for common dermatoses seen in HIV-infected patients:

(a) noninfectious;
(b) fungal;
(c) viral;
(d) bacterial, including methicillin-resistant *Staphylococcus aureus* (MRSA);
(e) parasitic;
(f) other (eosinophilic folliculitis [EF]).

III.19 REFERRAL — Discuss the need for referral to a dermatologist and the role of early skin biopsy in an afebrile patient and an acutely ill febrile patient with a skin eruption.

CHAPTER 23: DENTAL/ORAL AND ENT COMPLICATIONS

III.20 DENTAL/ORAL COMPLICATIONS — Describe the clinical presentation, diagnosis and therapy for common dental and oral manifestations of HIV infection.

III.21 ENT COMPLICATIONS — Describe the diagnosis and management of common ENT problems and their complications seen in HIV-infected patients.

CHAPTER 24: ENDOCRINE DISORDERS

III.22 SCREENING, DIAGNOSIS AND MANAGEMENT — Discuss screening, diagnosis and management of common endocrine manifestations of HIV disease, including but not limited to diabetes mellitus and adrenal dysfunction.

III.23 HYPOGONADISM AND ANABOLIC AGENTS — Discuss the prevalence, evaluation and management of hypogonadism among HIV-infected patients, including the appropriate use of anabolic agents in this context.

CHAPTER 25: GYNECOLOGIC COMPLICATIONS

III.24 COMMON GYNECOLOGIC INFECTIONS — Discuss the prevalence, diagnosis and management of the following common gynecologic infections in HIV-infected women:

(a) vaginal candidiasis;
(b) bacterial vaginosis;
(c) trichomoniasis;
(d) pelvic inflammatory disease (PID).

III.25 MENSTRUAL DISORDERS	Discuss the prevalence and differential diagnosis of amenorrhea and other menstrual disorders in HIV-infected women.

CHAPTER 26: RESPIRATORY COMPLICATIONS

III.26 COMMUNITY-ACQUIRED PNEUMONIA	Discuss the incidence, causes and management of community-acquired pneumonia in HIV-infected patients.
III.27 PNEUMONIA DIAGNOSIS AND MANAGEMENT	Formulate the differential diagnosis and discuss the management of cavitary pneumonia in HIV-infected patients.
III.28 TUBERCULOSIS	Describe appropriate diagnosis, management and drug therapy for latent, active pulmonary and extrapulmonary TB according to the most recent CDC/ATS guidelines.
III.29 LYMPHOCYTIC INTERSTITIAL PNEUMONITIS	Discuss lymphocytic interstitial pneumonitis in HIV-infected patients.
III.30 PULMONARY HYPERTENSION	Describe the occurrence, clinical presentation and management of primary pulmonary hypertension in HIV-infected patients.

CHAPTER 27: PSYCHIATRIC AND NEUROLOGIC COMPLICATIONS

III.31 PSYCHIATRIC DISORDERS	Identify the most common psychiatric disorders in HIV-infected patients, their basic management and when appropriate specialist referral is warranted.
III.32 NEUROCOGNITIVE DISORDERS	Discuss the clinical presentation, differential diagnosis and management of dementia and minor neurocognitive disorders in HIV-infected patients.
III.33 MYELOPATHY	Discuss the clinical presentation, differential diagnosis and management of myelopathy in HIV-infected patients.
III.34 INTRACRANIAL MASS LESIONS	Discuss the clinical presentation, differential diagnosis and treatment of an intracranial mass lesion in HIV-infected patients.
III.35 MENINGITIS	Discuss the clinical presentation, differential diagnosis and treatment of meningitis in HIV-infected patients.
III.36 DISTAL SYMMETRICAL POLYNEUROPATHY	Discuss the clinical presentation, differential diagnosis and management of distal symmetrical polyneuropathy in HIV-infected patients.
III.37 AIDP/CIDP	Discuss the clinical presentation, differential diagnosis and management of acute and chronic inflammatory demyelinating polyneuropathy (AIDP/CIDP) in HIV-infected patients.
III.38 CMV POLYRADICULOPATHY	Discuss the clinical presentation, differential diagnosis and management of cytomegalovirus polyradiculopathy in HIV-infected patients.
III.39 MONONEURITIS	Discuss the clinical presentation, differential diagnosis and management of mononeuritis multiplex in HIV-infected patients.

CHAPTER 28: GASTROINTESTINAL AND HEPATOBILIARY COMPLICATIONS

III.40 DIARRHEA	Describe the diagnosis and treatment of diarrhea in HIV-infected patients.

III.41 ESOPHAGEAL DISORDERS	Discuss the differential diagnosis and treatment of dysphagia, odynophagia and esophagitis in HIV-infected patients.
III.42 HEPATITIS	Discuss the following aspects of hepatitis in HIV-infected patients: (a) clinical presentation, diagnosis and treatment of nonalcoholic steatohepatitis (NASH); (b) clinical presentation, diagnosis, treatment and treatment complications of hepatitis B; (c) clinical presentation, diagnosis, treatment and treatment complications of hepatitis C; (d) other viral causes of hepatitis; (e) drug-induced hepatitis.
III.43 PANCREATITIS	Discuss the differential diagnosis and evaluation of an elevated serum amylase in HIV-infected patients, and causes and management of pancreatitis.
III.44 CHOLECYSTITIS AND CHOLANGIOPATHY	Describe the clinical presentation and management of cholelithiasis, cholecystitis, acalculous cholecystitis and cholangiopathy in HIV infection.

CHAPTER 29: OCULAR COMPLICATIONS

III.45 CYTOMEGALOVIRUS	Describe appropriate screening, diagnosis, management and referral for HIV-infected patients with CMV retinitis.
III.46 HIV RETINOPATHY	Distinguish between HIV retinopathy and CMV retinitis.
III.47 OTHER OPHTHALMOLOGIC INFECTIONS	Discuss the ocular manifestations of varicella zoster virus and retinal infection with *Toxoplasma gondii*, *Pneumocystis jiroveci (carinii)*, syphilis and *Candida*.

CHAPTER 30: HEMATOLOGIC COMPLICATIONS

III.48 CYTOPENIAS	Describe the etiology, evaluation and management of anemia, neutropenia and thrombocytopenia in HIV infection, including the use of agents such as erythropoietin and filgrastim.
III.49 PARVOVIRUS B19	Describe the manifestations, evaluation and treatment of parvovirus B19 infection in HIV-infected patients.
III.50 COAGULATION DISORDERS	Describe and discuss HIV-related venous thrombosis and coagulation disorders.
III.51 OTHER HEMATOLOGIC COMPLICATIONS	Discuss the differential diagnosis and management of hemolytic anemia with and without thrombocytopenia in HIV infection.

CHAPTER 31: CARDIAC COMPLICATIONS

III.52 CARDIOMYOPATHY	Review the prevalence, prognosis and management of cardiomyopathy in HIV infection.
III.53 PERICARDITIS	Formulate the differential diagnosis of pericardial disease in HIV-infected patients.

CHAPTER 32: RENAL COMPLICATIONS

III.54 NEPHROPATHY	Discuss risk factors, presentation, diagnosis and management of HIV-associated nephropathy.

→ **Denotes Recent Learning Objectives**

CHAPTER 33: MUSCULOSKELETAL COMPLICATIONS

III.55 SKELETAL AND RHEUMATOLOGIC DISORDERS	Discuss the diagnosis and management of significant skeletal and rheumatologic complications of HIV disease, including osteopenia, osteoporosis and avascular necrosis.
III.56 PYOMYOSITIS	Discuss pyomyositis and its therapy in HIV-infected patients.
III.57 MYOPATHY	Discuss myopathy in HIV-infected patients.

CHAPTER 34: SEXUALLY TRANSMITTED DISEASES

→ **III.58 SYPHILIS**	Discuss current epidemiology (including behavioral and clinical factors associated with transmission), screening, clinical manifestations, indications for cerebrospinal fluid analysis, treatment and follow-up for syphilis in HIV infection.
III.59 OTHER STDs	Discuss current epidemiology (including behavioral and clinical factors associated with transmission), screening, clinical manifestations, treatment and follow-up of other STDs in the context of HIV disease.

PART IV: PRINCIPLES OF ANTIRETROVIRAL THERAPY

CHAPTER 35: INITIATION OF THERAPY IN TREATMENT-NAIVE PATIENTS

➔ IV.1	TREATMENT OF ACUTE HIV	Debate the advantages and disadvantages of very early treatment of acute HIV infection.
➔ IV.2	INDICATIONS FOR INITIATING THERAPY	Summarize the latest guidelines for initiating HIV therapy by the Department of Health and Human Services (DHHS) and the International AIDS Society-USA (IAS-USA) Panel.
IV.3	TREATMENT GOALS	Discuss the rationale and goals for initiating antiretroviral therapy in HIV-infected patients who are treatment-naive.
➔ IV.4	DELAYING INITIATION	Discuss the advantages and disadvantages of delaying initiation of therapy in a patient with chronic HIV infection.

CHAPTER 36: SPECIFIC AGENTS

IV.5	MECHANISMS OF ANTIRETROVIRALS	Describe the mechanism and site of action for each of the different classes of FDA-approved antiretroviral agents: NRTI/NtRTIs, NNRTIs, protease inhibitors and entry inhibitors.
➔ IV.6	ANTIRETROVIRAL DOSING	Describe the usual dosing, dose modifications for weight or impaired renal or liver clearance, and contraindications for currently FDA-approved antiretroviral therapies.
➔ IV.7	PHARMACOGENOMICS	Discuss recent data on how pharmacogenomics may affect antiretroviral management in clinical practice, e.g., abacavir hypersensitivity reaction, atazanavir-induced hyperbilirubinemia and efavirenz pharmacokinetics..
➔ IV.8	COMMON ANTIRETROVIRAL TOXICITIES	Describe the important toxicities and their management for all current FDA-approved antiretroviral therapies.
➔ IV.9	ANTIRETROVIRAL INTERACTIONS WITH NON-ANTIRETROVIRAL DRUGS	Identify the important drug-drug interactions that may be seen with current FDA-approved antiretroviral therapies and other medications.
➔ IV.10	RESISTANCE MUTATIONS	Identify the most important mutations and patterns of mutations associated with resistance to each of the currently FDA-approved antiretrovirals, and describe the concept of high and low genetic barriers to resistance.
➔ IV.11	ONCE-DAILY REGIMENS	Discuss the advantages and disadvantages of once-daily regimens, and identify agents with pharmacokinetics favorable to once-daily administration.

CHAPTER 37: COMBINATION THERAPY

➔ IV.12	REGIMEN SELECTION	Discuss the principles of how to combine antiretroviral medications, including reference to the U.S. Public Health Service and the International AIDS Society-USA guidelines for therapy, noting changes from previous guideline versions.
IV.13	PATIENT FACTORS IN REGIMEN SELECTION	Discuss factors to be considered in the selection of antiretroviral therapy regimens, including pill burden, dosing frequency, side effects, and patient's lifestyle and preferences.
➔ IV.14	COFORMULATIONS	Name and describe all antiretroviral coformulated tablets and capsules currently available or soon to be available.

→ **IV.15 ANTIRETROVIRAL INTERACTIONS**	Describe the known interactions that occur between antiretroviral medications, and describe the recommended antiretroviral dose adjustment.
IV.16 PRINCIPALS OF PHARMACODYNAMICS AND PHARMACOKINETIC ENHANCEMENT	Describe the terms C_{min}, C_{max}, IC_{50}, area under the curve (AUC) and inhibitory quotient (IQ) and the principle of pharmacokinetic enhancement of protease inhibitor drug levels by inhibition of the cytochrome P450 isoenzymes and P-glycoprotein enzyme system using ritonavir or other agents.
→ **IV.17 BOOSTED PROTEASE INHIBITORS**	Discuss the advantages and specific dosage recommendations when combining ritonavir with other protease inhibitors.
→ **IV.18 NOT-RECOMMENDED ANTIRETROVIRAL COMBINATIONS**	Discuss which antiretroviral combinations are contraindicated and which should be coadministered with caution, and why.

CHAPTER 38: MONITORING AND RESISTANCE TESTING

IV.19 GUIDELINES ON LABORATORY MONITORING	Describe the U.S. Public Health Service and the International AIDS Society-USA guidelines on laboratory monitoring of HIV infection, including the use and interpretation of specific laboratory tests and the frequency with which they should be performed to track progression or regression of disease.
→ **IV.20 RESISTANCE TESTING**	Discuss the following aspects of genotypic, phenotypic and virtual phenotypic resistance tests: (a) evaluation of currently available resistance assays, including proper use, strengths and limitations, as well as interpretation and management of discordant phenotype and genotype resistance testing; (b) the role of resistance testing in selecting a drug regimen for a treatment-naive patient; (c) the role of resistance testing in selecting a drug regimen for a patient whose regimen is failing (in contrast to empiric selection of antiretroviral therapy based on the patient's treatment history).
IV.21 THERAPEUTIC DRUG MONITORING	Discuss the advantages and disadvantages of therapeutic drug monitoring.

CHAPTER 39: MODIFYING THERAPY

IV.22 PRECAUTIONS	Discuss the precautions and contraindications for modifying antiretroviral therapy due to allergy, toxicity and drug intolerance.
→ **IV.23 REGIMEN FAILURE/ INTOLERABILITY**	Define failure of an antiretroviral regimen, discuss possible etiologies including intolerability and discuss the significance of viral load "blips."
IV.24 TREATMENT GOALS IN ANTIRETROVIRAL-EXPERIENCED PATIENTS	Discuss the rationale and goals for antiretroviral therapy in patients at different stages of treatment.
IV.25 INTENSIFICATION	Describe the rationale for, approaches to and potential risks associated with intensification of an inadequately suppressive antiretroviral regimen.
→ **IV.26 ANTIRETROVIRAL CROSS-RESISTANCE**	Discuss antiretroviral cross-resistance resulting from previous therapy, including approach to agent selection based on resistance testing and treatment history.
IV.27 MULTIDRUG RESCUE THERAPY	Summarize the research on use of multidrug rescue therapy in patients who have failed numerous prior drug regimens.

IV.28 VIRAL FITNESS AND REPLICATION CAPACITY	Discuss the distinction between viral fitness and replication capacity and the potential utility of reduced fitness on treatment-enhancing strategies.
IV.29 TREATMENT INTERRUPTIONS	Discuss various approaches to, the rationale for and the risks and benefits of treatment interruption in: (a) HIV-infected patients who are on successful antiretroviral therapy; (b) HIV-infected patients for whom antiretroviral therapy is failing.
IV.30 TREATMENT CESSATION	Discuss the pharmacokinetic and resistance considerations and approaches to stopping antiretroviral regimens containing drugs with different half-lives.

CHAPTER 40: INVESTIGATIONAL ANTIRETROVIRAL MEDICATIONS AND STRATEGIES

IV.31 ACCESS TO CLINICAL TRIALS	Describe the differences between phase 1, 2, 3 and 4 research clinical trials and how to enroll as an investigator in an expanded/early-access program.
IV.32 INVESTIGATIONAL ANTIRETROVIRAL AGENTS	Describe the antiretroviral agents currently in advanced-phase clinical trials and expanded/early-access programs in terms of their class, resistance profile, toxicities and the means by which to access them prior to pharmacy availability.
IV.33 INVESTIGATIONAL STRATEGIES UTILIZING APPROVED ANTIRETROVIRALS	Discuss current data on investigational strategies utilizing of FDA-approved antiretroviral agents.

CHAPTER 41: PREGNANCY

IV.34 ANTIRETROVIRAL TREATMENT	Discuss CDC guidelines for antiretroviral treatment during pregnancy.
IV.35 ANTIRETROVIRAL AGENT TOXICITY AND CONTRAINDICATION IN PREGNANCY	Identify the toxicity of antiretroviral agents in pregnancy and those that are contraindicated in pregnancy and in reproductive-age women not actively avoiding pregnancy.
IV.36 ANTIRETROVIRAL TREATMENT DURING LABOR	Outline the antiretroviral treatment for an HIV-infected pregnant woman presenting in labor with no previous treatment.
IV.37 CESAREAN SECTION	Discuss the advantages, disadvantages and indications for cesarean section in decreasing mother-to-child transmission of HIV.
IV.38 PHARMACOKINETICS IN PREGNANCY	Discuss the variations in antiretroviral pharmacokinetics that may occur during pregnancy, as well as potential strategies to avoid the development of viral resistance or toxicity as a consequence.

CHAPTER 42: ADHERENCE ISSUES

IV.39 PRINCIPLES	Identify the degree of adherence necessary for successful antiretroviral therapy and discuss how various levels of adherence affect the probability of developing antiretroviral resistance.
IV.40 INITIATION STRATEGIES	List clinician knowledge and skills needed, and strategies used, to assess treatment readiness and enhance patient adherence when starting antiretroviral therapy.
IV.41 MEASUREMENT	Describe challenges in measuring patient adherence, as well as the potential use of questionnaires, pill counts, pharmacy medication fill data, electronic medication event monitoring system (MEMS®) cap monitoring and therapeutic drug monitoring to measure adherence.

IV.42 PSYCHIATRIC ISSUES	Explain the impact of untreated substance use, depression and other psychiatric disorders on a patientís adherence to antiretroviral therapy.
IV.43 MULTIDISCIPLINARY COUNSELING	Discuss the role and impact of multidisciplinary adherence counseling – including that of nurses, peers, counselors and physicians – on adherence success.
IV.44 ADHERENCE REMINDERS	Identify various reminder devices and strategies that can assist with patient adherence.
IV.45 ADDITIONAL SUPPORT	Describe the roles of community-based organizations, therapists, support groups and other alternatives in assisting with and enhancing patient adherence.
IV.46 DIRECTLY OBSERVED THERAPY	Summarize the findings of studies of directly observed antiretroviral therapy.

CHAPTER 43: COMPLICATIONS OF TREATMENT

→ **IV.47 MORPHOLOGIC CHANGES**	Describe morphologic changes (lipoatrophy and/or abnormal fat deposition) commonly observed in patients taking antiretroviral therapy and their association with antiretroviral agents.
IV.48 LABORATORY ABNORMALITIES	Discuss common perturbations that may be seen in routine blood hematology and chemistry testing as a result of being on certain antiretrovirals, e.g., a high mean corpuscular volume from zidovudine or stavudine, and hyperbilirubinemia from atazanavir or indinavir.
→ **IV.49 METABOLIC COMPLICATIONS**	Discuss the occurrence and management of metabolic complications of therapy, including but not limited to hyperlipidemia, insulin resistance and lactic acidosis.
→ **IV.50 CARDIOVASCULAR DISEASE**	Discuss the risk of cardiovascular disease associated with HIV and its treatment, and compare this with risk due to smoking, hypertension, diabetes, family history and other cardiac risk factors.
→ **IV.51 IMMUNE RECONSTITUTION INFLAMMATORY SYNDROME**	Discuss the clinical setting, manifestations and management of immune-reconstitution inflammatory syndrome secondary to opportunistic infections, including but not limited to MAC, TB, CMV, HBV, HCV, PML, HSV and VZV as a result of combination antiretroviral therapy.

CHAPTER 44: PRE- AND POSTEXPOSURE PROPHYLAXIS

→ **IV.52 OCCUPATIONAL POSTEXPOSURE PROPHYLAXIS**	Discuss the efficacy data and protocol of postexposure antiretroviral prophylaxis for occupational percutaneous and mucocutaneous exposure to HIV according to current CDC and OSHA guidelines.
→ **IV.53 NONOCCUPATIONAL EXPOSURE PROPHYLAXIS**	Discuss the use of pre- and postexposure antiretroviral prophylaxis for nonoccupational settings, including sexual exposure or rape.

CHAPTER 45: IMMUNE-BASED AND GENETIC THERAPIES

IV.54 INTERLEUKIN-2	Discuss the advantages and disadvantages of interleukin-2 as treatment in HIV disease.
IV.55 ALPHA INTERFERON	Describe the advantages and disadvantages of alpha interferon as a treatment in HIV disease.
IV.56 THERAPEUTIC HIV VACCINES	Describe the potential therapeutic use of HIV vaccines in HIV-infected patients.
→ **IV.57 GENETIC APPROACHES TO HIV THERAPY**	Describe new genetic approaches in research to find new treatments for HIV, such as gene therapy and RNA interference.

PART V: RESEARCH ISSUES

CHAPTER 46: RESEARCH DESIGN AND ANALYSIS

V.1 RESEARCH PLANNING

Discuss the rationale for determining specific end points and analytical methods for performing power calculations prior to initiating research studies.

V.2 EVALUATING THE STATISTICAL ANALYSIS OF CLINICAL TRIALS

Differentiate between an on-treatment analysis and an intent-to-treat analysis, time-to-loss of virologic response (TLOVR), noninferiority analysis and average area under the curve minus baseline (AAUCMB).

V.3 DETERMINING CAUSE-AND-EFFECT ASSOCIATIONS

Discuss the difficulties in drawing cause-and-effect conclusions about associated factors identified in a research studies, including the limitations of observational studies and cross- study comparisons.

CHAPTER 47: ETHICAL ISSUES IN PERFORMING HIV RESEARCH

V.4 INFORMED CONSENT

Describe the FDA/DHHS Good Clinical Practice guidelines and key elements required for obtaining informed consent for study participants.

V.5 IRBs AND OTHER ETHICAL ISSUES

Describe the essentials of institutional review-board processes and approval procedures, informed consent and other ethical issues related to research in HIV medicine.

INTERNATIONAL ISSUES (NOT REQUIRED FOR CARE IN UNITED STATES)

The AAHIVM Core Curriculum focuses on what an HIV specialist needs to know to practice up-to-date, state-of-the-art HIV medical care. To do this, it is not essential to have extensive knowledge of or interest in the international HIV/AIDS epidemic and care delivery internationally. However, many HIV specialists in the United States are increasingly interested in learning about how antiretroviral therapy can be delivered to the millions who need it internationally.

With this in mind, we include this international section as appendix to the AAHIVM Core Curriculum. It is an appendix only; the focus of this section will not be used to create questions for the credentialing examination, but is included as these issues are of such major importance internationally and of considerable interest to may of our members.

PART I: OVERVIEW OF HIV

GLOBAL EPIDEMIOLOGY — Discuss the geographic prevalence and implications of various HIV clades.

AIDS DEFINITION — Describe the WHO definition of AIDS.

TRANSMISSION — Identify factors shown to facilitate and retard HIV transmission in resource-limited settings.

PART II: APPROACH TO THE PATIENT WITH HIV

INTERNATIONAL: BASELINE EVALUATIONS — Identify important baseline laboratory evaluations for a new patient with HIV infection in a resource-limited setting.

INTERNATIONAL: BREAST-FEEDING — Discuss issues surrounding breast-feeding by HIV-infected women in resource-limited settings.

INTERNATIONAL: MOTHER-TO-CHILD TRANSMISSION — Discuss contemporary issues, including efficacy and drug resistance, related to the use of antiretrovirals to prevent mother-to-child transmission in resource-limited settings.

INTERNATIONAL: TESTING AND PREVENTION — Discuss cultural, political and economic challenges in HIV prevention and testing in resource-limited settings.

PART III: CLINICAL MANIFESTATIONS OF HIV INFECTION AND ASSOCIATED CONDITIONS

INTERNATIONAL: SYNDROMIC MANAGEMENT — Discuss syndromic management of opportunistic diseases in resource-limited settings.

INTERNATIONAL: OPPORTUNISTIC INFECTION PREVALENCE — Identify global geographic differences in the prevalence of opportunistic infections associated with HIV.

INTERNATIONAL: OPPORTUNISTIC INFECTION PROPHYLAXIS — Propose a strategy of monitoring clinical and laboratory thresholds in a resource-limited setting to guide the decision of when to initiate prophylaxis for opportunistic infections.

INTERNATIONAL: GENITAL ULCERATIVE DISEASE — Discuss the reciprocal impact on transmission risk of HIV and genital ulcerative disease (GUD), and describe evaluation and syndromic management of GUD in a resource-limited setting.

PART IV: PRINCIPLES OF ANTIRETROVIRAL THERAPY

INTERNATIONAL: PROVIDING ANTIRETROVIRALS	Describe factors affecting the provision of antiretroviral therapy in resource-limited settings.
INTERNATIONAL: ANTIRETROVIRAL INITIATION	Discuss WHO recommendations for initiation of antiretroviral therapy and first-line recommended regimens in resource-limited settings.
INTERNATIONAL: ANTIRETROVIRALS TO PREVENT PERINATAL TRANSMISSION	Discuss use of short-course antiretroviral prophylactic regimens for prevention of perinatal transmission and their effectiveness and disadvantages.
INTERNATIONAL: EFFICACY OF GENERIC ANTIRETROVIRALS	Describe potential complications resulting from use of generic antiretrovirals with pharmacokinetic or activity profiles that differ from their trademarked counterparts, and list known generic agents with demonstrated nonequivalency.
INTERNATIONAL: ANTIRETROVIRAL SEQUENCING	Propose a strategy of sequential antiretroviral regimens, based on known probable resistance development, for application in settings without access to resistance testing.
INTERNATIONAL: MONITORING	Describe a strategy of laboratory and clinical evaluation for monitoring HIV-infected patients on and off of HIV therapy in a resource-limited setting.
INTERNATIONAL: RESISTANCE	Describe strategies to monitor antiretroviral resistance on a population level, and how population results may be used to allocate resources for performing resistance testing in individuals and modifying individuals' antiretroviral treatment.

INDEX

H

I

J

K

L

M

S

T

U

V

W

XYZ